Microsurgery for Fertility Specialists

Jay I. Sandlow
Editor

Microsurgery for Fertility Specialists

A Practical Text

Springer

Editor
Jay I. Sandlow, MD
Department of Urology
Medical College of Wisconsin
Milwaukee, WI, USA

ISBN 978-1-4614-4195-3 ISBN 978-1-4614-4196-0 (eBook)
DOI 10.1007/978-1-4614-4196-0
Springer New York Heidelberg Dordrecht London

Library of Congress Control Number: 2012942083

Printed on acid-free paper

Springer is part of Springer Science+Business Media (www.springer.com)

To my wife, Bridget, and my daughters, Samantha, Jacquelyn, and Rachel: your patience and understanding always remind me of what is important in life.

Preface

"*Microsurgery for Fertility Specialists: A Practical Text*" is designed as a resource for physicians who specialize in the surgical treatment of infertility. This book will outline some of the basics of microsurgery, the indications, as well as various surgical techniques. It is intended for all providers who practice microsurgery in the field of andrology. The field has evolved over the years, from the use of loupe magnification to state-of-the art operating microscopes. Although improvements in assisted reproductive technology (ART), specifically intracytoplasmic sperm injection, has rendered some microsurgical procedures to become secondary to ART, many fertility specialists continue to provide excellent outcomes, as well as the restoration of fertility and sexual function, to their patients. This book is designed to provide these specialists with detailed operative descriptions of these surgical procedures, from vasectomy reversals to sperm acquisitions, tubal re-anastomosis, and even penile surgery. Furthermore, it is intended to help teach the next generation of microsurgeons, as I believe that it is incumbent upon us, as physicians, to pass on our knowledge. Each chapter is cowritten by both a junior and a senior author in order to allow more junior-level experts to gain valuable experience and knowledge. There are chapters that are specifically dedicated to the education of residents and fellows, as they are the future of fertility surgery. Finally, the role of microsurgery in non-infertility procedures is covered as well.

"*Microsurgery for Fertility Specialists*" will allow providers with a basic knowledge of infertility surgery to become better prepared in the field, while those with more advanced knowledge will be able to utilize this resource to maintain and advance their microsurgical practice, as well as assist in the education of others.

Milwaukee, WI, USA Jay I. Sandlow

Acknowledgments

I would like to gratefully acknowledge the many people who have helped me prepare this book, as well as those who have helped my career along the way. This book would not have been possible without the outstanding contributions of each of the authors. Springer's Developmental Editor, Maureen Alexander has been invaluable in helping with the organization of this book. Finally, my administrative assistant, Cindy Ziebell, has worked tirelessly to collect, format, and prepare the various chapters.

I would also like to thank all those who have influenced my career and teaching philosophy. I inherited a strong desire to teach from my father, Dr. Les Sandlow, who had a long and distinguished career in academic medicine. My former chair, Dr. Richard Williams, nurtured my academic career and gave me the tools necessary to succeed. I have had many mentors, both formal and informal, who have taught me the clinical and research aspects of male infertility, and to them I am grateful for their guidance and wisdom.

Acknowledgments

Contents

Contributors

Karen Baker, MD Center for Male Fertility, Glickman Urological and Kidney Institute, Cleveland Clinic, Cleveland, OH, USA

Joshua A. Bodie, MD Department of Urology, University of Minnesota Medical Center, Minneapolis, MN, USA

Jamin V. Brahmbhatt, MD Department of Urology, University of Tennessee Health Science Center, Memphis, TN, USA

Robert E. Brannigan, MD Department of Urology, Feinberg School of Medicine, Northwestern University, Chicago, IL, USA

Arthur L. Burnett, MD Department of Urology, The Johns Hopkins Hospital, Baltimore, MD, USA

Tommaso Falcone, MD Ob/Gyn and Women's Health Institute, Cleveland Clinic, Cleveland, OH, USA

Jeffrey M. Goldberg, MD Department of Obstetrics and Gynecology, Cleveland Clinic, Cleveland, OH, USA

Marc Goldstein, MD Department of Urology, Center for Male Reproductive Medicine and Microsurgery, Weill Cornell Medical College, Cornell University, New York, NY, USA

Ethan Grober, MD, MEd Division of Urology, Mount Sinai and Women's College Hospital, University of Toronto, Toronto, ON, Canada

Ahmet Gudeloglu, MD Department of Urology, Winter Haven Hospital and University of Florida, Winter Haven, FL, USA

Michael A.S. Jewett, MD, FRCSC FACS Division of Urology, Departments of Surgery and Surgical Oncology, Princess Margaret Hospital and the University Health Network, University of Toronto, Toronto, ON, Canada

Peter N. Kolettis, MD Department of Surgery/Urology, University of Alabama-Birmingham, Birmingham, AL, USA

Philip S. Li, MD Department of Urology, Center for Male Reproductive Medicine and Microsurgery, Weill Cornell Medical College, Cornell University, New York, NY, USA

Akanksha Mehta, MD Department of Urology, Weill Cornell Medical College, Cornell University, New York, NY, USA

Ajay K. Nangia, MBBS Department of Urology, University of Kansas Medical Center, Kansas City, KS, USA

Sijo J. Parekattil, MD Department of Urology, Winter Haven Hospital and University of Florida, Winter Haven, FL, USA

Ranjith Ramasamy, MD Department of Urology, Center for Male Reproductive Medicine and Microsurgery, Weill Cornell Medical College, Cornell University, New York, NY, USA

Kalen Rimar, BA, BS Department of Urology, Feinberg School of Medicine, Northwestern University, Chicago, IL, USA

Jeffrey Lee Rosenblum, MD The Rosenblum Center for Urologic Care, Exton, PA, USA

Edmund Sabanegh Jr, MD Center for Male Fertility, Glickman Urological and Kidney Institute, Cleveland Clinic, Cleveland, OH, USA

Jay I. Sandlow, MD Department of Urology, Medical College of Wisconsin, Milwaukee, WI, USA

Peter N. Schlegel, MD Department of Urology, Weill Cornell Medical College, New York Presbyterian Hospital, Weill Cornell Medical Center, New York, NY, USA

Anand Shridharani, MD Department of Urology, Medical College of Wisconsin, Milwaukee, WI, USA

James F. Smith, MD, MS Department of Urology, Obstetrics, Gynecology, and Reproductive Sciences, UCSF, San Francisco, CA, USA

Oleksandr Stakhovskyi, MD Division of Urology, Departments of Surgery and Surgical Oncology, Princess Margaret Hospital and the University Health Network, University of Toronto, Toronto, ON, Canada

Landon Trost, MD Department of Urology, The Mayo Clinic, Rochester, MN, USA

Chapter 1
Male Infertility Microsurgical Training

Philip S. Li, Ranjith Ramasamy, and Marc Goldstein

Abstract *Microsurgical training is important for urologists and clinical andrologists specializing in male infertility* [1, 2]. *Like* "pure microvascular," *plastic, and other reconstructive microsurgeries, microsurgery for male infertility ranks among the most technically and mentally challenging of surgical procedures*. Most male infertility microsurgeries are performed under 10–25× magnification. Under the operating microscope, tiny movements are magnified by 15–40×. There are few surgical fields where outcomes are so dependent on technical performance in the operating room. *Success in male infertility microsurgery is therefore heavily dependent on the quality and extent of practice and training in the microsurgical laboratory* [3, 4]. Coordination, dexterity, and steadiness of one's hands and fingers can be developed with extensive practice in the laboratory. The purpose of this chapter is to review the basic male infertility microsurgical skills for working with microsurgical instruments, needles, and sutures at different magnifications. *Male infertility microsurgery should be learned in the laboratory, not on patients.*

Keywords Male • Infertility • Microsurgery • Training • Urology

Introduction

Microsurgical training is important for urologists and clinical andrologists specializing in male infertility [1, 2]. *Like* "pure microvascular," *plastic, and other reconstructive microsurgeries, microsurgery for male infertility ranks among the most technically and mentally challenging of surgical procedures*. Most male infertility

P.S. Li, M.D. (✉) • R. Ramasamy, M.D. • M. Goldstein, M.D.
Department of Urology, Center for Male Reproductive Medicine and Microsurgery,
Weill Cornell Medical College, Cornell University, 525 East 68th Street,
Box 269, New York, NY 10065, USA
e-mail: psli@med.cornell.edu

J.I. Sandlow (ed.), *Microsurgery for Fertility Specialists: A Practical Text*,
DOI 10.1007/978-1-4614-4196-0_1,

microsurgeries are performed under 10–25× magnification. Under the operating microscope, tiny movements are magnified by 15–40×. There are few surgical fields where outcomes are so dependent on technical performance in the operating room. *Success in male infertility microsurgery is therefore heavily dependent on the quality and extent of practice and training in the microsurgical laboratory* [3, 4]. Coordination, dexterity, and steadiness of one's hands and fingers can be developed with extensive practice in the laboratory. The purpose of this chapter is to review the basic male infertility microsurgical skills for working with microsurgical instruments, needles, and sutures at different magnifications. *Male infertility microsurgery should be learned in the laboratory, not on patients.*

Surgical instruction for urology residents is often based on the "see one, do one, teach one" model of apprenticeship. If the trainee has been experienced in basic surgical principles, this method of teaching generally works well. However, urologic procedures that employ optics such as microsurgery and minimally invasive techniques such as laparoscopic or robotic surgery may require additional skills, not necessarily because they are more complex than conventional techniques but because they utilize principles to which most trainees have had no prior exposure, such as altered spatial perception. In addition, for microsurgery, the scale of the surgery is so dramatically different that even common tasks such as suturing require the use of different muscles in hands and fingers as well as specific ergonomic considerations. In recognition of the need for additional training to acquire specialized surgical skills, it is important that residency programs around the country establish laboratories for microsurgical training.

Basic Equipment and Materials for Microsurgery Training

1. *Operating microscope*. There are a variety of microscopes available for use in the laboratory and the operating room. A good operating microscope provides bright illumination, smooth focusing, zooming, and easy operation. The basic components of an operating microscope consist of the objective lens, eyepieces, binocular tube, and microscope body that house the magnification changer. The objective lens determines the focal length or working distance.

   A 200 mm objective lens is commonly used for male infertility microsurgery, which focuses on the surgical field 200 mm away from the objective lens. It is important to set up the correct focal length or working distance. If the working distance is too close to the surgical field, it can result in instrument contamination or difficulty in manipulating the instruments, whereas a working distance that is too far away from the surgical field can result in strain on muscles in the back. Although there are many available magnification ranges (10×, 12.5×, 15×, and 20×) for the eyepieces, the higher power eyepieces result in smaller fields of view. As such, *10× and 12.5× are commonly used for male infertility microsurgery.* The microsurgeon should be familiar with his or her operating microscope and create a comfortable working environment.

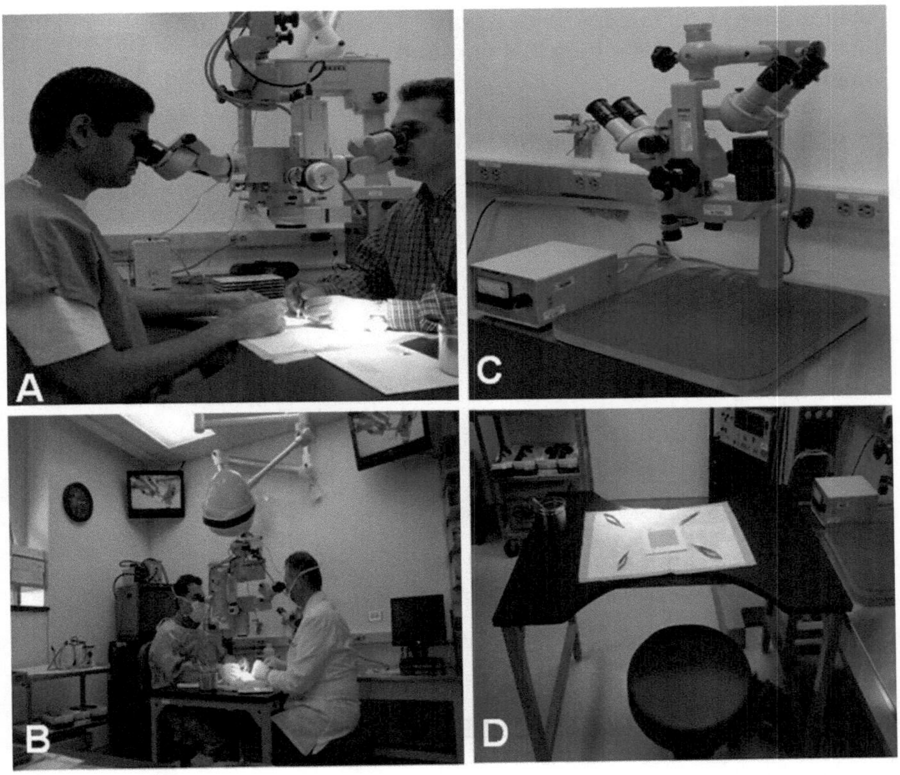

Fig. 1.1 Zeiss OPMI/S3/S4 Surgical Microscope Systems (**a, b**) with motorized zoom and focus and Zeiss OPMI-1 binocular diploscope (**c**) with manually controlled zoom and focus are used for male infertility microsurgery training. Microsurgical bench table (**d**)

In our microsurgical laboratory, we use the Zeiss OPMI/S3 and Zeiss OPMI Cs/S4 Surgical Microscope Systems with motorized zoom and focus (Fig. 1.1a, b) as well as the Zeiss OPMI-1 binocular diploscope with manually controlled zoom and focus system (Fig. 1.1c) for microsurgery training.

2. *Microsurgical table*. The bench table should be solid and stable, with a height around 30 in. to allow for comfortable placement of the operators' knees below the table (Fig. 1.1d). Workspace dimensions of at least 30–35 in. in length and 24 in. in width will provide ample working space.
3. *Microsurgical instruments.* There are only a few instruments required to perform virtually all urologic microsurgical procedures (Fig. 1.2):

Basic Microsurgical Set

(a) A straight fine-tip forceps (Solomon's forceps) with and without a suture platform (10–13.5 cm long with flat or round handle).
(b) A non-locking needle holder with a rounded, fine curved tip (13.5 or 15 cm long).
(c) A curved-blunt tip dissecting scissor.
(d) A sharp iris scissor.

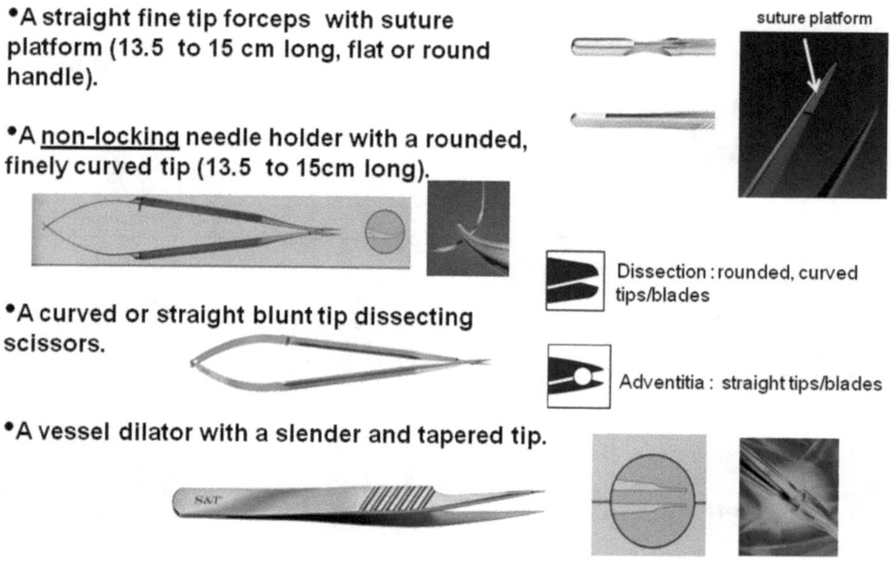

Fig. 1.2 Basic microsurgical instrument set for male infertility microsurgery

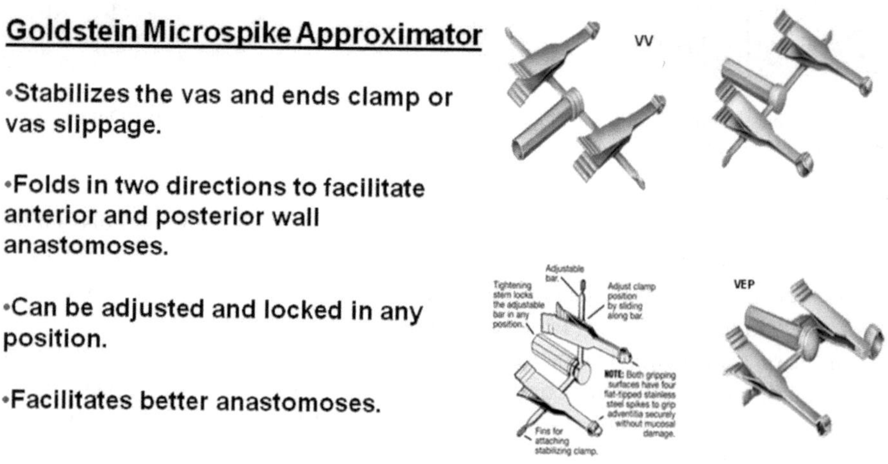

Fig. 1.3 Goldstein Microspike approximator

(e) A vessel dilator with a slender and tapered tip.
(f) A small straight approximator double vascular/tubal clamps (ASSI, #ST-ATCC-22) or Goldstein Microspike approximator clamp for vasovasostomy (Fig. 1.3).
(g) Microsurgical bipolar cautery with fine-tipped forceps.

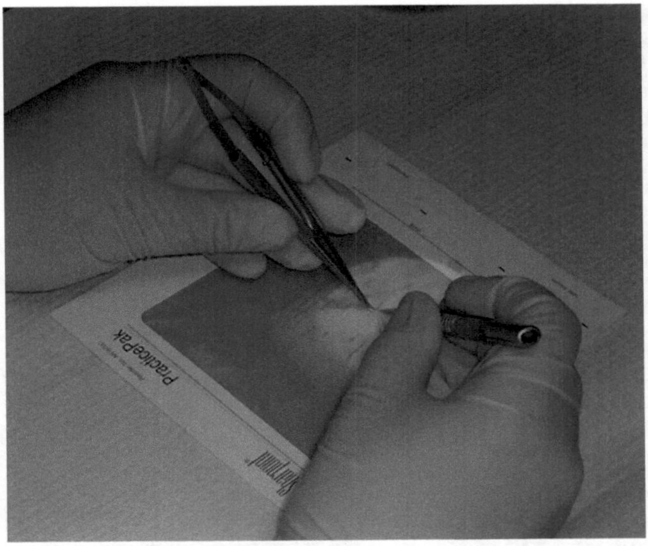

Fig. 1.4 Sharpoint suture practice card. Reprinted with permission of Angiotech Pharmaceuticals Inc. © 2012 Angiotech Pharmaceuticals, Inc

4. *Non-microsurgical set and microsuture materials*

(a) A basic set of surgical instruments for small animal surgery (e.g., small needle holder, small smooth and toothed forceps, small suture scissors, small curved or blunt dissecting scissors, and clip applier).
(b) Operating board, 35×35 cm^2.
(c) Microsurgical suture (Sharpoint Laboratory Pack/Non-sterile, double-armed or single-armed 10-0 sutures, #AK-0100, #AK-0101) and Microsurgical Suturing Practice Cards (Sharpoint #AK-9000), soft silicone tubing (Fig. 1.4).
(d) Tape for fixing practice objects to the board.
(e) 10 cc irrigating syringe (with heparin or saline solution) attended to a blunt rounded 27 1/2 gauge needle.
(f) Background material: Deep blue is the most satisfactory background color.
(g) Silicone tubing or segments of vas deferens.
(h) Spasmolytics—such as 1 or 2% lidocaine hydrochloride (20 mg/ml), papaverine heparinized (100–150 units/ml) solution, Ringer's lactate solution, or saline.

5. *Microsurgical instrument maintenance. Good performance requires properly maintained microsurgical instruments. Working with damaged instruments can be laborious and frustrating for beginners as well as experienced microsurgeons* [5]. When not in use, microsurgical instruments should be stored in an instrument case with their fine tips fully protected by plastic covers or segments of silicone tubing (Fig. 1.5). Grasping more than one instrument at a time increases the chances of damage to the tips. Each instrument should be examined under the microscope prior to use and repaired as needed. Simple repairs can be accomplished by

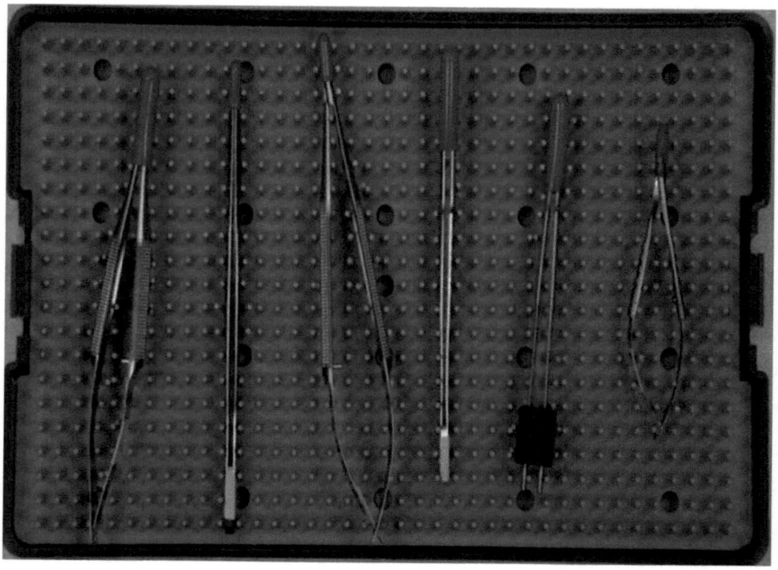

Fig. 1.5 Microsurgical instruments should be protected by plastic covers in a microsurgical instrument case

sharpening the instrument tips with Arkansas white stone, emery paper, and nail file. Microsurgical instruments are often damaged during cleaning; therefore, great care must be taken during the cleaning process. Instruments should be soaked and cleaned immediately after use in a hemolytic enzyme solution such as Haemo-Sol (Haemo-Sol, Inc., Baltimore, MD). After soaking, the instruments should be rinsed in tap water and placed on paper towels to dry. Instruments must be dry prior to storage. Covering the tips of the instruments not only avoids damage to the fine instruments but also prevents magnetization from coming in contact with each other.

Basic Preparation for Microsurgery Training

Learning male infertility microsurgery requires extensive practice and patience. Laboratory training allows for acquisition of basic skills such as microscope adjustment, instrument handling, and knot tying prior to clinical application. The following suggestions may help to structure the laboratory training routine:

1. *Set up flexible but sufficient practice time.* As a resident, fellow, or practicing surgeon, time is valuable and limited. However, the minimum practice time should be at least twice a week for 1–2 h per session until basic skills are mastered.
2. *Minimize mental stress.* Try to get adequate sleep the night before a practice session.
3. Accept that mastery of microsurgery cannot be achieved overnight. The process involves many steps with intricate details, each of which requires attention and

concentration. Frustration is common especially during the first week of training, but do not be discouraged.

4. *Find a comfortable sitting position and eliminate outside distractions.* Your arms should be bent at a 90° angle at the elbows. Your wrists and hands should be in a relaxed anterior position. Use supportive objects, such as towels or soft material like foam to support your hands and forearms. Adjust your stance to allow yourself easy access to the controls of the operating microscope.
5. *Use appropriate magnification and sharp focus with maximum illumination.* High magnification is only needed to prepare the ends of the vas deferens or the epididymal tubule and to pass the needle through the lumen of the vas deferens or the epididymal tubule. Low magnification is used to dissect tissue and to manipulate the needle to the correct position in the needle holder. The surgeon's knot is best tied under low power.

Learning to Use the Operating Microscope

No matter what kind of operating microscope you have, you should completely understand how to operate it before learning microsurgery.

1. *Adjust your seat level until you have a comfortable position.* Having the level too high or low can result in a sore neck or back. Your head should sit straight on your neck, and your eyes should look straight ahead, perpendicular to your spine.
2. *Adjust the interocular distance of the eyepieces until the two images fuse together.*
3. *Maximize the light source to provide adequate light for the entire field.* However, follow the instructions on the microscope and your own common sense about light intensity and the distance between the light source and the specimen to avoid burn injury.
4. *Choose a correct focal length or working distance.* A working distance of 200 mm is optimal for male infertility microsurgery.
5. *Focus each eyepiece with the microscope at the highest magnification.* Start with the eyepiece at the "0" position and adjust until a sharp image is obtained for each eye. Focus at the highest magnification should ensure focus at all lower magnifications.

Learning to Handle Microsurgical Instruments

1. Holding the instruments: Although many surgeons have developed their own way of holding the forceps and needle holder, the pencil-holding position with the instrument resting in the index and thumb web space is recommended (Fig. 1.6).

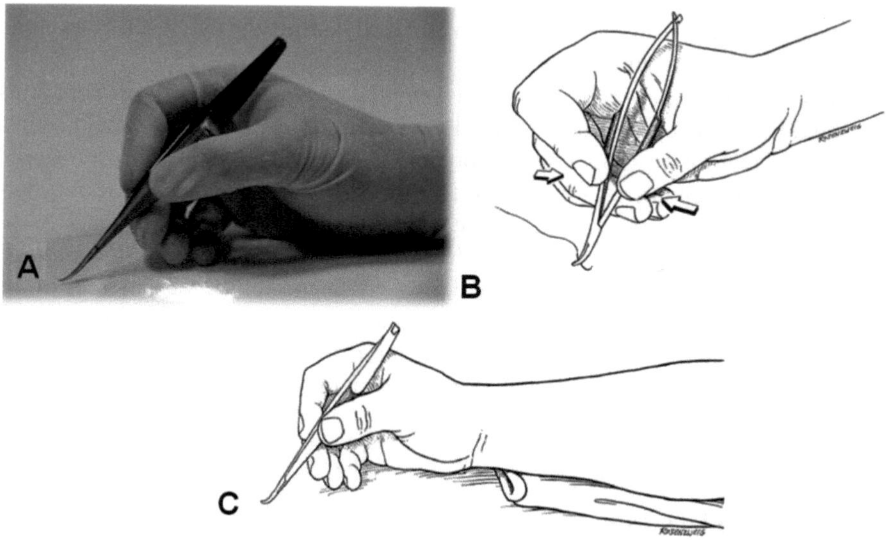

Fig. 1.6 Pencil-holding position (**a**) is demonstrated with a needle holder. The tips of the needle holder are parallel to the surface with the needle at a 30° angle. A needle is held by the tips of the needle holder using gentle pressure between thumb and index finger (**b**). To control hand or finger tremor, a folded surgical towel is placed to support the hand and forearm (**c**)

Most microsurgical skills, including suturing and knot tying, require only a slight movement of the fingers. The rest of the hand must be perfectly still. The thumb, index, and middle fingers must support each other precisely. Moreover, the weight of the hand must rest on its base to maintain stability. The thumb and index finger must hold the instrument so that its weight is transmitted through the middle finger to the work surface below. Holding the needle or cutting a suture is precisely controlled by a slight motion between the thumb and index finger (Fig. 1.6b).

2. *Controlling hand tremor*. It is extremely difficult even for surgeons with considerable microsurgical experience to coordinate hand and instrument movement and to prevent tremors without proper hand support. Therefore fingers must support each other during micromanipulation. We prefer to use folded surgical towels to support the hand and forearm (Fig. 1.6c).
3. "Light touch": Microsurgical needles and sutures are easily damaged if held too firmly. A "light or gentle touch" is needed to accurately control the instrument with minimal hand pressure. *One distinction of a good microsurgeon is the ability to preserve the original shape and condition of the needle throughout the operation.* Once the needle is grasped between the fine tips of the needle holder, fine adjustments to the angle of the needle can be made by gently touching the needle with the tips of the forceps (Fig. 1.7a). The best way to stabilize the needle is to hold it at a point roughly one-half to two-thirds of the way back from the tip of the needle. The needle will wobble if held too close to the suture end (Fig. 1.7b) or too near the tip (Fig. 1.7c). Keeping the needle pointing in the right direction can take practice.

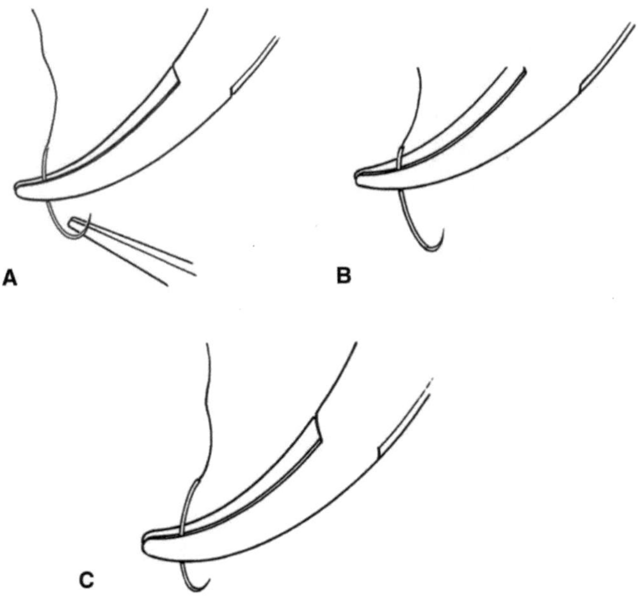

Fig. 1.7 Learn how to control the needle; and how to position the needle with the needle holder and forceps. Use the tips of the forceps to adjust the position of the needle in the needle holder (**a**). The needle will be unstable if held too close to the suture end (**b**) or too near the tip (**c**)

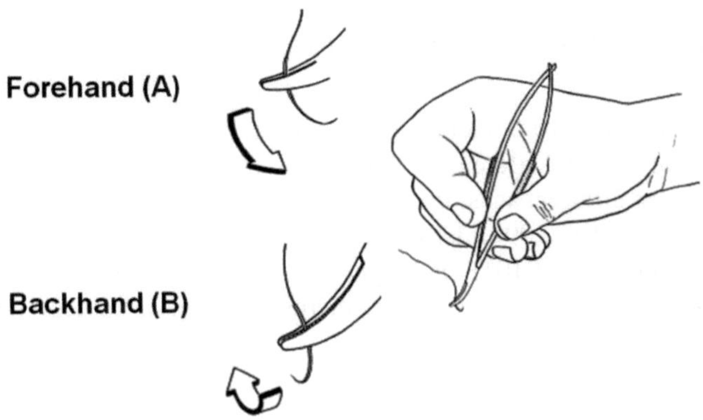

Fig. 1.8 Needle holding positions for forehand (**a**) and backhand (**b**) suturing require only a slight rotational movement of the fingers

4. Forehand or backhand: How the needle is loaded on the needle holder depends on the direction of the needle stroke to be made. For right-handed surgeons, a needle stroke from right to left or towards the surgeon is made with the needle in the forehand position (Fig. 1.8a). A needle stroke from left to right or away from the surgeon requires the needle in the backhand position (Fig. 1.8b). Most microsurgeons are better able to control the needle using a forehand hold. Unless one is ambidextrous, both forehand and backhand holds are important to learn. One must learn to rotate the needle in various directions.

Fig. 1.9 Sharpoint Laboratory Suture Practice Card 10-0 microsuture. Reprinted with permission of Angiotech Pharmaceuticals Inc. © 2012 Angiotech Pharmaceuticals, Inc

Preparation of Microsurgical Sutures

Currently, we use only 10-0 microsurgical sutures for male infertility microsurgical anastomoses of the vas deferens or epididymis in our lab. There are a variety of needle shapes for different anastomoses. We commonly use non-sterile 10-0 laboratory pack (Fig. 1.9), 100 micron, nonabsorbable black nylon with double-armed (Sharpoint #AK-0101) or single-armed needles (Sharpoint #AK-0100). Animal studies suggested that nylon microsutures may be less reactive than polypropylene [6].

Preparation of Microsuturing Practice Card

Passing the needle through tissue—A practice microsuturing card (e.g., Sharpoint Latex card, #AK-9000) is a simple and effective tool for developing suturing skills under the operating microscope.

A small incision is made on the card with a scalpel. It is important to visualize the entrance and exit points before passing the needle through the card. The entrance should be made at a point two times the wall thickness of the tissue. The needle should be perpendicular to the tissue at its entry point. Forceps provide counter-pressure to help the needle pass through the tissue edge between the tips of the

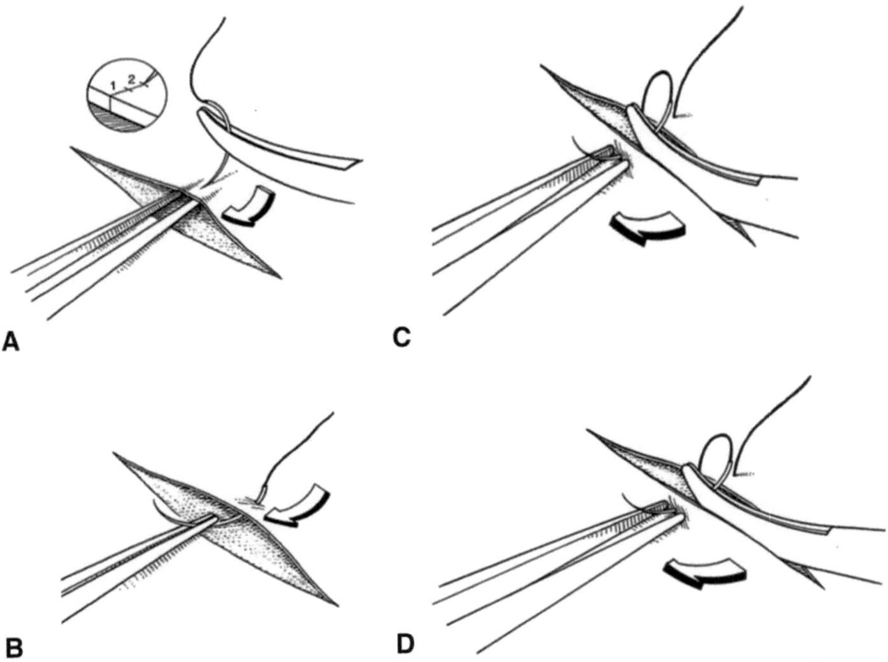

A C B D

Fig. 1.10 The entrance should be perpendicular at a point twice the wall thickness from the edge and the tips of the forceps provide counter-pressure, helping the needle pass through the tissue (**a**). The needle is slowly pulled out from the edge following its curvature (**b**). Then, the needle is gently passed through the edge by a slight movement of the fingers with needle's own curvature (**c** and **d**)

forceps (Fig. 1.10a). Under low power magnification, the needle is passed perpendicular to the tissue plane through the left tissue edge from the inside, between the tips of the forceps, with a bite equal to that on right edge (Fig. 1.10b). The movement of the hand must follow the curvature of the needle (Fig. 1.10c). The needle should never be pulled through the tissue in one straight movement. One rough, straight pull can bend the needle and weaken the edge of the tissue by enlarging the needle hole. The needle holder keeps the suture end parallel to the exit hole as the needle is guided out of the tissue. Stop pulling the suture when a 1–2 cm length of the suture tail remains. Pull the needle and redundant length of suture away from the suture site before tying the knot (Fig. 1.10d).

Learning to Tie a Microsurgical Knot

Because so many microsurgical knots must be tied during a single male infertility microsurgical procedure, *learning how to tie a secure microsurgical knot tying is essential. Indeed, knot tying may consume up to 70% of total anastomotic time.* Therefore, *male infertility microsurgery is greatly facilitated by the surgeon's*

Fig. 1.11 Microsurgical knot

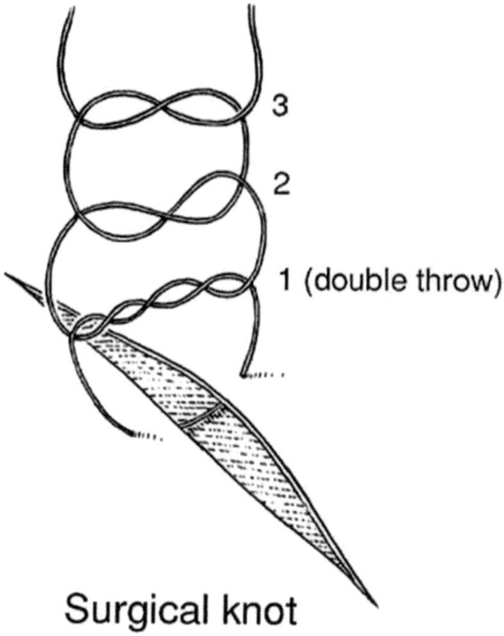

facility to tie knots with speed and accuracy under the operating microscope. In male infertility microsurgery, discrepant luminal diameters, thick muscular wall, and elastin content of the vas deferens make the surgeon's knot the choice of most microsurgeons [7–9]. Excellent microsurgical knot tying skills should be developed through extensive practice in the microsurgical lab.

Good microsurgical suturing skills can significantly reduce the operating time, which benefits both the patient and surgeon. The surgeon's knot starts with a double throw and completes with two to three additional throws (Fig. 1.11):

(a) Making a double loop and picking up the suture tail: When the suture is passed through the tissue from right to left, the short end of the suture on the right side should be about 1–2 cm in length. The long end of the suture is grasped using the forceps in the left hand at a point 3–4 cm from the exit point (Fig. 1.12a). The suture is looped with a clockwise movement above the suture site around the needle holder (Fig. 1.12b). The loop must be large enough to accommodate the tips of the needle holder and the suture long enough so that the loop of suture does not drop off the tips of the needle holder (Fig. 1.12c). After two loops are made, the tips of the forceps holding the suture should touch those of the needle holder, preventing the double loops from falling off the tip of the needle holder (Fig. 1.12d). The short tail of the suture is grasped with the needle holder (Fig. 1.13a). It can be difficult to pick up the suture tail when it sticks to the tissue. A piece of rubber glove laced around the suture site can help prevent this phenomenon.

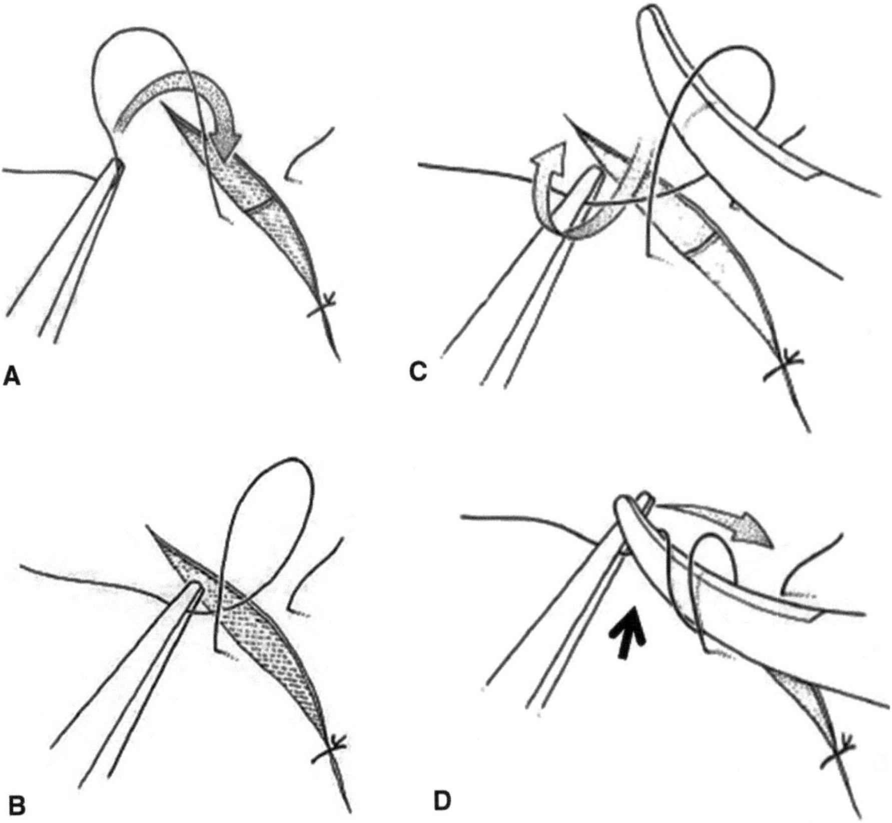

Fig. 1.12 It is critical to leave the suture end long enough to facilitate making a double loop under microscopic guidance .With the tips of the forceps grasping the suture, a single loop is made using a clockwise motion (**a**), in a half-circle towards the suture site (**b**). While a single loop is made (**c**), the tips of the needle holder are encircled clockwise around the tips of the forceps to make the second loop (**d**)

(b) Completing the first knot: Once the suture tail is grasped by the tips of the needle holder, the surgeon's knot is completed by drawing the instruments apart with an even motion along a flat plane (Fig. 1.13b). The knot should be tightened until the tissue edges are just apposed, not strangulated. The proper tension for each knot can be difficult to judge with delicate suture material (9-0 or 10-0).

(c) Completing the second and third knots: After the first knot is completed, the short end of the suture is placed so that it sticks up in the air. A single loop is made by the forceps around the tips of the needle holder and the suture tail is grasped and pulled through the loop to complete the second knot. With the same sequence of movements, the third knot is finished providing a secure knot (Fig. 1.13c).

(d) Cutting the suture: Once the knot has been completed, hold both ends of the suture on gentle traction with the forceps. The suture is cut with microscissors leaving the ends long enough (2 mm) to prevent unraveling of the knot (Fig. 1.13d). The needle is finally removed from the operative field and placed on a needle pad.

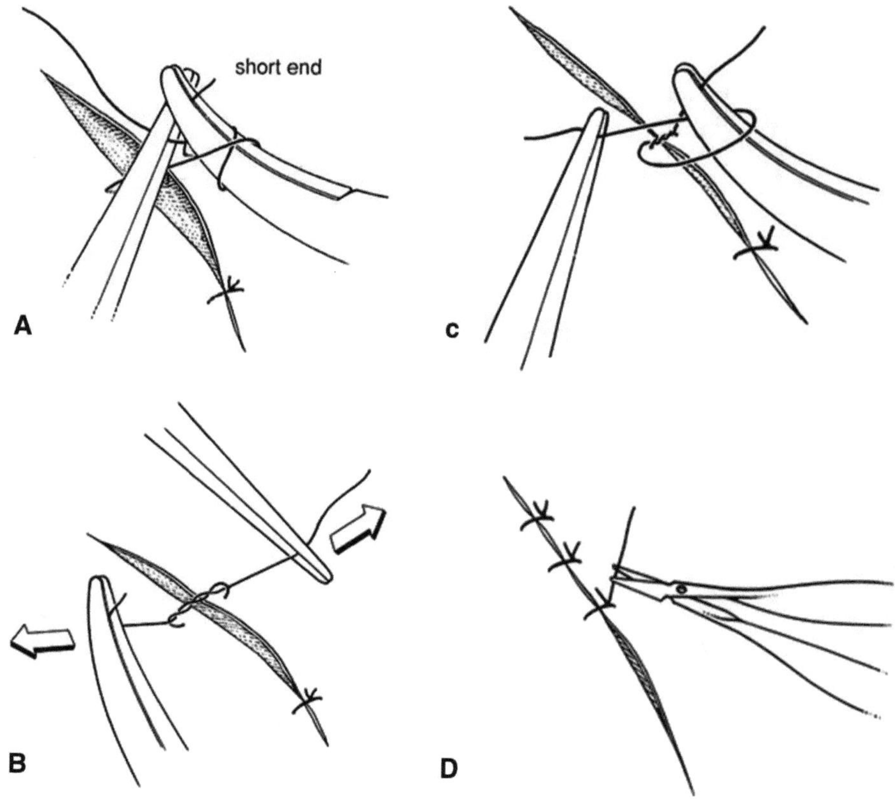

Fig. 1.13 After the double (second) loop is made, the tips of the needle holder are held close together and moved to pick up the short suture end (**a**). The first double-throw knot is completed by pulling the needle holder and forceps apart flat (**b**). The second single loop is made and a surgeon's knot is completed by typing the second and third throws (**c**). Suture is cut with a pair of microscissors (**d**)

Silicone Tubing and Vasectomized Segments in Vasovasostomy Training

We have found the use of silicone tubing and vasectomy specimens to be inexpensive and readily available models for training of urology residents and fellows [3].

1. *Preparation of silicone tubing*. A 5–10 cm length of soft silicone medical grade tubing (0.062 in. inner diameter and 0.125 in. outer diameter) is held with a Microspike approximator [10]. The inner layer of the silicone tubing simulates the mucosal suturing. The silicone tubing is divided in a perpendicular plane with a scalpel or a razor blade between the arms of the approximator (Fig. 1.14). The approximator is fixed in place with tape to prevent movement under the

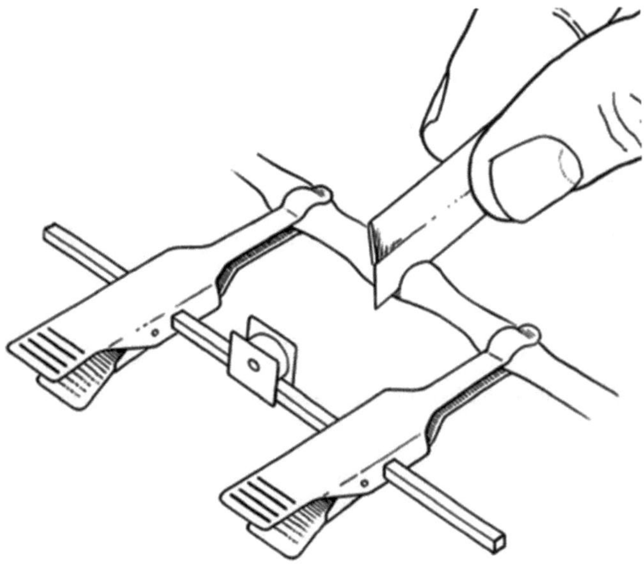

Fig. 1.14 A sharp razor blade is used to cut the silicone tubing between the two arms of the Microspike approximator or a vascular clamp

microscope. The Microspike approximator holds the tubing in place and allows the anterior and the posterior walls of the anastomosis to be exposed.

(a) *End-to-end anastomosis with one-layer technique*. Although multilayer techniques are generally used in clinical settings, the one-layer anastomosis is useful for learning microsurgical vasovasostomy. Trainees can practice with this technique to familiarize themselves with proper positioning, order, and placement of sutures for a one-layer or a two-layer end-to-end anastomosis [8]. A (10-0 or 9-0) single-armed needle is perpendicularly placed at a point twice the wall thickness from the edge on the posterior wall of the tubing from the outside. The tips of the forceps provide counter-pressure on the wall of the silicone tubing as the needle is passed through the wall between the tips of the forceps (Fig. 1.15a). The needle tip is passed through the wall from inside out on the other side. The needle is carefully pulled through the wall of the tubing following the curve of the needle, with small gentle motion (Fig. 1.15b). Two to four additional sutures are placed on the top half of the tubing. The approximator is turned over and folded in the opposite direction to expose the back wall of the anastomosis. The identical procedure is repeated on the backside. Eight to twelve interrupted 9-0 or 10-0 monofilament nylon sutures are required to complete the anastomosis of the silicone tubing.

(b) *End-to-end anastomosis with two-layer technique*. Preparation is the same as for the single-layer anastomosis. Two to three interrupted sutures of 10-0 monofilament nylon, single or doubled armed, are placed through only the inner one-half of the tubing (Fig. 1.16a). Right-handed surgeons can use the

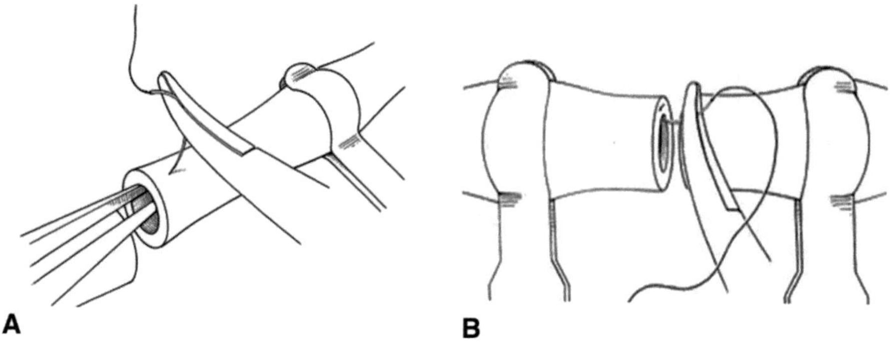

Fig. 1.15 The initial suture of an end-to-end anastomosis using silicone tubing. The tip of forceps must support the wall of silicone tubing with counter-pressure to assist the needle pass through the anterior wall between the tips of the forceps (**a**). Then, the needle pierces upward through the other side of the silicone tubing following its own curvature (**b**)

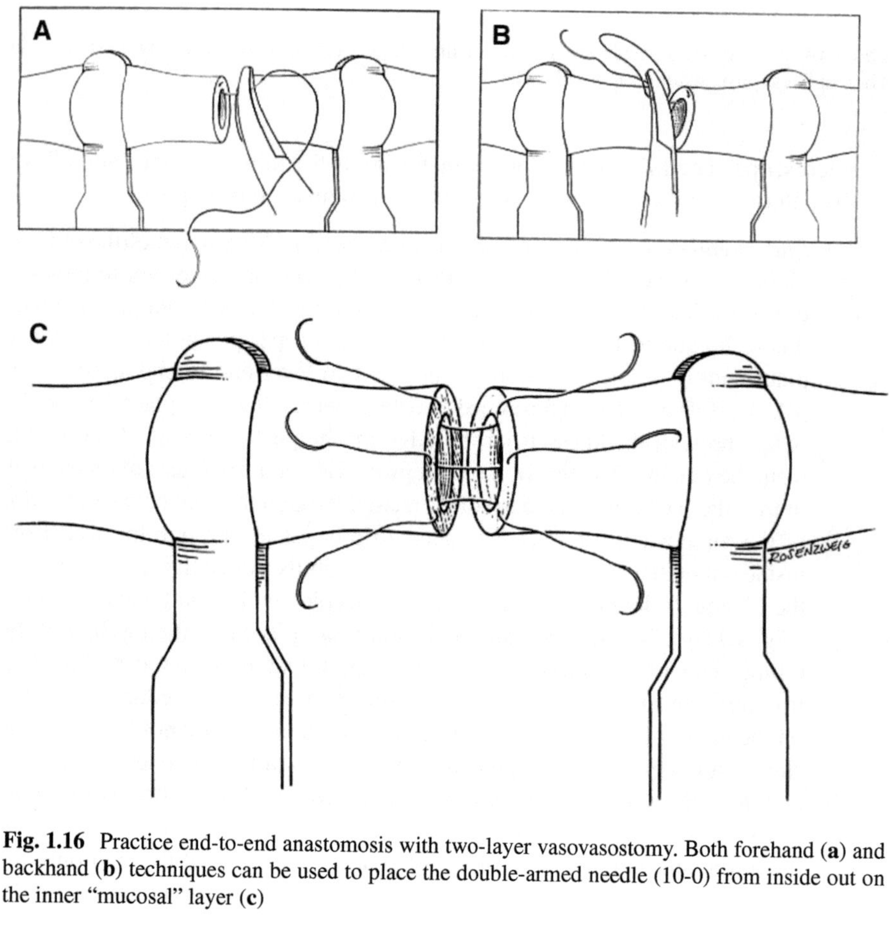

Fig. 1.16 Practice end-to-end anastomosis with two-layer vasovasostomy. Both forehand (**a**) and backhand (**b**) techniques can be used to place the double-armed needle (10-0) from inside out on the inner "mucosal" layer (**c**)

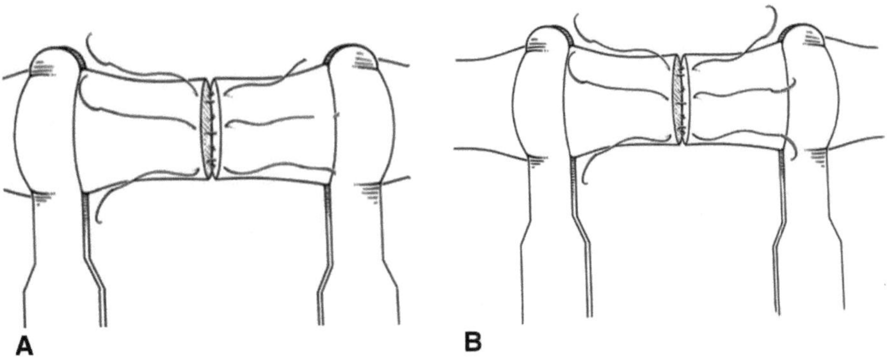

Fig. 1.17 After completion of the "mucosal" layer, several interrupted sutures are placed and tied exactly between the two previous sutures in the "mucosal" layer. Then, the approximator is turned over and folded in the opposite direction to expose the back wall of anastomosis. Identical procedures are repeated on the second side. (a) Single-armed needle. (b) Double-armed needle

backhand needle hold to place the needle from inside out on the inner layer of the right-sided tubing (Fig. 1.16b). Once the first 2–3 mucosal sutures are placed and tied with the surgeon's knot, a 9-0 monofilament nylon single-armed needle is placed exactly in between the two previous "mucosal" sutures in the outer layer of the tubing without penetrating the lumen of the tube, simulating the placement of the muscularis and adventitial layer suture (Fig. 1.16c). The approximator is turned over and folded in the opposite direction to expose the back wall of the anastomosis (Fig. 1.17a, b). The inner layer of tubing is approximated with 6–8 interrupted 10-0 monofilament nylon sutures. Eight to twelve interrupted 9-0 sutures are placed to close the outer layer.

2. *Vasectomy segments*. Use of vasectomy specimens for training was originally reported by Belker et al. as an effective method for learning two-layer vasovasostomy in the laboratory [11]. Long segments of vas deferens can also be harvested from radical prostatectomy specimens. After vasectomy, the segment is placed in a saline-moistened gauze sponge in a small capped jar and immediately refrigerated until use for practice in the laboratory (Fig. 1.18a). Although refrigerated human vasal specimens preserved in saline may be usable for up to 8 weeks, fresh segments always provide a more realistic tissue consistency. After practicing the one-layer and two-layer anastomoses on silicone tubing, the trainee can apply the technique on vasal segments.

End-to-end anastomosis with multilayer technique: The Microspike approximator is used to stabilize the segment on the operating board. The segment must be kept moist with saline at all times during the procedure. The segment is perpendicularly divided between the arms of the approximator. The cut surface of both ends of the vasectomized segment is inspected under 8–10 power magnification. If the lumen of the vas deferens is not clearly visible, a fine microvessel dilator with a rounded tip is gently inserted into the lumen (Fig. 1.18b). After dilation, a mucosal ring should

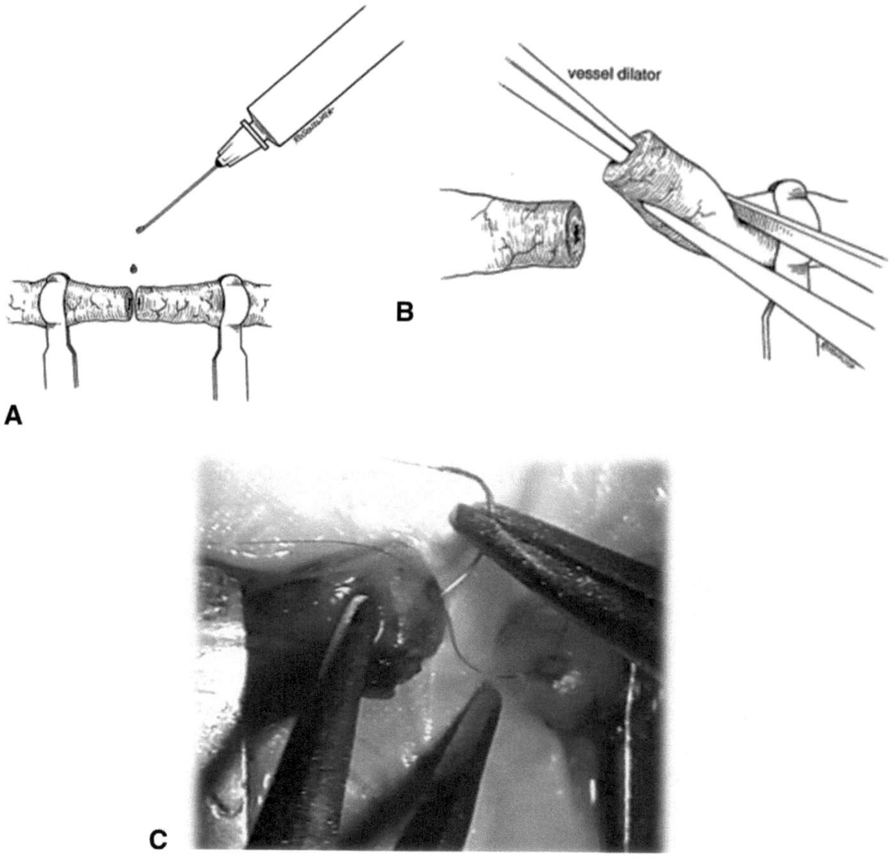

Fig. 1.18 The vas segment should be kept moist with saline solution at all time during the anastomosis practice (**a**). If the lumen of the vas is not clearly visible, a fine microvessel dilator with a rounded tip is gently inserted into the lumen without damaging the mucosa and muscularis (**b**). A mucosal ring should be seen after dilation. Both ends of the vas should be inspected carefully. A mucosal suture is placed from inside to outside if a double-armed suture is used (**c**)

be seen (Fig. 1.18c). Blue tape is placed under the anastomotic site as a contrast background. The double-armed 10-0 monofilament nylon suture is placed through the mucosa on each side, from inside out. The 10-0 nylon double-armed fishhook-shaped mucosal needles minimize mucosal manipulation and trauma (Fig. 1.19a). After the first two or three mucosal sutures are placed and tied anteriorly, slightly deeper muscularis sutures are placed in between each pair of previously placed mucosal sutures (Fig. 1.19b). Finally, two to four superficial adventitial 9-0 sutures are placed outside the mucosal sutures. The approximator is turned over and folded in the opposite direction to expose the mucosa (Fig. 1.19c). The mucosal and muscularis layers are completed in a fashion identical to that just described (Fig. 1.19d).

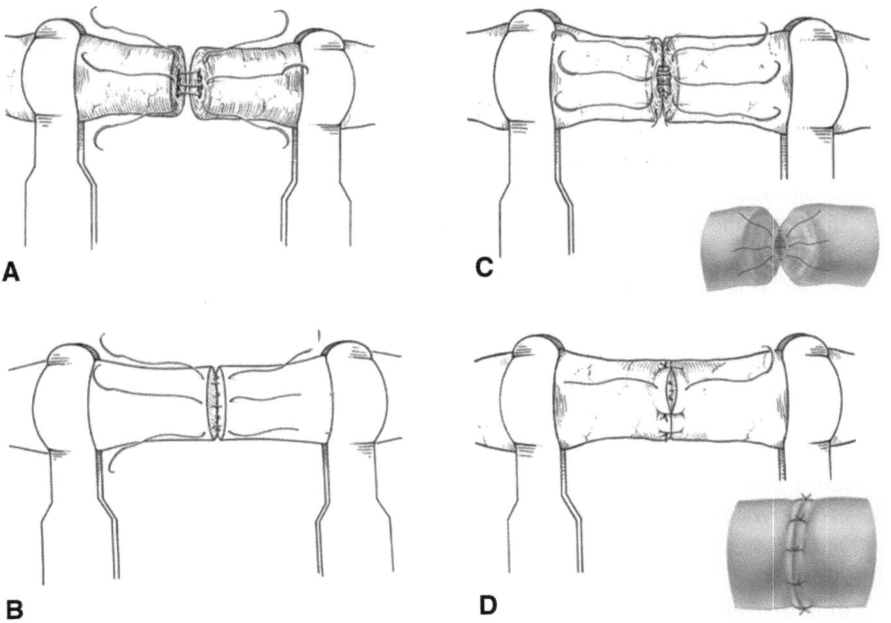

Fig. 1.19 Three mucosal sutures (double-armed, 10-0) are placed from inside to outside on the mucosal (**a**). After all of the mucosal sutures are tied with surgeon's knots, several 9-0 (single-armed) sutures are placed through the muscularis and adventitia in between each pair of mucosal sutures (**b**). When the anterior layer is completed, the approximator is then turned over and folded to expose the mucosa in order to perform the posterior mucosal and muscularis anastomosis (**c**). Several interrupted sutures complete the anastomosis of muscularis and adventitial layers (**d**)

Evaluation of the Anastomosis

A technically accurate anastomosis using silicone tubing or vasal segments should be leakproof when injected with fluid. In addition, the lumen of the silicone tubing or vasal segment should be exposed by longitudinally cutting open the inner (mucosa) and the outer (muscularis) layers of the anastomosis under the operating microscope to assess for evenness of suture placement.

Use of Rats for Microsurgical Training and Research

Six-to-eight-week-old (200–300 g) male, Sprague-Dawley rat is ideal for male infertility microsurgical training and research. A vasal obstruction animal model can be prepared by occlusion of the vas deferens with two small metal clips without dividing the vas deferens resulted in the lowest incidence of sperm granuloma formation (50%). Maximal epididymal tubule dilation is observed 7 days after vasal occlusion and maintained thereafter. Currently, we use an unobstructed rat model for male infertility microsurgical training. Anesthesia for all microsurgical procedures was induced using intraperitoneal injection of Xylazine (10 mg/kg) mixed with ketamine chloride (100 mg/kg).

1. *Rat vasovasostomy*. The rat vas deferens can be challenging to work with because of its small size. The rat vas deferens measures approximately 1.5–2 mm in outer diameter and approximately 0.15–0.25 mm in luminal diameter for rats weighing 250–300 g. Dilation of the testicular end to a 0.5 mm luminal diameter can be achieved with the technique described, mimicking the discrepant luminal diameters seen in vasectomized patients seeking reversal. Rat vasovasostomy is performed as an end-to-end anastomosis using either a one-layer or a two-layer technique, as previously described (Fig. 1.18a–c). Hemostasis can be precisely accomplished with microsurgical bipolar cautery, which allows current flow only between the two fine blades of the bipolar cautery forceps. *It is important to learn how to use the bipolar cautery correctly in the lab. The bipolar cautery creates a much smaller area of tissue damage than monopolar cautery. Surgeons should avoid to use a monopolar cautery for male infertility microsurgeries.* Although the surgical steps are similar to those used for practice with silicone tubing, tissue feel in the rat model more accurately reflects actual clinical experience.
2. *Rat vasoepididymostomy. Vasoepididymostomy (VE) represents the most technically challenging microsurgical procedure for the treatment of obstructive male infertility.* Success for this type of surgery is heavily dependent on the quality and extent of practice and training in the lab. Rat vasoepididymostomy may be performed with the end-to-side intussusception technique. In this chapter, we describe the double-armed 2-suture end-to-side longitudinal intussusception VE technique as well as the single-armed 2-suture longitudinal VE technique. *Since 2002, the longitudinal 2-suture VE has been our standard technique at Cornell.*

Preparation of the animal is similar regardless of vasoepididymostomy technique. Through a midline incision in the post-vasectomy rat, the reproductive organs are delivered and examined. The gubernaculum is divided for complete mobilization of the epididymis and testis. The location of tubular dilatation is found. The cauda and corpus of the epididymis are gently dissected free from the testis. The epididymis can be transected above the level of obstruction or an opening in the tunic can be made which allows for dissection of an individual epididymal tubule. The ideal location to create a window in the tunic is an avascular area with visible dilated epididymal tubules (Fig. 1.20a). The size of the tunical opening should approximate the outer dimension of the cut surface of the vas deferens. The end-to-side technique requires a small opening on an epididymal tubule that has been dissected free from its neighboring tubules in the open tunical window (Fig. 1.20a,b). The tubular opening is created by elevating the free tubule and incising it with microscissors. Two 10-0 mucosal sutures are placed to bring together the lumen of the epididymal tubule with the mucosa of the vas deferens (Figs. 1.20c and 1.21b). This method eliminates the possibility of inadvertent transection of the tubule from

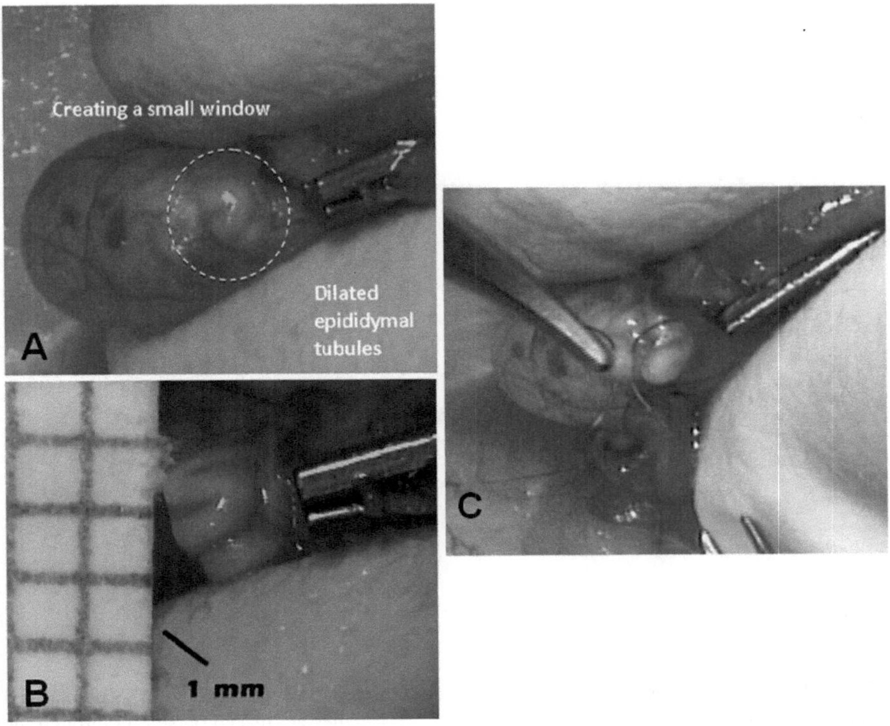

Fig. 1.20 Creating a small window in the tunica in order to free a dilated epididymal tubule in the region of the cauda (**a**). Measurement of cauda epididymal tubule (**b**). Two microsutures are placed on the epididymal tubule longitudinally (**c**)

direct lateral placement of suture. Ten to twelve 10-0 sutures are used to close the outer layer. This results in a watertight connection between the epididymal tunic window and the outer sheath of the vas deferens.

1. *Longitudinal single-armed suture intussusception end-to-side vasoepididymostomy* (Fig. 1.21) [12]. The single-armed suture longitudinal intussusception vasoepididymostomy is performed using two of the same single-armed 10-0 nylon sutures (Sharpoint AK-0100; Surgical Specialties Corp.). The first suture is placed in an outside-in fashion through the mucosal layer of the vas at position a1 (Fig. 1.21a). The needle pierces the lateral aspect of the epididymal tubule, in and out longitudinally. However, the needle is not pulled through, but rather left in the wall to prevent collapse of the tubule (Fig. 1.21b). The second 10-0 single-armed nylon suture is placed identically through position b1 on the vas but parallel to the first suture on the contralateral side of the vas and epididymal tubule (Fig. 1.21a and 1.21b). The epididymis is carefully opened with a pair of ophthalmic microscissors longitudinally in between the two needles and the extruded content is examined for sperm. The needles from sutures a and b are pulled through the wall of the epididymis and placed inside out through the mucosal

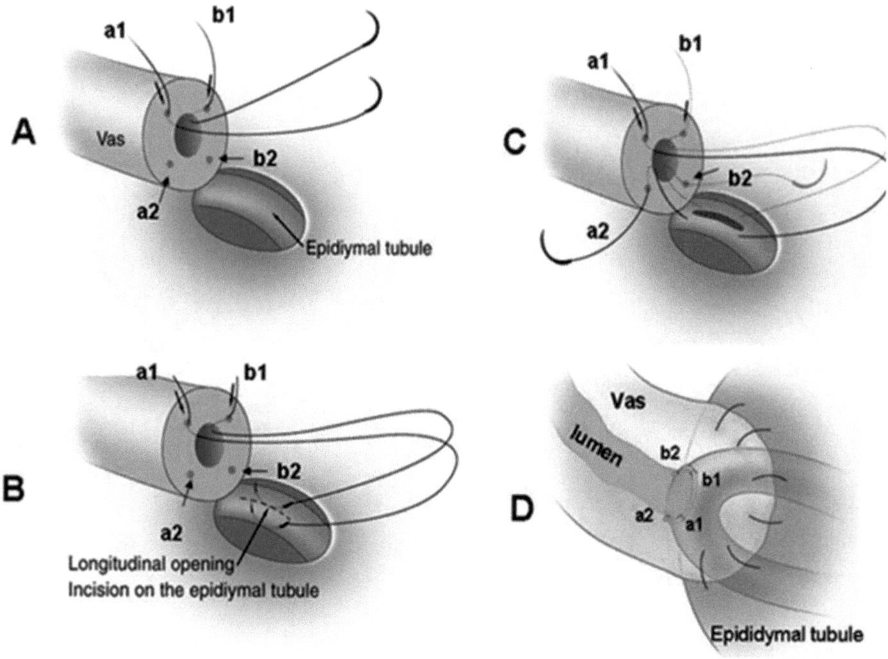

Fig. 1.21 Longitudinal single-armed 2-suture intussusception VEP technique: Single-armed 2-suture placement in the mucosa of the vas deferens. Needles are placed outside-in through the vasal lumen at positions a1 and b1 (**a**). Needles are placed longitudinally through the wall of the epididymal tubule, but not pulled through (**b**). The epididymal tubule is opened longitudinally and examined for motile sperm Needles are placed inside out through the vasal lumen at positions a2 and b2 (**c**). Sutures "a" and "b" are tied down (a1–a2 and b1–b2) and the epididymal tubule intussuscepts into the lumen of the vas. Watertight closure of the anastomosis and the epididymal tubule intussuscepts into the lumen of the vas (**d**)

layer of the vas at positions a2 and b2, respectively, at the base of the vasal lumen. All of the sutures are placed approximately 1 mm into the vasal lumen. When the sutures are tied down (a1–a2 and b1–b2), the epididymal tubule gently intussuscepts into the lumen of the vas (Fig. 1.21c). The epididymal tunic is secured to the vasal muscle and adventitia with eight to ten interrupted 10-0 nylon sutures using the remaining length of the single-armed sutures (Fig. 1.21d).

2. *Longitudinal double-armed two-suture intussusception end-to-side vasoepididymostomy* (Fig. 1.22) [13]. The setup is identical to that for the single-armed suture technique described above in which the abdominal side of the vas is anchored to the epididymal tunic with a single 10-0 nylon suture. However, two 10-0 nylon double-armed sutures are used (Sharpoint AK-0101, Surgical Specialties Corp.) with a different suture placement pattern (Fig. 1.22a). In the initial step, one needle from each of the two sutures is placed longitudinally along both edges of the selected epididymal tubule parallel to each other in the same configuration as above, without pulling the needles through, and then, the

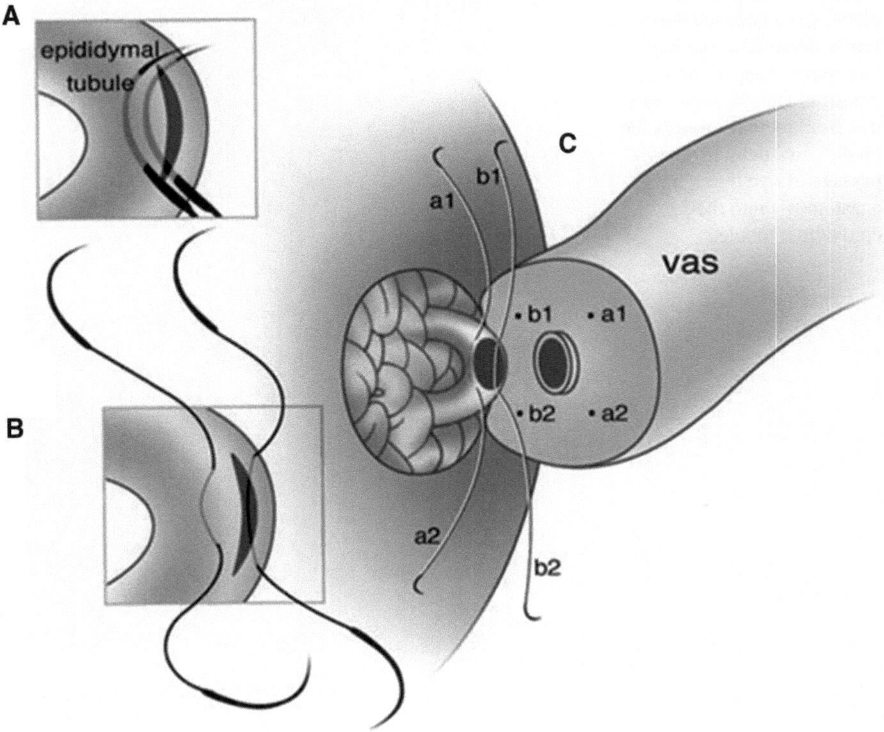

Fig. 1.22 Longitudinal double-armed 2-suture intussusception VEP technique. Two double-armed 10-0 sutures are placed on the epididymal tubule longitudinally. The epididymal tubule is then opened using microscissors between the two needles (**a**). The needles are pulled through and prepared to be placed through the vas (**b**). The first suture is passed inside out through the vas lumen (a1) while the needle on the other end is passed inside out through position a2. The second suture will follow the same suture placement pattern as the first suture, where b1 from the epididymal tubule will pass inside out through the vas lumen and the needle on the other end is passed inside out through position b2 from the epididymal tubule to the vas lumen b2 (**c**)

epididymal tubule is opened longitudinally between the two needles. The needles are pulled through and prepared for placement through the vas (Fig. 1.22b). Starting with the first suture, the needle on one end is passed inside out through the mucosal layer of the vas at position a1 while the needle on the other end is passed inside out through position a2 (Fig. 1.22c). The same maneuver is performed with the second suture. One needle is passed inside out through the mucosal layer of the vas at position b1 and the needle on the other end of the suture is passed inside out through position b2. The two sutures are tied down (a1–a2 and b1–b2), resulting in intussusception of the epididymal tubule into the vasal lumen (Fig. 1.21d).

3. *Postoperative evaluation techniques*. The reproductive organs are exposed to evaluate the anastomosis for any complications. Patency is defined using two

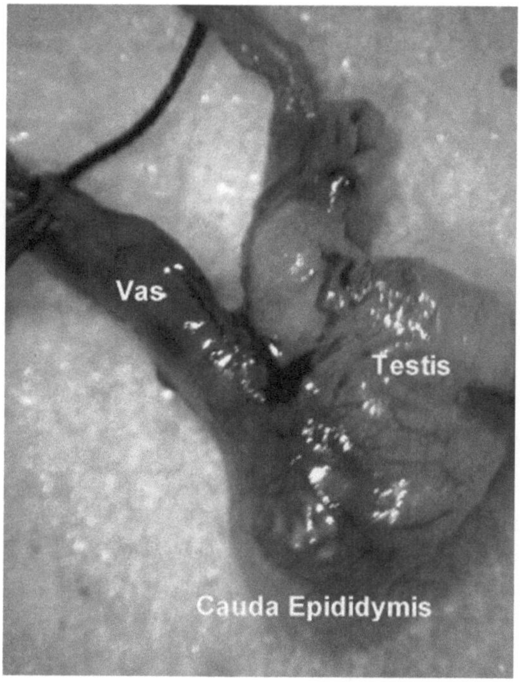

Fig. 1.23 Mechanical patency is achieved when a retrograde methylene-blue vasogram, using a 24-G angiocatheter sheath to inject dye from the vas towards the epididymis, demonstrates passage of dye through the anastomosis into the epididymal tubules

criteria: (a) functional patency is achieved when motile sperm are found in the vasal fluid microscopically at 400× magnification on phase contrast microscopy; (b) mechanical patency is achieved when a retrograde methylene-blue vasogram, using a 24-G angiocatheter sheath to inject dye from the vas towards the epididymis, demonstrates passage of dye through the anastomosis into the epididymal tubules (Fig. 1.23).

Male Infertility Microsurgical Pearls

- Success in male infertility microsurgery is heavily dependent on the quality and extent of practice and training in the microsurgical laboratory.
- Microsurgery should be learned in the microsurgical lab, not on the patient.
- Adjust your seat level until you have a comfortable sitting position. Having the sitting level too high or low can result in a sore neck or back. Your head should sit straight on your neck, and your eyes should look straight ahead, perpendicular to your spine.
- Learning how to tie a secure microsurgical knot tying is essential; it may take up to 70% of total operative time. Male infertility microsurgery is greatly facilitated

by the surgeon's ability to tie knots with speed and accuracy under the operating microscope.
- Good microsurgical suturing skills can significantly reduce the operating time, which benefits both the patient and surgeon.
- One distinction of a good microsurgeon is the ability to preserve the original shape and condition of the needle throughout the operation.
- Like pure microvascular, plastic, and other reconstructive microsurgeries, microsurgery for male infertility ranks among the most technically and mentally challenging of surgical procedures.
- We have found the use of suture practice card, silicone tubing, and vasectomy specimens to be inexpensive and readily available models for training of urology residents and fellows.

Other Learning Sources

Online microsurgical videos are a great educational source for understanding and learning male infertility microsurgery. For more information about our microsurgical training course and our online microsurgical videos, please visit our Web site at http://www.maleinfertility.org.

References

1. Silber SJ. Microsurgery for male infertility. Microsurgery. 1988;9:251.
2. Gilbert BR, Goldstein M. New directions in male reproductive microsurgery. Microsurgery. 1988;9:281.
3. Li PS, Schlegel PN, Goldstein M. Use of silicone medical grade tubing for microsurgical vasovasostomy training. Urology. 1992;39:556.
4. Goldstein M. The making of a microsurgeon. J Androl. 2006;27:161.
5. Acland RD. Instrumentation for microsurgery. Orthop Clin North Am. 1977;8:281.
6. Sheynkin YR, Li PS, Magid ML, et al. Comparison of absorbable and nonabsorbable sutures for microsurgical vasovasostomy in rats. Urology. 1999;53:1235.
7. Sharlip ID. Vasovasostomy: comparison of two microsurgical techniques. Urology. 1981;17:347.
8. Southwick GJ, Temple-Smith PD. Epididymal microsurgery: current techniques and new horizons. Microsurgery. 1988;9:266.
9. Belker AM. Technical aids for vasovasostomy. Urology. 1982;20:635.
10. Goldstein M. Microspike approximator for vasovasostomy. J Urol. 1985;134:74.
11. Belker AM, Acland RD, Sexter MS, et al. Microsurgical two-layer vasovasostomy: laboratory use of vasectomized segments. Fertil Steril. 1978;29:48.
12. Monoski MA, Schiff J, Li PS, et al. Innovative single-armed suture technique for microsurgical vasoepididymostomy. Urology. 2007;69:800.
13. Chan PT, Li PS, Goldstein M. Microsurgical vasoepididymostomy: a prospective randomized study of 3 intussusception techniques in rats. J Urol. 2003;169:1924.

Chapter 2
Microsurgery Training: What Should a Resident Know? Should All Microsurgeons be Fellowship Trained?

Ethan Grober and Peter N. Kolettis

Abstract Surgery for male infertility has evolved into a highly specialized endeavor within the specialty of Urology. Most procedures in this field, including vasectomy reversal, varicocele ligation, and sperm retrieval are performed with microsurgery. In some Urology residency programs, training in male infertility may not be viewed as a priority and many Urology departments do not have a faculty member dedicated to this field. As a result, there is a perception among male infertility specialists that many urologists' training is deficient in this area. This chapter outlines the need and scope of microsurgical training in residency and reviews the impact of fellowship training on the practice of urologic microsurgery.

Keywords Microsurgery • Training • Fellowship • Education • Residency

Surgery for male infertility has evolved into a highly specialized endeavor within the specialty of Urology. Most procedures in this field, including vasectomy reversal, varicocele ligation, and sperm retrieval are performed with microsurgery. In some Urology residency programs, training in male infertility may not be viewed as a priority and many Urology departments do not have a faculty member dedicated to this field. As a result, there is a perception among male infertility specialists that many urologists' training is deficient in this area.

Along with this perceived deficiency in male infertility training is a concern regarding a deficiency in microsurgery training. In US residency training programs,

---

E. Grober, M.D., M.Ed. (✉)
Division of Urology, Mount Sinai and Women's College Hospital, University of Toronto, 60 Murray Street, 6th Floor, Toronto, ON, Canada M5T 3L9
e-mail: egrober@mtsinai.on.ca

P.N. Kolettis, M.D.
Department of Surgery/Urology, University of Alabama-Birmingham, 1530 Third Avenue South, Birmingham, AL 35294-3411, USA
e-mail: peter.kolettis@ccc.uab.edu

J.I. Sandlow (ed.), *Microsurgery for Fertility Specialists: A Practical Text*, DOI 10.1007/978-1-4614-4196-0_2, © Springer Science+Business Media New York 2013 it is not possible to gather data on the number of microsurgical cases performed by a particular resident. Infertility microsurgery procedures are included in the category of "scrotal surgery" which would also include hydrocelectomy and spermatocelectomy, among others. This concern has implications for which practitioners should be allowed to perform microsurgical procedures such as vasectomy reversals. Vasovasostomy (VV) can be performed without an operating microscope but it is generally acknowledged that outcomes for vasectomy reversal are superior with microsurgery [1]. Despite this generally accepted information, considerable variability in practice patterns exists. In a study of practicing urologists who perform vasectomy reversals, 56% of community urologists, 65% of academic, non-fellowship-trained urologists, and 93% of fellowship-trained urologists used an operating microscope [2]. In some cases, vasoepididymostomy (VE) is required for vasectomy reversal [3]. Given the dimensions of the epididymis, it would be impossible to perform VE without an operating microscope. It seems unlikely and few would disagree that one could receive sufficient microsurgery training in residency to adequately perform VE. Thus, most male infertility specialists would say fellowship training is required to perform VE.

Some investigators, with justifiable concern, have suggested that vasectomy reversals should be performed only by those able to perform VE. In their study, Chawla et al. reported that 48% of failed anastomoses were due to untreated epididymal obstruction where a vasovasostomy rather than vasoepididymostomy was performed. The possibility of selection bias exists, as these patients were all seen at a tertiary center for redo reversals after an initial failed reversal elsewhere [4]. Nonetheless, other studies clearly describe a significant chance for failed reversals secondary to epididymal obstruction if only VV is performed.

The probability of epididymal obstruction and the need for VE increases with increasing time since the vasectomy. For example, in the study by the Vasovasostomy Study Group, the patency rate for VV was 70% for obstructive intervals of at least 15 years [5]. This suggests that the prevalence of bilateral epididymal obstruction is 30% (assuming 100% patency) for this obstructive interval. Similarly, Fuchs and Burt demonstrated that with an obstructive interval of 15 years, over 60% of men required a VE on at least one side [6].

Predicting with certainty when VE is required is not possible but the probability of requiring VE can be estimated based on the discussion above. One must determine what failure rate would be tolerated if VV were performed for everyone, regardless of need for VE, and determine a maximum obstructive interval that corresponds to this failure rate. For example, if one accepts a possible 30% technical failure rate, then only surgeons who can perform VE should perform reversals for obstructive intervals greater than 15 years. The alternative is to allow only those capable of performing VE (likely only those with fellowship training) to perform vasectomy reversals.

A recent study by Nangia et al. examined the distribution of male infertility specialists in the USA. Data were obtained from the membership directories of two subspecialty societies devoted to the study and treatment of male infertility, The Society for the Study of Male Reproduction (SSMR) and the Society for Male Reproduction and Urology (SMRU). Their study suggested that large areas of the country are underserved with respect to care for male infertility. For example, 13 states had no male reproductive specialists [7]. These data would therefore suggest that there simply are not enough fellowship-trained urologists to provide all the male infertility care, so general urologists, by necessity, should be able to perform the basic evaluation and procedures in this subspecialty.

What should be considered basic evaluation and procedures? It is the authors' opinion that the general urologist should be able to perform the initial history, physical and laboratory evaluation. With respect to procedures for male infertility, the general urologist could perform diagnostic testis biopsy, varicocele ligation and possibly VV. Given our capability to distinguish between obstructive and nonobstructive azoospermia in most instances based on history, physical examination and serum FSH level, a testis biopsy is rarely required for diagnostic purposes only. As described above, VV outcomes are generally superior with microsurgery. In addition, there is literature that suggests microsurgical varicocele ligation has superior results and fewer complications than non-microsurgical techniques. Therefore, residency training programs should provide education that allows the graduating resident to be able to perform the basic evaluation and basic procedures. In our residency, we have offered a 1 week laboratory course as an introduction to microsurgery. Residents also rotate through the outpatient clinic and participate in the evaluation of male infertility patients.

Even if one takes the position that only fellowship-trained urologists should do microsurgery, residency training should still at least expose the resident to male infertility and microsurgery. Without this exposure during residency, it seems unlikely that one would be stimulated to pursue additional fellowship training in the field.

More specialized procedures, such as microsurgical sperm retrieval, require more specialized training and collaboration with reproductive endocrinologists that perform in vitro fertilization [8]. Thus, it seems unlikely that the general urologist who did not complete fellowship training would have the required training to perform these procedures. Therefore, microsurgical sperm retrieval is probably best performed by those urologists with fellowship training in male infertility and microsurgery. Based on the above discussion, then, microsurgical training is important for providing optimal care for male patients with infertility and general urologists should be able to provide at least basic care. It follows then that basic male infertility and microsurgical training should be included in residency training. Training programs that do not have a specialist dedicated to this field would hopefully recognize this need and recruit a faculty member with expertise in male infertility and microsurgery.

Should all Urologic Microsurgeons be Fellowship Trained?

While fundamentally a philosophical question, it is worth exploring the impact of specialized fellowship training on our profession as urologic microsurgeons.

Over the few past decades, surgery has undergone significant evolution fueled by a forever-expanding quest for knowledge and incorporation of innovative surgical technologies [9–11]. In the face of such rapid evolution, issues concerning education and training have become paramount. Longer and more advanced training programs with increased specialization for urological surgeons have emerged as coping strategies in both education and practice. Throughout the urological community in Canada and the USA, increasing emphasis is being placed on surgical fellowships that provide periods of highly specialized and advanced surgical training, following the completion of formal residency training [9, 12–14]. Moreover, there continues to be a trend towards "credential inflation" to the point where new faculty positions within academic surgical programs almost universally require specialized fellowship training and a commitment towards research or teaching. Increasingly, many community and private practice positions are seeking urologists with unique and specialized skills sets and fellowship experience.

For the trainee, fellowships offer a period of focused training with high-volume surgical exposure allowing for the development of specialized technical skill sets and sound intraoperative judgment. They allow trainees to develop algorithms for the delivery of evidence based clinical care and cultivate the seeds towards a future program of research and scholarship. Fellowships stimulate networking among specialists with common interests and often lead to strong mentoring relationships with more established surgical faculty [9].

For the fellowship training programs and faculty, fellows contribute to the academic and financial productivity of the department, provide a high level of clinical service to patients, teach residents and medical students, share in the on-call duties, and represent a vehicle for national and international dissemination of program expertise and reputation [9].

Urologic microsurgery has evolved to become a highly specialized discipline that typically falls within the domain of the male infertility specialist. The surgical repertoire includes procedures like microsurgical vasectomy reversal (including both vasovasostomy and vasoepididymostomy), microsurgical varicocelectomy, microsurgical testicular sperm extraction (micro-TESE), and microsurgical spermatic cord denervation for chronic orchialgia. While many of these surgeries can and have been performed without microsurgical magnification, best evidence to date suggests that a microsurgical approach significantly enhances technical precision and leads to better patient outcomes [8, 15–17].

Better patient outcomes are also achieved with increased surgical volume and experience [18, 19]. However, exposure to microsurgery during urology residency is limited in many programs. Not all training programs have faculty dedicated to the practice of male infertility and microsurgery. Consequently there is a deficiency in both practical knowledge and skill among graduating urologists that can adversely impact patient care and surgical outcomes.

Urologic microsurgery is particularly challenging due to the inherent size and unique characteristics of the male reproductive anatomy. The microsurgical vasoepididymostomy (VE) best exemplifies this concern. In an analysis of patients undergoing a redo vasectomy reversal, Chawla et al. [20] demonstrated that 48% of vasectomy reversal failures were due to unrecognized epididymal obstruction. This finding likely reflects the inability of the original surgeon to perform a VE or a deficiency in their knowledge that a VE was indicated. The authors of this study concluded that all surgeons offering vasectomy reversal should be able to offer VE if indicated in order to best serve patients and their future fertility. Few urology residency graduates would be equipped to perform a VE without fellowship training in microsurgery.

Specific to vasectomy reversal, Crain et al. [21] highlighted important differences in practice patterns between fellowship-trained and non-fellowship-trained urologists. In particular, fellowship-trained infertility specialists performed significantly more vasectomy reversals and were more likely to perform procedures for patients with an obstructive interval >15 years. Moreover, surgeons with fellowship training were more likely to use an operating microscope, examine the vasal fluid intraoperatively and use finer suture material compared to surgeons without fellowship experience.

Currently there are ten established fellowship training programs devoted exclusively to the practice of male infertility and microsurgery within North America [22]. Training periods range from 1 to 2 years. Some offer a dedicated basic science research experience. All are supervised by specialists with extensive microsurgery experience. All fellowships offer high-volume clinical and surgical patient exposures that are complimented by the opportunity for repetitive, deliberate practice in the microsurgical skills laboratory.

The importance of good microsurgical fellowship training prior to independent surgical practice was recently reviewed by Williams et al. [23] who reported on the microsurgical vasectomy reversal outcomes of ten recently graduated (within 2 years) fellowship-trained microsurgeons. Analyzing a total of 310 microsurgical vasectomy reversals, overall patency rates (91%) and postoperative semen parameters were consistent with those reported by experienced microsurgeons. Unfortunately, there is no comparable data available on the operative outcomes of non-fellowship-trained specialists as it relates to urologic microsurgery.

Some insight on the impact of fellowships on the "surgical learning curve" is offered by Bianco et al. [24] who investigated the effects of fellowship training on cancer control following open radical prostatectomy. Overall, fellowship-trained surgeons had significantly lower rates of biochemical recurrence and positive surgical margins as compared to non-fellowship-trained surgeons. Interestingly, such findings were mitigated as the surgical experience of the non-fellowship-trained surgeons increased. The authors concluded that the surgical volumes that come as part of fellowship training could modify the slope of the surgical learning curve.

The duration of fellowship training that is required to achieve a sufficient degree of microsurgical competence is debatable and depends largely on the motivation and talents of the individual trainee together with the structure, objectives and opportunities provided within the fellowship training program. A minimum training period of 6–12 months seems reasonable. Quality microsurgical training opportunities outside of established fellowship programs are rare. Weekend microsurgery training courses may offer the opportunity to learn new techniques and brush up on established skill sets; however they are unlikely to be comprehensive enough to provide sufficient set skills, knowledge and judgment required of a contemporary urologic microsurgeon. Moreover, in the authors' view, it is critical that surgical skills training be achieved in the context of real patient clinical care. Despite the numerous testimonials of surgeons throughout the World Wide Web, weekend microsurgery training courses, microsurgery observerships, or short "mini" fellowships are not the same as formalized fellowship training in microsurgery. Even the most experienced microsurgeons continually reinforce that successful microsurgery is dependent upon much more than technical skill. There are critical judgments intraoperatively as well as decisions as to the best type of procedure for each patient that only come with practical experience and being involved in cases in real time. Mastery in microsurgery is a truly lifetime endeavor.

So back to the original question—*Should all urologic microsurgeons be fellowship trained?* Ideally yes. However, it is important to keep in mind that many of the pioneers in this field, those that have made some of the most important advancements, discoveries and contributions to urologic microsurgery, were not formally fellowship trained, but self-taught. Nonetheless, few would argue that a fellowship-trained specialist in urologic microsurgery represents the highest standard of surgical training and education. Such standards may be achieved without fellowship training as experience is obtained over time, however fellowships may serve to facilitate a surgeons progress and trajectory on the surgical learning curve [24, 25]. As access to medical information and self-advocacy increases, our patients will realize and demand such high standards of their surgeons. Our profession should promote and protect such high standards.

References

1. Middleton RG, Belker AM. Macrosurgery or microsurgery for vasovasostomy? Contemp Urol. 1995; 55–60.
2. Crain DS, Roberts JL, Ambling CL. Practice patterns in vasectomy reversal surgery: results of a questionnaire study among practicing urologists. J Urol. 2004;171:311–5.
3. Silber SJ. Epididymal extravasation following vasectomy as a cause for failure of vasectomy reversal. Fertil Steril. 1979;31:309–15.
4. Chawla A, O'Brien J, Lisi M, Zini A, Jarvi K. Should all urologists performing vasectomy reversals be able to perform vasoepididymostomies if required? J Urol. 2004;172:1048–50.
5. Belker AM, Thomas Jr AJ, Fuchs EF, Konnak JW, Sharlip ID. Results of 1,469 microsurgical vasectomy reversals by the Vasovasostomy Study Group. J Urol. 1991;145:505–11.
6. Fuchs EF, Burt RA. Vasectomy reversal performed 15 years or more after vasectomy: correlation of pregnancy outcome with partner age and with pregnancy results of in vitro fertilization with intracytoplasmic sperm injection. Fertil Steril. 2002;77:516–9.
7. Nangia AK, Likosky DS, Wang D. Distribution of male infertility specialists in relation to the male population and assisted reproductive technology centers in the United States. Fertil Steril. 2010;94:599–609.
8. Schlegel PN. Testicular sperm extraction: microdissection improves sperm yield with minimal tissue excision. Hum Reprod. 1999;14:131–5.
9. Grober ED, Elterman DS, Jewett MAS. Fellow or foe: the impact of fellowship training programs on the education of Canadian urology residents. Can Urol Assoc J. 2008;2:1–38.
10. Hemal AK, Menon M. Robotics in urology. Curr Opin Urol. 2004;14:89–93.
11. Reznick RK. Virtual reality surgical simulators: feasible but valid? J Am Coll Surg. 1999;189:127–8.

12. Endourological Society. Recognized fellowship programs. http://www.endourology.org/fellowship/fellowship.php. Accessed 17 July 2012.
13. Society of Pediatric Urology. Participating fellowship programs. http://www.spuonline.org/fellowships_pp.cgi. Accessed 17 July 2012.
14. Society of Urologic Oncology. Approved fellowship programs. http://suonet.org/fellowships/default.aspx. Accessed 17 July 2012.
15. Fox M. Vasectomy reversal-microsurgery for best results. Br J Urol. 1994;73(4):449–53.
16. Al-Said S, Al-Naimi A, Al-Ansari A, Younis N, Shamsodini A, A-Sadiq K, Shokeir AA. Varicocelectomy for male infertility: a comparative study of open, laparascopic and microsurgical approaches. J Urol. 2008;180(1):266–70.
17. Al-Kandari AM, Shabaan H, Ibrahim HM, Elshebiny YH, Shokeir AA. Comparison of outcomes of different varicocelectomy techniques: open inguinal, laparoscopic, and subinguinal microscopic varicocelectomy: a randomized clinical trial. Urology. 2007;69(3):417–20.
18. Klein EA, Bianco FJ, Serio AM, Eastham JA, Kattan MW, Pontes JE, Vickers AJ, Scardino PT. Surgeon experience is strongly associated with biochemical recurrence after radical prostatectomy for all preoperative risk categories. J Urol. 2008;179(6):2212–6.
19. Vickers AJ, Bianco FJ, Serio AM. The surgical learning curve for prostate cancer control after radical prostatectomy. J Natl Cancer Inst. 2007;99:1171–7.
20. Chawla A, O'brian J, Lisi M, Zini A, Jarvi K. Should all urologists performing vasectomy reversals be able to perform vasoepididymostomies if required? J Urol. 2004;172(3):1048–50.
21. Crain DS, Robert JL, Amling CL. Practice patterns in vasectomy reversal surgery: results of a questionnaire study among practicing urologists. J Urol. 2004;171(1):311–5.
22. American Society for Reproductive Medicine. Fellowship opportunities. http://www.asrm.org/detail.aspx?id=926. Accessed 17 July 2012.
23. Williams IV DH, Karpman E, Grober ED, Schrepferman CG, Crain DS, Chuang WW, Shin D, Khera M, Kuang W, Tanrikut C. Early vasectomy reversal experience and outcomes of fellowship-trained microsurgeons. J Urol. 2009;181:4–729.
24. Bianco FJ, Cronin AM, Klein EA, Pontes JE, Scardino PT, Vickers AJ. Fellowship training as a modifier of the surgical learning curve. Acad Med. 2010;85(5):863–8.
25. Oliak D, Owens M, Schmidt HJ. Impact of fellowship training on the learning curve for laparascopic gastric bypass. Obes Surg. 2004;14(2):197–200.

Chapter 3
Microsurgical Subinguinal Varix Ligation: Techniques and Technical Pearls

Joshua A. Bodie and Jay I. Sandlow

Abstract Varicocele can be defined as dilatation or tortuosity (varicosity) of the veins of the pampiniform plexus. Varicoceles are present in approximately 15% of unselected men, in 40% of men presenting with primary infertility, and a much higher percentage of couples with secondary infertility [1, 2]. Varicoceles are the most commonly seen and correctable cause of male-factor infertility [3]. Tulloch's report in 1955 [4] brought to the forefront the proactive treatment and study of varicoceles in the subfertile male. Previously, many investigators felt that varicocele repair was cosmetic or only halted testicular injury at best. Since this time, many studies have demonstrated that improvement in semen parameters and chance of pregnancy are very possible with surgical repair of varicoceles.

Keywords Varicocele • Subinguinal • Microsurgical • Infertility

Introduction/Background

Varicocele can be defined as dilatation or tortuosity (varicosity) of the veins of the pampiniform plexus. Varicoceles are present in approximately 15% of unselected men, in 40% of men presenting with primary infertility, and a much higher percentage of couples with secondary infertility [1, 2]. Varicoceles are the most commonly seen and correctable cause of male-factor infertility [3]. Tulloch's report in 1955 [4] brought to the forefront the proactive treatment and study of varicoceles in the subfertile male.

J.A. Bodie, M.D. (✉)
Department of Urology, University of Minnesota Medical Center,
MMC 394, 420 Delaware St. SE, Minneapolis, MN 55455, USA
e-mail: bodieja@umn.edu

J.I. Sandlow, M.D.
Department of Urology, Medical College of Wisconsin,
9200 W. Wisconsin Avenue, CLCC Bldg, 4th Floor, Milwaukee, WI 53226, USA
e-mail: jsandlow@mcw.edu

J.I. Sandlow (ed.), *Microsurgery for Fertility Specialists: A Practical Text*,
DOI 10.1007/978-1-4614-4196-0_3, © Springer Science+Business Media New York 2013

Previously, many investigators felt that varicocele repair was cosmetic or only halted testicular injury at best. Since this time, many studies have demonstrated that improvement in semen parameters and chance of pregnancy are very possible with surgical repair of varicoceles.

The exact mechanism by which varicoceles affect spermatogenesis or testicular function remains unclear. Suggested causes of testicular dysfunction due to varicoceles includes disruption of the countercurrent heat exchange in the spermatic cord resulting in decreased cooling of the testis compared to body core/rectal temperature, and the presence of reactive oxygen species/oxidative stress. Additional theories include autoimmunity and the venous reflux of adrenal hormones into the pampiniform plexus. Of these mechanisms, heat is probably the largest contributor, and there is evidence showing decrease of testis temperature post-varicocelectomy [5–7].

Varicoceles typically become evident around puberty. They are most commonly left sided but can be found bilaterally in at least 10%, and up to 50%, of men. The etiology may be a longer left spermatic vein with its right-angle insertion into the left renal vein and/or absence of valves, which causes a higher hydrostatic pressure in the left spermatic vein, causing dilatation [8, 9]. The nutcracker phenomenon is also a possible etiology [10], although this is less likely. Significant solitary right varicoceles are less common, likely due to the right internal spermatic vein's drainage directly into the inferior vena cava, but in rare cases could be the presenting symptom of an occult retroperitoneal malignancy.

Indications

There are three potential consequences of varicoceles: decreased sperm quantity/quality, loss of endocrine function of the testicle over time, and pain.

The majority of men undergoing varicocele ligation are approximately 20–45 years of age, most typically for fertility or pain issues. There is some evidence that testosterone production may improve after microscopic varicocele ligation but varicocele repair strictly for endocrine hypofunction is a debated topic [11]. The insult of the varicoceles is felt to be cumulative over time, and testicular atrophy may occur in adults. The majority of the testicular volume is made up by germ cells, so significant size loss of the testicle is typically caused by decreased germ cells/spermatogenesis, rather than loss of Leydig cells. Varicoceles in adolescents are associated with a smaller ipsilateral testis as well, but hypotrophy may be present, rather than atrophy. Those adolescents with objective evidence of testis size loss ipsilateral to the varicocele should be considered for varicocele repair [12]. Varicocele repair in adolescents has been shown to result in "catch-up" growth in boys with ipsilateral loss of testicular volume [13, 14].

Treatment of a varicocele for fertility reasons is indicated only for clinically detectable varicoceles [12]. This signifies varicoceles that are palpable on physical exam, not solely diagnosed by ultrasound, radiography or other means. The exception may be use of trans-scrotal ultrasonography to compliment a difficult physical exam, such as in an obese man or in one with an abnormally thick scrotal wall. Ultrasound may be helpful in rare cases where it is difficult to determine on physical exam whether a thickened spermatic cord is due to a varicocele versus a lipomatous cord. Men with varicoceles commonly show abnormalities in sperm concentration or motility. Men with larger varicoceles tend to have lower sperm concentration and motility than those with smaller varicoceles, though not all studies have shown this association [15–17].

Surgical Technique

Some of the earliest reports of varicocele repair describe a scrotal approach. This route has since been abandoned due to high rates of complications and recurrence. Palomo, in 1948, reported the high retroperitoneal method of varicocele repair. The retroperitoneal approach involves ligation of the internal spermatic vein as it exits the internal inguinal ring with preservation of the internal spermatic artery. In modern times, a slightly modified approach of this type can also be performed laparoscopically, i.e., ligating veins above the internal ring. Cons of the retroperitoneal approach include relatively higher rates of recurrence and postoperative hydrocele formation [18–21]. An inguinal approach has also been described and can be performed microscopically or non-microscopically. Although the microsurgical approach generally takes longer and requires additional surgeon training and equipment, this technique minimizes complications and recurrences.

Percutaneous embolization or sclerotherapy is also a potentially curative option for varicocele repair as well, though not as successful an approach as modern microsurgical techniques. Decreased success is due to technical difficulties that can be present in remotely maneuvering catheters into the internal spermatic vein under fluoroscopic guidance, and a higher chance of varicocele recurrence/persistence postoperatively [8]. Moreover, right-sided varicoceles are more difficult to access due to the acute angle of insertion of the right gonadal vein into the inferior vena cava.

Most current urologic reproductive surgeons utilize microscopic methods/techniques for varicocelectomy [19]. Microscopic subinguinal varicocele is a same-day operation performed under local, regional, or general anesthesia, and is well suited to be performed in either an ambulatory surgery center or hospital setting. The patient is positioned supine on the operating room table, with arms abducted. Standard precautions are taken regarding padding, perioperative antibiotics, and venous thromboembolism prophylaxis, based on patient age and risk factors. Intravenous antibiotics with coverage primarily for gram positive skin organisms are routinely administered before incision, but postoperative oral antibiotics are not routinely required for uncomplicated cases.

Anesthesia is general, and can be administered with a laryngeal mask airway or an endotracheal tube. General anesthetic is strongly preferred over regional or local/sedation due to the need to have the patient completely motionless during fine microscopic dissection, as even small movements are greatly magnified under the microscope.

The incision (Fig. 3.1) is typically 2–3 cm and is made in a subinguinal location, just lateral to the base of the penis, a few centimeters caudal to the external ring. This is a slightly semicircular incision as it follows Langers' lines around the lateral border of the base of the genitals (Fig. 3.1).

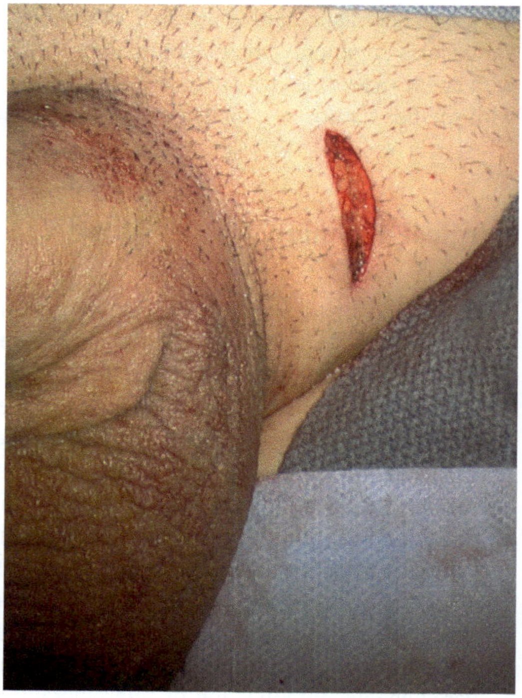

Fig. 3.1 A 2–3 cm incision is typically made in a subinguinal location, just lateral to the base of the penis, a few centimeters caudal to the external ring

Skin is incised sharply, and the deep dermal layer and subcutaneous adipose tissue are divided with electrocautery, taking care to stay superficial to avoid inadvertent injury to the spermatic cord. The authors prefer an insulated needle-tip for the monopolar electrocautery. Twenty watts works well for performing the initial skin incision, and power is reduced to 15 W when later working on gross structures in the spermatic cord. Bipolar cautery is mandatory to have as well, when later isolating individual structures in the vascular portion of the cord.

Retraction with Army-Navy retractors can then be used to bluntly dissect tissue down to Scarpa's fascia (Fig. 3.2), which is then entered bluntly with the retractors or by spreading with the tips of a Metzenbaum scissors. Retraction parallel to the spermatic cord should then quickly identify the cord. Slight traction on the ipsilateral testis will show motion in the cord to aid identification if needed. The lateral and medial aspects of the cord are then exposed by spreading with a Metzenbaum scissors. Spreading is most effective and less traumatic to the cord if it is done parallel to the cord, rather than perpendicular. Once freed from attachments to tissues in the prepubic space, the cord can be atraumatically grasped with a Babcock or spermatic cord clamp and brought up into the incision. Some blunt finger dissection along the surface of the cord in the cranial and caudal direction is usually required to further release any attachments between the cord and prepubic adipose tissues, allowing the cord to be brought up above the level of the skin. Palming the Babcock in the dominant hand, hooking the dominant index finger underneath the cord, and then using a 4″x 8″ sponge for blunt, gentle, sweeping will help isolate the cord circumferentially from the surrounding tissues (Fig. 3.3). The isolated cord is

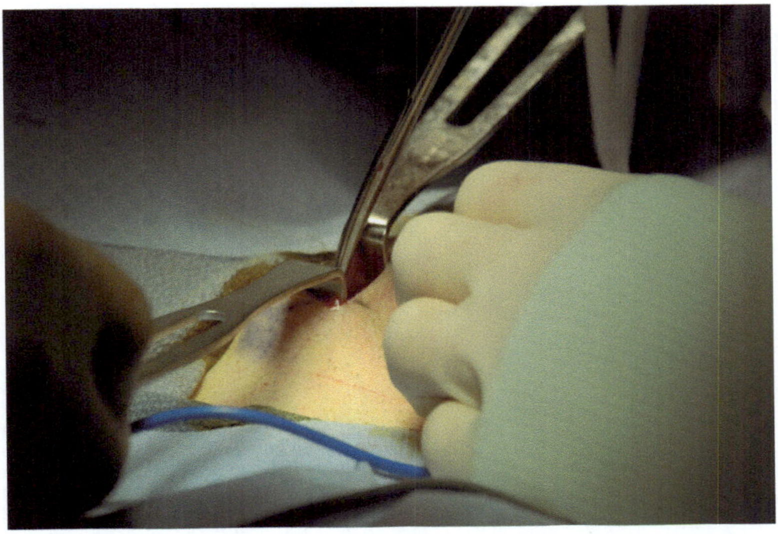

Fig. 3.2 Army-Navy retractors are used to bluntly dissect tissue down to Scarpa's fascia, which is then entered bluntly with the retractors or by spreading with the tips of a Metzenbaum scissors

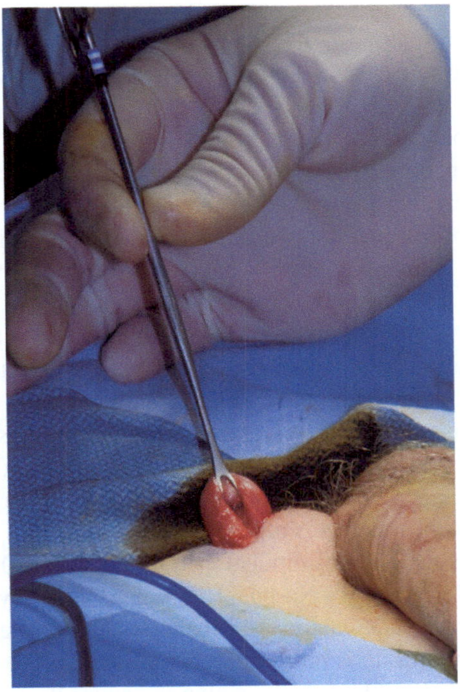

Fig. 3.3 A Babcock clamp is used to bring the spermatic cord up through the skin inclsion

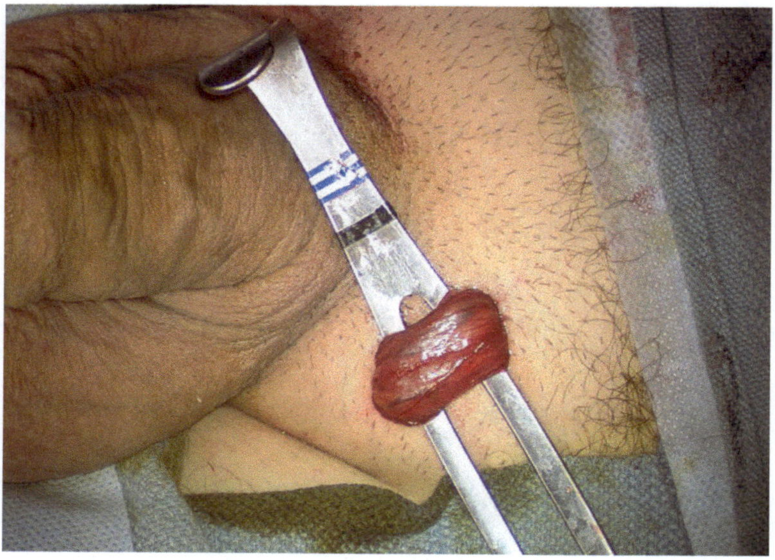

Fig. 3.4 After isolating the cord, it is suspended above the skin level by passing the Army-Navy under the cord

elevated with a Penrose or Army-Navy and the prepubic space is inspected for any external cremasteric veins, which are then ligated. Loupes may be of help in identifying these veins.

After isolation of the cord, we find that suspension of the cord above the skin level is best performed by passing the Army-Navy under the cord (Fig. 3.4). Other surgeons may prefer an empty scalpel handle or Penrose to similarly keep the cord elevated. In cases of bilateral varicocelectomy, a Penrose drain tagged around the cord works well to maintain control of the cord while the contralateral incision is performed, prior to bringing in the operative microscope.

Under microscopic view, the external spermatic fascia, cremasteric muscle fibers, and internal spermatic fascia are then opened along the direction of the cord with electrocautery (Fig. 3.5). Often, these three layers essentially separate out as one. A bundle of spermatic fasciae and cremasteric muscle fibers is then isolated medially and laterally, and these are retracted perpendicularly from the cord in opposite directions with blue microvessel loops (Fig. 3.6). This maneuver helps expose the vas deferens and vascular elements of the cord.

Before further dissection or manipulation of the cord, the 20 MHz microvascular Doppler (Vascular Technology—Nashua, NH) is used to survey the cord for arteries (Fig. 3.7). Significant manipulation of the cord can cause vasospasm of the artery(ies), so Doppler exam is performed first to identify the number and relative position of arteries before the fine dissection is begun. If vasospasm occurs or is suspected during the dissection, application of papaverine (30 mg/mL) diluted in a

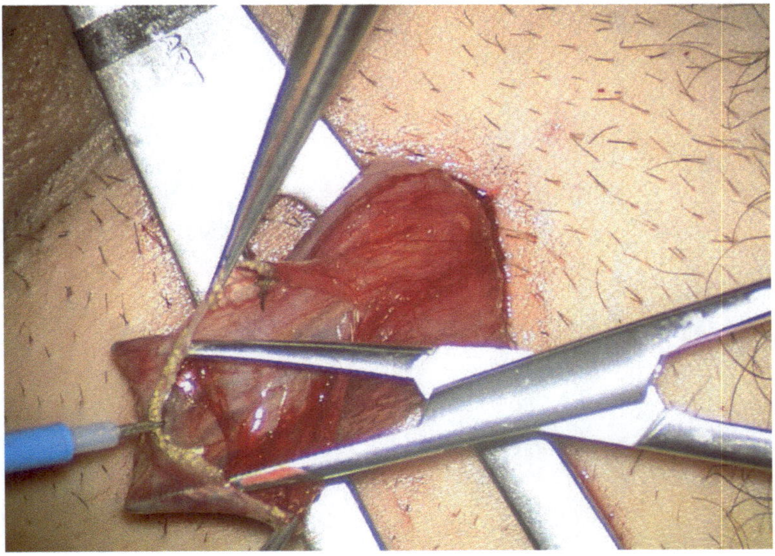

Fig. 3.5 Under microscopic view, the external spermatic fascia, cremasteric muscle fibers, and internal spermatic fascia are then opened along the direction of the cord with electrocautery

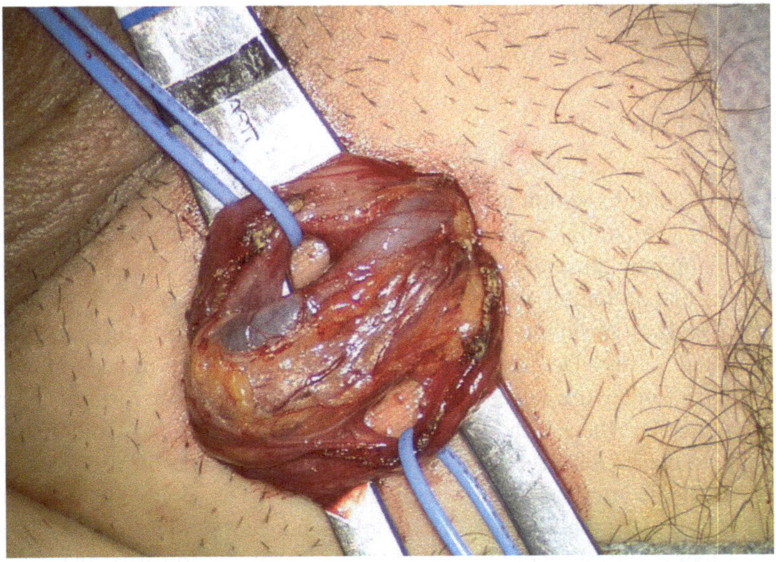

Fig. 3.6 A bundle of spermatic fasciae and cremasteric muscle fibers is isolated medially and laterally, and retracted perpendicularly from the cord in opposite directions with blue microvessel loops

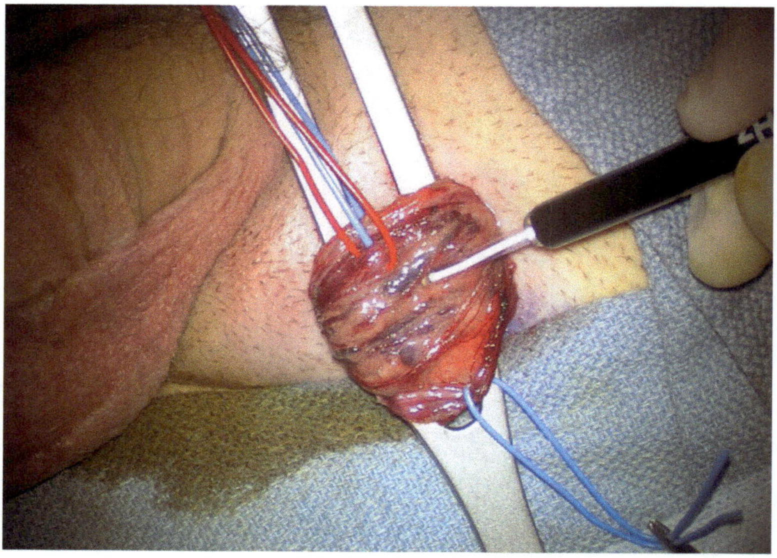

Fig. 3.7 A 20 MHz microvascular Doppler (Vascular Technology—Nashua, NH) is used to survey the cord for arteries

1:5 ratio with saline to the operative field via a 5 cc syringe with 24 G angiocatheter will help dilate the arteries to aid in Doppler identification.

Technical Pearls

The goals of cord dissection are to: (1) identify and preserve the vas deferens and vasal vessels, (2) identify and preserve any internal spermatic arteries, (3) preserve adequate lymphatic channels, and (4) ligate and divide any veins of the pampiniform plexus and preferably cremasteric layer as well.

A fine Jacobson mosquito is the authors' preferred dissection instrument. Some surgeons find a fine Detrich right angle useful for blunt dissection as well. Microsurgical forceps are a necessity; we prefer the 8″ Pierse microsurgical forceps. We prefer to isolate the vas and vasal vessels first (Fig. 3.8), as to avoid inadvertent later injury to these vital structures. Microdissection is then performed to isolate the internal spermatic arteries, during which obvious veins are double ligated with 4-0 silk ties or vascular titanium clips (Horizon™) and sharply divided using Westcott scissors. Liberal utilization of the Doppler probe is advised to verify that any vessel or tissue about to be ligated is not arterial, and also to periodically identify the patency of the arterial supply elsewhere in the cord. Any packets of vascular elements that have a Doppler-identified arterial wave pulse are looped with a red vessel loop, and retracted for later meticulous dissection. The internal spermatic artery(ies) invariably lie within the venous plexus, and very commonly have closely associated

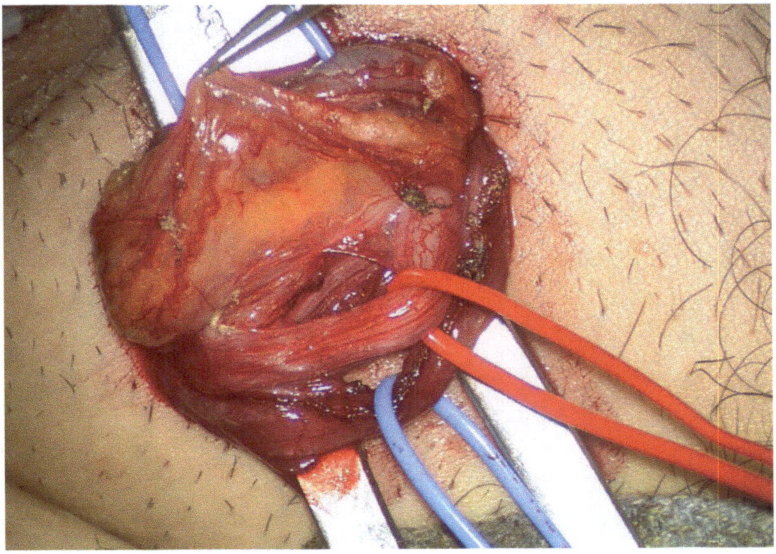

Fig. 3.8 The vas and vasal vessels are isolated to avoid inadvertent later injury to these vital structures

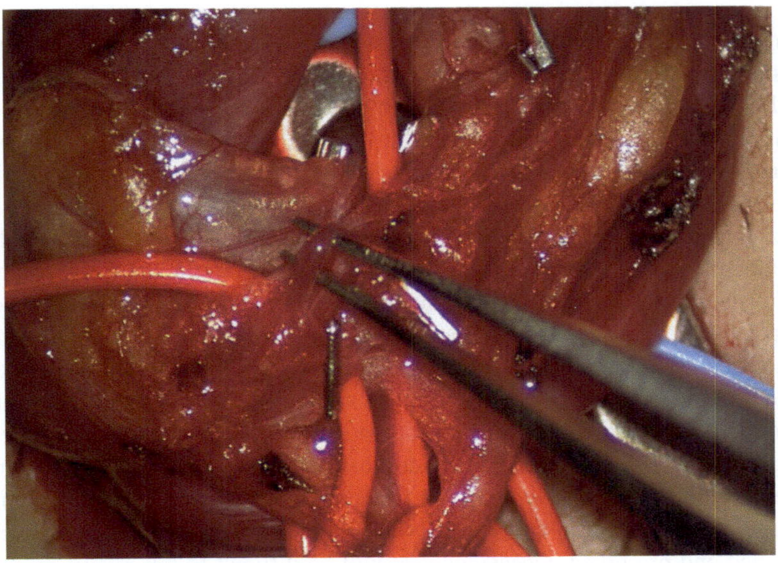

Fig. 3.9 A micro-forceps can tease an adherent vein off the artery

veins or lymphatic structures. Once artery-containing vascular bundles are isolated and the whole spermatic cord is superficially/grossly dissected, fine dissection of individual packets is then performed.

To separate other structures off the artery of interest, a few technical aspects have been found to be very useful. A very fine-tipped instrument such as a curved micro-forceps can tease an adherent vein off the artery (Fig. 3.9). This should only

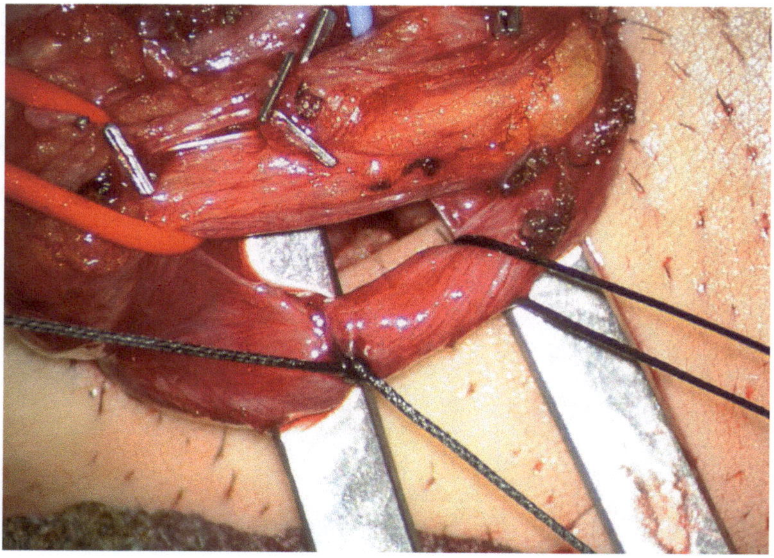

Fig. 3.10 The cremasteric fibers are ligated and divided. These are typically doubly suture-ligated with silk ties and sharply divided

be done under situations of fine dissection where all structures are well seen, because the sharp-tipped instrument may easily disrupt the arterial wall. Fine veins separated off the artery are then ligated with bipolar electrocautery. Care must be taken to NEVER to use monopolar cautery in this setting, as the current will conduct down the artery when such fine structures have been isolated. A fine-tipped bipolar cautery forceps can be used for fine dissection of structures off the artery as well, which then allows bipolar cauterization of the structure without the need to change instruments. Any small-caliber lymphatics separated from the artery are spared.

Constant watch for lymphatic channels is performed while dividing veins of the pampiniform plexus and isolating and preserving any arteries. Lymphatics are frequently identified superficially just below the internal spermatic fascia or often are found near the internal spermatic arteries. A minimum of 1–2 lymphatics are all that is probably necessary to prevent a postoperative hydrocele, but the authors prefer to isolate at least 4–5, after which any additional obvious lymphatics are spared, but extremely fine dissection looking for further lymphatics is not typically pursued because of the low rate of hydrocele formation once multiple lymphatics have been identified and preserved. Occasionally it will be difficult to tell a very small lymphatic vessel from a vein, in which case moving on to another portion of the dissection and then later reexamination of the vessel may be elucidative; otherwise it should be ligated as long as significant lymphatics have otherwise been spared.

After dissection of the vascular structures of the cord beneath the internal spermatic fascia, with preservation of the vas deferens and vasal vessels, lymphatic vessels, and internal spermatic arteries, the layers of spermatic fasciae and the cremasteric muscle fibers are then addressed. These bundles had previously been retracted laterally and medially with blue vessel loops. The Doppler device can be used to identify any significant arterial wave pulses, but these are often not able to be identified. An occasional sizeable cremasteric artery can be identified and preserved. Provided that sufficient internal spermatic arteries are identified and preserved, the cremasteric fibers can then be ligated and divided. These are typically doubly suture-ligated with silk ties and sharply divided (Fig. 3.10). The authors will commonly leave 1/3–½ of the cremasteric fibers doubly ligated but not divided. The theory is this will maintain a bit of cremasteric reflex for the ipsilateral testicle, and will provide some support so the arterial structures are theoretically less at risk for traction injury. Significant venous collaterals can be found in the cremasteric layer, so ligation of this layer should reduce the incidence of recurrence of the varicocele. Some surgeons routinely deliver the testicle to ensure that any gubernacular collaterals are also disrupted, but this may not be necessary given the low baseline recurrence rates with modern microscopic techniques. Data exist to support equivalent outcomes with and without delivery of the testis [22, 23].

Complications

Potential complications from varicocelectomy occur infrequently and are rarely severe. Complications may include wound infection, hydrocele formation, persistence or recurrence of the varicocele, and rarely, atrophy of the testis. An inguinal incision may be associated with scrotal numbness or prolonged pain [2].

A recent randomized trial between open inguinal, laparoscopic, and microscopic subinguinal varicocelectomy demonstrated similar rates of pregnancy and improvement in the semen parameters between the three surgical methods, but microscopic subinguinal repair had the lowest rate of complications of hydrocele or varicocele recurrence, as observed by other authors [24, 25]. With the microscopic subinguinal technique as described above, varicocele recurrence rates are 1% or less, hydrocele formation is similarly rare, less than 1%. The most common complications of non-microscopic varicocelectomy include postoperative persistence/recurrence of the varicocele (5–20%), and hydrocele formation (3–39%) [17, 26, 27] Even with microscopic technique, injury to internal spermatic arteries has been reported to occur on rare occasions, and can be associated with worsening of semen parameters with or without testis atrophy [28, 29]. The quality/availability of collateral arterial supply from the deferential and cremasteric arteries to the testis may explain heterogeneity in degree of injury/effect resulting from known internal spermatic artery injury.

Outcomes

Success of varicocelectomy can be measured by improvement in semen parameters and ultimately by achievement of spontaneous pregnancy. Commonly, varicoceles induce what is classically referred to as a "stress pattern" on the parameters of the semen analysis, with many or all of the main parameters depressed. Postoperative improvements in sperm concentration, motility, and morphology have been studied in men with varicoceles. A retrospective study by Boman et al. in 2008 examined the effect of varicocelectomy in 69 infertile men with isolated asthenospermia, and found significant improvement in total motile sperm count (39 million vs. 30 million) and also a doubling of the spontaneous pregnancy rate(65% vs. 32%) when compared to 49 similar men who declined varicocelectomy [30]. A great number of studies have been published demonstrating the improvement in sperm count/concentration after varicocelectomy. Sixteen studies were reviewed in by Schlesinger in 1994, twelve of which showed statistically significant improvements in sperm concentration after varicocele repair. Earlier reviews such as this are more likely to include some men with normal semen parameters, however. There exist several studies that suggest a decreased chance of improved semen parameters when men are moderately to severely oligospermic (5–10 or less million sperm/mL) [17, 31, 32] Other prospective studies [33] have examined men with preoperative sperm concentrations of 5–20 M/mL and have noted statistically significant improvements in sperm concentration, motility, and morphology, as well as improved pregnancy rates over the control population (up to 60% vs. 10%) in men undergoing immediate high (Palomo) ligation versus observation.

Regarding pregnancy after varicocelectomy, Marmar et al. published a recent modified meta-analysis examining spontaneous pregnancy rates in men with clinical varicocele and abnormal semen parameters. Pregnancy rates were significantly higher in the surgical varicocelectomy group (33%) versus 15.5% chance of pregnancy in couples where the man did not undergo varicocelectomy [27] At the present time, a randomized study examining the effect of modern microsurgical varicocelectomy on men with a clinically palpable varicocele(s) and abnormal semen parameters has not been completed.

Another measure of sperm quality is sperm DNA fragmentation assay (SDFA). There are studies that suggest varicoceles are associated with abnormal SDFA [34, 35], and that repair may improve SDFA parameters [36–38]. The impact of varicocele repair on sperm DNA damage is an interesting area of study and a growing area of interest.

Conclusions

Despite the continued challenge from skeptics, there is significant evidence for the role of varicocelectomy in male infertility. Appropriate patient selection is critical. Following the available evidence, infertile men with palpable varicocele and at least one abnormal semen parameter should be considered for surgical management. Complications from modern microsurgical subinguinal varicocelectomy are low, and a majority of men will see improvement in the semen parameters and hopefully spontaneous pregnancy as well.

References

1. Gorelick JI, Goldstein M. Loss of fertility in men with varicocele. Fertil Steril. 1993;59(3):613–6.
2. Medicine, A.U.A.a.A.S.f.R. Report on varicocele and infertility. http://www.auanet.org (2001). Accessed 9 Jan 2011.
3. Dubin L, Amelar RD. Etiologic factors in 1294 consecutive cases of male infertility. Fertil Steril. 1971;22(8):469–74.
4. Tulloch WS. Varicocele in subfertility; results of treatment. Br Med J. 1955;2(4935):356–8.
5. Wright EJ, Young GP, Goldstein M. Reduction in testicular temperature after varicocelectomy in infertile men. Urology. 1997;50(2):257–9.
6. Dada R, Gupta NP, Kucheria K. Spermatogenic arrest in men with testicular hyperthermia. Teratog Carcinog Mutagen 2003; Suppl 1:235–43.
7. Jung A, Schuppe HC. Influence of genital heat stress on semen quality in humans. Andrologia. 2007;39(6):203–15.
8. Pryor JL, Howards SS. Varicocele. Urol Clin North Am. 1987;14(3):499–513.
9. Braedel HU, et al. A possible ontogenic etiology for idiopathic left varicocele. J Urol. 1994;151(1):62–6.
10. Graif M, et al. Varicocele and the testicular-renal venous route: hemodynamic Doppler sonographic investigation. J Ultrasound Med. 2000;19(9):627–31.
11. Tanrikut C, Goldstein M. Varicocele repair for treatment of androgen deficiency. Curr Opin Urol. 2010;20(6):500–2.
12. ASRM, A.a. Report on varicocele and infertility. http://www.auanet.org (2001). Accessed 9 Jan 2011
13. Kass EJ, Belman AB. Reversal of testicular growth failure by varicocele ligation. J Urol. 1987;137(3):475–6.
14. Paduch DA, Niedzielski J. Repair versus observation in adolescent varicocele: a prospective study. J Urol. 1997;158(3 Pt 2):1128–32.
15. Steckel J, Dicker AP, Goldstein M. Relationship between varicocele size and response to varicocelectomy. J Urol. 1993;149(4):769–71.
16. Sigman M, Jarow JP. Ipsilateral testicular hypotrophy is associated with decreased sperm counts in infertile men with varicoceles. J Urol. 1997;158(2):605–7.
17. Dubin L, Amelar RD. Varicocelectomy: 986 cases in a twelve-year study. Urology. 1977;10(5):446–9.
18. Rothman CM, Newmark 3rd H, Karson RA. The recurrent varicocele–a poorly recognized problem. Fertil Steril. 1981;35(5):552–6.
19. Lipshultz L, TAJ, Khera M. Surgical management of male infertility. In: Campbell-Walsh urology. 9th ed. Chapter 20. New York: W.B. Saunders; 2007 pp. 659.
20. Homonnai ZT, et al. Varicocelectomy and male fertility: comparison of semen quality and recurrence of varicocele following varicocelectomy by two techniques. Int J Androl. 1980;3(4):447–58.
21. Niedzielski J, Paduch DA. Recurrence of varicocele after high retroperitoneal repair: implications of intraoperative venography. J Urol. 2001;165(3):937–40.
22. Goldstein M, et al. Microsurgical inguinal varicocelectomy with delivery of the testis: an artery and lymphatic sparing technique. J Urol. 1992;148(6):1808–11.
23. Ramasamy R, Schlegel PN. Microsurgical inguinal varicocelectomy with and without testicular delivery. Urology. 2006;68(6):1323–6.
24. Al-Kandari AM, et al. Comparison of outcomes of different varicocelectomy techniques: open inguinal, laparoscopic, and subinguinal microscopic varicocelectomy: a randomized clinical trial. Urology. 2007;69(3):417–20.
25. Watanabe M, et al. Minimal invasiveness and effectivity of subinguinal microscopic varicocelectomy: a comparative study with retroperitoneal high and laparoscopic approaches. Int J Urol. 2005;12(10):892–8.

26. Szabo R, Kessler R. Hydrocele following internal spermatic vein ligation: a retrospective study and review of the literature. J Urol. 1984;132(5):924–5.
27. Marmar JL, DeBenedictis TJ, Praiss D. The management of varicoceles by microdissection of the spermatic cord at the external inguinal ring. Fertil Steril. 1985;43(4):583–8.
28. Silber SJ. Microsurgical aspects of varicocele. Fertil Steril. 1979;31(2):230–2.
29. Steinberger E, Tjioe DY. Spermatogenesis in rat testes after experimental ischemia. Fertil Steril. 1969;20(4):639–49.
30. Boman JM, Libman J, Zini A. Microsurgical varicocelectomy for isolated asthenospermia. J Urol. 2008;180(5):2129–32.
31. Matkov TG, et al. Preoperative semen analysis as a predictor of seminal improvement following varicocelectomy. Fertil Steril. 2001;75(1):63–8.
32. Kamal KM, Jarvi K, Zini A. Microsurgical varicocelectomy in the era of assisted reproductive technology: influence of initial semen quality on pregnancy rates. Fertil Steril. 2001;75(5):1013–6.
33. Madgar I, et al. Controlled trial of high spermatic vein ligation for varicocele in infertile men. Fertil Steril. 1995;63(1):120–4.
34. Blumer CG, et al. Effect of varicocele on sperm function and semen oxidative stress. BJU Int. 2012;109(2):259–65.
35. Blumer CG, et al. Sperm nuclear DNA fragmentation and mitochondrial activity in men with varicocele. Fertil Steril. 2008;90(5):1716–22.
36. La Vignera S, et al. Effects of varicocelectomy on sperm DNA fragmentation, mitochondrial function, chromatin condensation, and apoptosis. J Androl. 2012;33(3):389–96.
37. Smit M, et al. Decreased sperm DNA fragmentation after surgical varicocelectomy is associated with increased pregnancy rate. J Urol. 2010;183(1):270–4.
38. Werthman P, et al. Significant decrease in sperm deoxyribonucleic acid fragmentation after varicocelectomy. Fertil Steril. 2008;90(5):1800–4.

Chapter 4
Vasovasostomy Techniques for Microsurgery Specialists

Kalen Rimar, Landon Trost, and Robert E. Brannigan

Abstract Every year, roughly 500,000 vasectomies are performed in the USA, and it is estimated that up to 6% of these men will eventually request a reversal [1, 2]. Surgical technique has evolved since Dr. William Quinby performed the first vasovasostomy in 1919 [3], and microsurgical repair with the aid of stenting or loupe magnification has largely been replaced by microsurgical approaches. The improved visualization and stabilization the operating microscope provides are well suited for re-approximating a delicate, 0.3 mm diameter structure like the vas deferens. This chapter provides a brief history of vasal repair, an overview of the authors' preferred technique for microsurgical vasovasostomy, and evidence-based recommendations for preoperative and postoperative care.

Keywords Vasovasostomy • Vasectomy reversal • Microsurgery • Surgical techniques

Introduction

Every year, roughly 500,000 vasectomies are performed in the USA, and it is estimated that up to 6% of these men will eventually request a reversal [1, 2]. Surgical technique has evolved since Dr. William Quinby performed the first

K. Rimar, B.A., B.S.
Department of Urology, Feinberg School of Medicine, Northwestern University, 251 East Huron St, Chicago, IL 60611, USA

L. Trost, M.D.
Department of Urology, The Mayo Clinic, 200 First St SW, Rochester, MN 55905, USA

R.E. Brannigan, M.D. (✉)
Department of Urology, Feinberg School of Medicine, Northwestern University, Galter, Suite 20-150, 675N. Saint Clair St, Chicago, IL 60611, USA
e-mail: r-brannigan@northwestern.edu

J.I. Sandlow (ed.), *Microsurgery for Fertility Specialists: A Practical Text*, DOI 10.1007/978-1-4614-4196-0_4, vasovasostomy in 1919 [3], and microsurgical repair with the aid of stenting or loupe magnification has largely been replaced by microsurgical approaches. The improved visualization and stabilization the operating microscope provides are well suited for re-approximating a delicate, 0.3 mm diameter structure like the vas deferens. This chapter provides a brief history of vasal repair, an overview of the authors' preferred technique for microsurgical vasovasostomy, and evidence-based recommendations for preoperative and postoperative care.

Brief History of Vasectomy Reversal

Dr. Edward Martin documented the first human vasal repair, an epididymovasostomy, in 1902 [4]. Martin had a strong interest in male infertility, and he continued to perform this procedure for men with obstructive azoospermia secondary to epididymitis [5]. Martin incised the epididymis and, after visualization of milky fluid, he created the vasal–epididymal anastomosis using four fine silver wire sutures [4]. In a small series, he performed epididymovasostomies on 11 men with epididymal obstruction, achieving patency and pregnancy rates of 64 and 27%, respectively [4].

In 1919 Quinby documented the first successful vasovasostomy in a man with a history of vasal resection 8 years prior [6]. The vasal anastomosis was created over a strand of silk gut that was placed in the lumen and was later removed [6]. Decades later, Quinby's assistant O'Conor reported a patency rate of 64% in a series of 14 vasectomized patients utilizing the same technique [6]. Possibly realizing the limitations of these small single surgeon series, O'Conor was also determined to gauge national clinical practices. In the same paper described above, O'Conor reported the results of his survey of 1,240 urologists regarding vasectomy reversal. 750 responded, with only 135 having any experience with the procedure. The mean patency rate of 38% was much lower than previous reported rates [6].

In the 1960s, an increasing number of vasectomies were performed which subsequently resulted in an increased number of vasectomy reversals [7, 8]. As more surgeons became comfortable with vasovasostomy, subtle differences in technique began to emerge. The use of loupe magnification was increasingly utilized and provided improved visualization of the vasal lumen and a more accurate approximation of the mucosa. Its use is described in techniques by Amelar, Dubin, and Schmidt [9–11]. Similarly, stents were frequently employed in an attempt to assure vasal patency. Dorsey described the placement of a monofilament dermalon suture as an anastomotic stent which was subsequently removed in 12–14 days [11]. Despite the increased risk of infection associated with the use of a foreign body, stenting was shown to have superior patency and pregnancy outcomes in a number of small series and was the method of choice for three decades [12–14]. However, with the advent of the microsurgical vasovasostomy in the late 1970s, the need for stenting was largely eliminated.

Microsurgical Technique

The first microsurgical vasovasostomy technique for clinical use is attributed to Owen and Silber who individually published operative techniques in 1977, with Silber describing its first use in humans in 1975 [15–17]. Although animal studies frequently employed a one-layer anastomotic technique, Silber strongly supported a two-layer anastomosis as he noted that dilation of the proximal vas from prior obstruction resulted in incongruent vasal diameters [18]. As such, a two-layer anastomosis would help ensure approximation and prevent leak. Silber's reported technique included dilation of the proximal vas deferens with jeweler's forceps with subsequent anastomosis using 9-0 nylon sutures under 16× to 25× magnification. Six or seven mucosal sutures were placed followed by meticulous inspection for tears, gaps, or discordant approximation of the lumen. The seromuscular layer was then sutured to help ensure a watertight anastomosis. Through this technique, Silber reported a 91% patency rate in 42 patients [16]. Though these results were promising, similar patency rates had been achieved in single surgeon series using macroscopic techniques [19, 20].

In a direct comparison of the macroscopic and microscopic techniques, Lee and McLoughlin reported on 87 patients undergoing vasectomy reversal [21]. Realizing that the learning curve for microsurgery was not insignificant, their goal was to determine if the technique resulted in a true clinical benefit. The macroscopic repair was a single-layer anastomosis performed with a monofilament internal stent removed 7–14 days postoperatively and resulted in patency and pregnancy rates of 90 and 46%, respectively [21]. The microscopic repair was a two-layer anastomosis with patency and pregnancy rates of 96 and 54% respectively [21]. Since Lee's landmark paper, numerous additional studies comparing these techniques have confirmed the superior patency and pregnancy rates achieved with microscopic repair [22–24].

Indications

Vasectomy currently remains the most common cause of vasal obstruction, with other less common etiologies including accidental injury or inflammation resulting in obstruction [2, 8].

Though microsurgical vasovasostomy has been shown to be more cost effective than assisted reproductive techniques like IVF with ICSI, it may not be appropriate for all men with obstructive azoospermia [25–29]. The current AUA best practice statement on infertility identifies clinical characteristics associated with reduced chances for pregnancy with microsurgical vasovasostomy, including a vasal obstructive interval of greater than 15 years, female partner age over 37 years, or female partner with a history of tubal disease or ligation. Patients presenting with these factors are encouraged to also carefully consider assisted reproductive techniques, given poorer relative outcomes in this patient population. [30].

As female fecundity declines significantly after age 35, it is important to counsel patients on appropriate expectations for surgical and assisted reproductive technique outcomes. Given that the average time to pregnancy following vasectomy reversal is 12 months, this may be factored into the decision on which infertility treatment is most appropriate [31, 32]. Similarly, success rates with assisted reproductive techniques including IVF and ICSI are significantly reduced after age 40 [33, 34].

Patient Demographics

Age at the time of vasectomy is the strongest predictor of eventual reversal, and young men (age 20–29) are consistently identified as the group at highest risk [2, 8, 35]. The vast majority of vasectomy reversals occur in the setting of remarriage, and divorced men inquiring about vasectomy should be counseled about this fact. Other less common presentations include the death of a child or the desire for more children. These findings indicate the need for thorough counseling at the time of vasectomy, particularly in the young male and divorced male populations.

Clinical Evaluation

Healthy men with proven fertility require little preoperative evaluation. A complete history and physical is always recommended as findings may influence the type of surgery performed, as well as expected outcomes. The duration of occlusion is the most important component of the history because it is currently the best predictor of outcomes [32]. Patients with a history of pelvic surgery, inguinal surgery, or vasectomy-related complications (hematoma, infection) are at increased risk for secondary sites of vasal obstruction. These individuals may require a more technically challenging repair including possible epididymovasostomy (EV). Parekattil and colleagues created an EV prediction model based on patient historical information including age and obstructive interval in an attempt to preoperatively identify patients who are likely to require EV [36, 37]. Although the model demonstrated 100% sensitivity and 58% specificity, its clinical utility is limited as the decision to perform VV or EV is based predominantly on intraoperative factors.

Integral aspects of the physical exam include palpation of the testicles, epididymis, and vasal segments. Men with evidence of atrophic testicles should have a serum follicle stimulating hormone level obtained, which when elevated preoperatively might suggest some baseline, spermatogenic dysfunction. As noted by Hsiao et al. patients with increased FSH levels should be counseled that they will have an increased likelihood of needing assisted reproduction to achieve a pregnancy after vasectomy reversal [38]. Patients presenting with vasal obstruction and large varicoceles may be considered for concomitant repair at the time of vasectomy reversal, as reported by Mulhall et al. in 1997 [39]. Increased testicular vasal segment length and the presence of sperm granulomas are important positive prognostic signs, as it is hypothesized that they may relieve pressure in the epididymis and reduce the likelihood of secondary epididymal damage due to backpressure from the more distal vasal obstruction [40–43]. Induration or fullness of the epididymis indicates possible epididymal obstruction and the possible need for EV.

Laboratory

Routine laboratory testing is typically not required. However, FSH and testosterone levels should be checked in patients with a history of an abnormal semen analysis, impaired sexual function, testicular atrophy, or other clinical findings suggestive of endocrinopathy. The association between anti-sperm antibodies (ASA) and fecundity remains controversial. Serum ASA testing is not routinely performed as a large percentage of men will form antibodies following vasectomy [31, 44]. Additionally, the clinical importance of the presence of ASA remains indeterminate.

Imaging

Most men with known vasal obstruction following vasectomy do not require preoperative radiographic evaluation. However, in men with suspected inflammatory obstruction or iatrogenic injury, intraoperative vasography to further evaluate the more distal vas deferens, the ipsilateral seminal vesicle, and the ipsilateral ejaculatory duct may assist in identifying additional regions of suspected obstruction. As vasography may result in scarring, it is only performed at the time of a planned reconstruction. An alternative to formal vasography involves injection 10 cc of normal saline into the abdominal vasal lumen after vasal transection. If resistance is encountered, indigo carmine is added to the solution, with a formal vasography performed if no indigo carmine is observed in the patient's catheterized urine specimen. Patients with suspected ejaculatory duct obstruction should undergo transrectal ultrasonography preoperatively [45].

Female Factor

Simultaneous gynecologic workup is recommended for the female partner prior to vasovasostomy, particularly in women with unproven fertility, advanced maternal age (>35 years old), or a history of pelvic/abdominal surgery. Women with preexisting tubal disease should be evaluated for IVF with ICSI in lieu of vasectomy reversal as previously noted [30].

Operative Technique

Anesthesia and Positioning

While local, regional, and general anesthetics are all options for vasectomy reversal, most subspecialists use general anesthesia to minimize patient movement and to optimize patient comfort during the procedure. The decision is typically surgeon and patient-dependent. This is especially relevant given the length of the procedure and the precision required. A single prophylactic dose of IV antibiotics is typically given to patients approximately 1 h prior to incision.

The patient should be placed in the supine position with pressure points appropriately padded. To allow proper positioning of the operating microscope, the patient's arm ipsilateral to the base should be tucked. Foot extenders should be used to position the patient in an area of the bed where both the surgeon and assistant can sit with their knees comfortably under the table. The scrotum and penis should be shaved and prepped in the usual sterile fashion. The penis may be placed cephalad out of the operative field if required. The microscope headpiece is placed perpendicular to the bed and approximately 8 in. from the scrotum. Ensure that the foot pedals are within reach of the surgeon or assistant. The surgeon's elbows or wrists should gently rest on an object in the surgical field to help stabilize their movements.

Incision and Exposure

A vertical incision is made in the anterior aspect of the hemiscrotum overlying the vasectomy site and extended more deeply with sharp dissection and electrocautery. In some instances, an incision as short as 1 cm will be sufficient to isolate both vasal ends. In other instances, such as cases where the vasal ends are difficult to palpate or are separated by a large gap, a longer incision with delivery of the testicle he may be needed. The vasectomy site is identified with finger palpation. A towel clamp is then placed around the testicular side of the vas with careful downward traction. A pair of curved iris scissors is passed behind the vas creating space for the assistant to place a mosquito. Careful dissection of the vasal adventitia should be performed at this site, making sure to spare perivasal vasculature. Hemostasis is best achieved with the bipolar cautery device in order to avoid injury to the vas. A 5–0 chromic holding stitch is placed 1–2 cm inferior to the planned transection site. The vas is placed in a 2 mm slotted nerve holder, avoiding tension, and swiftly transected at a 90° angle with a Dennis blade through the slot. It is imperative, particularly in the convoluted vas, that the site is carefully selected and placed in the nerve holder to avoid creating an oblique lumen. The abdominal vas should be exposed and divided in a similar fashion. The vas deferens on the side corresponding to the previous vasectomy site is then ligated with a 4-0 chromic tie. The distal vas is held in place and triangulated using three 0.12 pickups, and the exposed lumen is gently dilated using the dilating jewelers forceps. Next, a 24-French angiocatheter is used to cannulate and flush the distal vas and confirm distal patency. If resistance is met, indigo carmine should be added to the flushing solution. If no indigo carmine is seen in the patient's urine, formal vasography should be performed. Additionally, an 0-nylon suture may be advanced through the abdominal vasal lumen up to the point of blockage to help define its distance from the vasectomy site.

Table 4.1 Sperm grading and associated success rates (Adapted with permission from Belker et al. [32])

Sperm grade	Grade description	Return of sperm to ejaculate (%)	Pregnancy rate (%)
Grade 1	Mainly normal motile sperm	94	63
Grade 2	Mainly normal nonmotile sperm	91	54
Grade 3	Mainly sperm heads	96	50
Grade 4	Sperm heads only	75	44
Grade 5	No sperm	60	31

This table was published in The Journal of Urology, [32]. Copyright Elsevier. 1991

Vasovasostomy Versus Epididymovasostomy

After transection and confirmation of patency, the testicular vasal fluid is inspected to determine whether vasovasostomy or epididymovasostomy is indicated. Fluid should be milked from the vas and placed on a glass slide. If the fluid is particularly thick it can be diluted with saline. Epididymovasostomy is typically performed if the vasal fluid is thick/creamy or if vasal fluid is absent. An epididymovasostomy may also be appropriate in the setting of thick fluid with only sperm heads present; however, pregnancy and patency rates in this particular case are comparable to vasovasostomy [46]. A summary of the system used by The Vasovasostomy Study Group (VVSG) to grade the gross and microscopic appearance of the vasal fluid, along with associated patency and pregnancy rates, can be found in Table 4.1 [32].

Sperm cryopreservation is an option at the time of reversal; however, two studies have shown that routine cryopreservation for all vasectomy reversals is neither necessary nor beneficial cost effective [47, 48]. The authors' of the first study suggested protocol has been to encourage cryopreservation at the time of reversal if the patient is unwilling to undergo further procedures, if there is a high likelihood for epididymovasostomy, or if the patient is definitively planning to pursue IVF/ICSI [47]. The authors of the second study encouraged sperm banking in men undergoing bilateral epididymovasostomy, and in select patients undergoing vasovasostomy with epididymovasostomy based on preoperative counseling and intraoperative findings [48].

Anastomosis

If the decision is made to proceed with VV, the new cut ends of the vas are approximated. Surgeon preference dictates the technique used (adventitial holding stitch or vas approximating clamp). A 5-0 PDS suture placed through the loose adventia on each vasal end is effective at laying the foundation for a tension-free anastomosis. Symmetry of the vasal ends should also be one of the surgeon's priorities because this will help ensure patency.

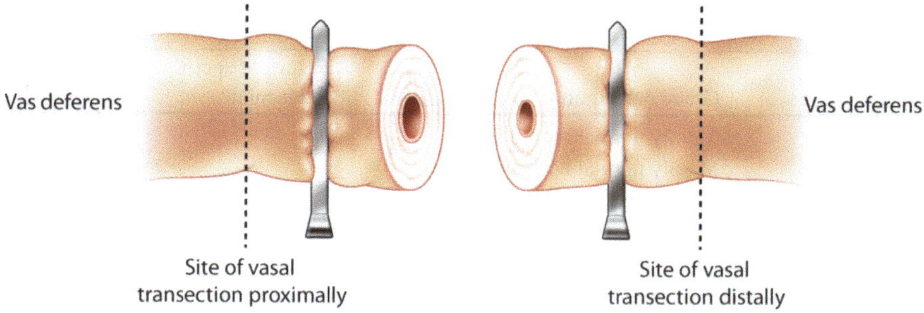

Fig. 4.1 The vasovasostomy anastomotic site is prepared by transection of each end of the vas deferens at the vasectomy site

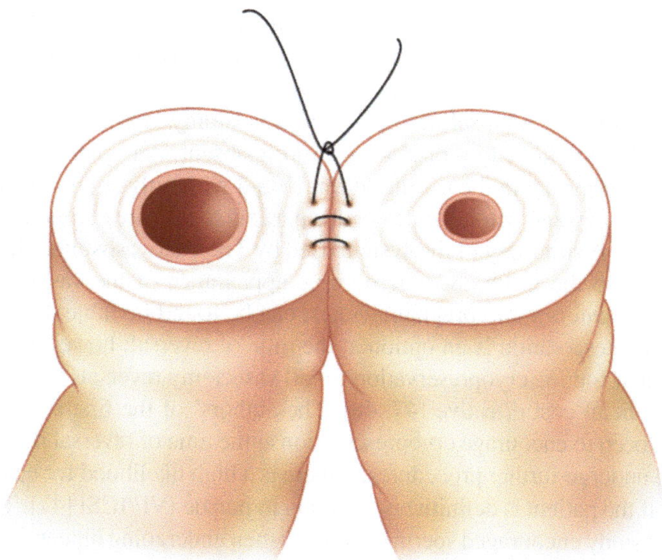

Fig. 4.2 The first three outer layer anastomotic stitches

The tradition method of anastomosing the vasal ends is a two-layer technique. The vasovasostomy anastomotic site is prepared by transection of each end of the vas deferens at the vasectomy site (Fig. 4.1). The outer layer of the anastomosis is started by placing three, 9-0 nylon interrupted sutures at the 5, 6, and 7 o'clock positions through the vasal muscularis and adventitia (Fig. 4.2). The inner layer of the anastomosis is then performed by placing three, 10-0 nylon interrupted sutures at the 5, 6, and 7 o'clock positions through the mucosal layer (Fig. 4.3). Each of these is cut immediately after it is placed and tied. The remaining inner layer sutures are placed but not tied for a total of six to eight 10-0 nylon sutures (Fig. 4.4). These are sequentially tied and cut (Fig. 4.5). A small portion of muscularis should be incorporated into the inner layer sutures to help prevent tearing of the vas. If the mucosa

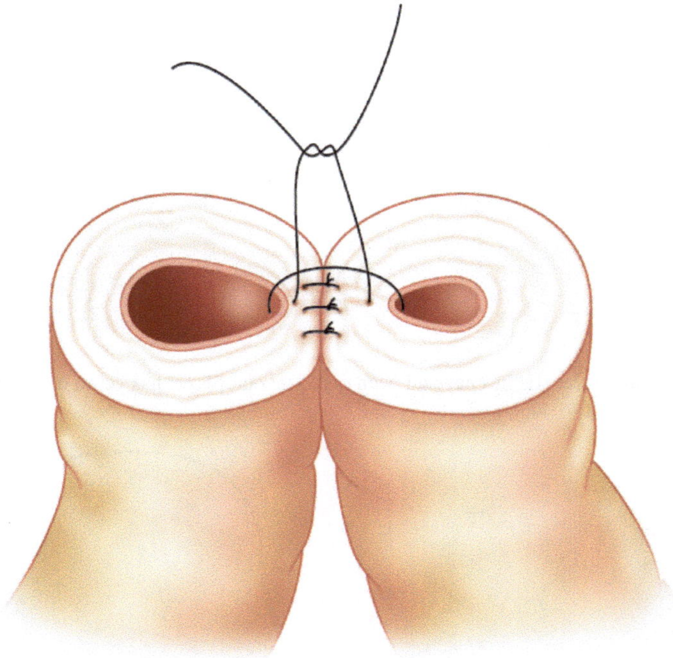

Fig. 4.3 The first three outer layer stitches have been placed and tied. The first inner layer stitch is then placed and tied

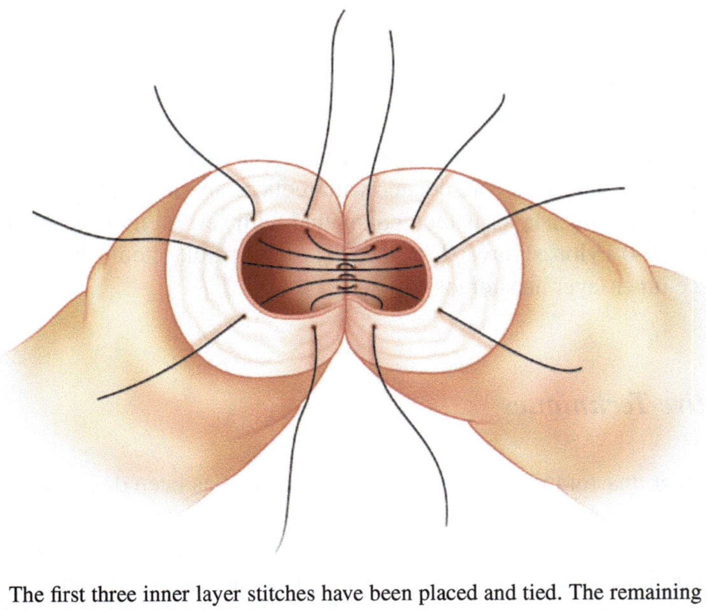

Fig. 4.4 The first three inner layer stitches have been placed and tied. The remaining inner layer stitches are then all placed before tying

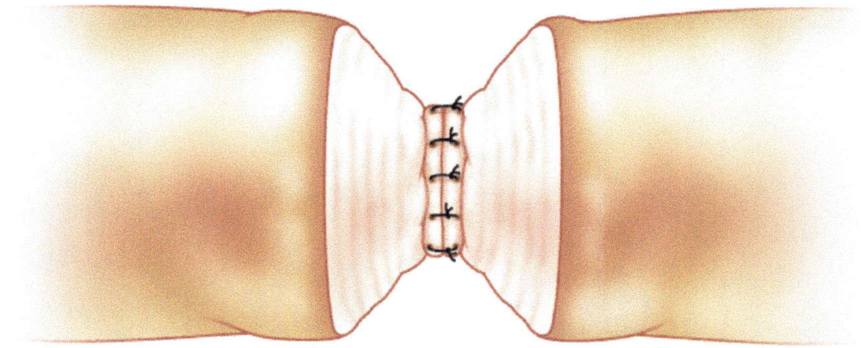

Fig. 4.5 The inner layer stitches have all been tied. The outer layer has yet to be completed

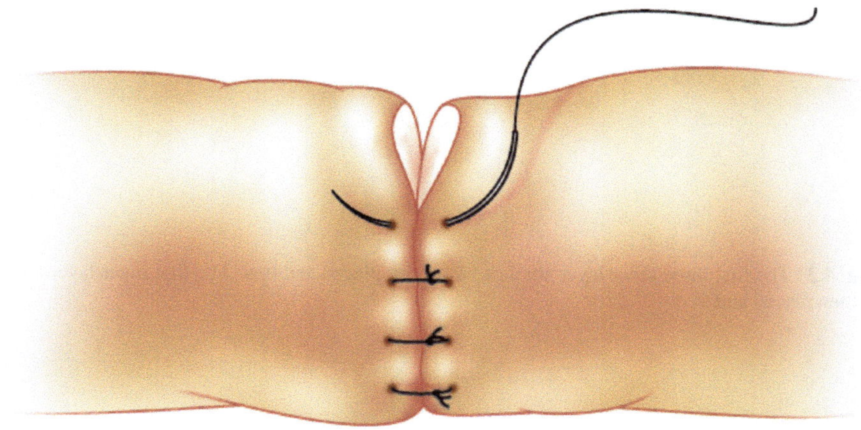

Fig. 4.6 The completion of the outer layer of the anastomosis

is difficult to visualize, a drop of indigo carmine can assist in highlighting this tissue. Methylene blue has been associated with reduced sperm motility and should be avoided [49]. The outer layer is then completed with several more interrupted, circumferential 9-0 nylon sutures (Fig. 4.6). The end result should be a watertight, tension-free inner layer anastomosis.

Alternative Techniques

A single-layer anastomotic vasovasostomy technique has been described in the literature [50]. The purported advantages of this technique include its relative simplicity and reduced operative time [51]. Retrospective analysis comparing microsurgical modified one-layer versus two-layer microsurgical vasovasostomy reported similar patency and pregnancy results [32, 52]. To date, though, there have been no prospective, randomized, controlled trials comparing single-layer versus two-layer microsurgical repair, and the decision regarding which approach to use is thus based largely on surgeon preference.

The microdot technique, first described by Goldstein and colleagues [52], is a microsurgical technique developed to aid in accurate suture placement. Microdots are placed at the 3, 6, 9, and 12 o'clock positions midway between the mucosa and serosal margin of both the abdominal and testicular vas. Four more dots are then placed evenly between the initial four dots. The anastomosis is then completed using eight inner layer 10-0 sutures and eight outer layer 9-0 sutures. Care is taken to ensure that the inner layer sutures exit from the center of the microdots. The vasal sheath is also re-approximated using 6-8 interrupted 6-0 sutures. The purported advantage of this technique is the separation of suture planning and placement. Goldstein et al. report that this approach may be particularly helpful when dealing with markedly discrepant luminal diameters. No studies to date have investigated this assertion; however, patency and pregnancy rates with the microdot technique have been comparable to those found with traditional microsurgical vasovasostomy [52].

Intraoperative Factors

Several intraoperative findings may necessitate small alterations in surgical technique. A large vasal gap will require extra distal and proximal mobilization to ensure a tension-free anastomosis. Blunt dissection can be used to separate the vas from cord structures up to the level of the superficial inguinal ring. Testicular vasal length is added by dissection of the vas away from the epididymis, taking care to avoid the nearby vasal, epididymal, and testicular blood vessels. In rare patients, no vas is located in the inguinal canal, and retroperitoneal mobilization may be required. Isolation of the deep inferior epigastric artery and vein is performed to locate the vas curving beneath these vessels toward the seminal vesicles. This portion of the vas is mobilized and placed over the pubic symphysis. Utilizing this technique, Buch et al. demonstrated an increase in vasal segment length of 5.83 ± 0.65 cm [53].

The proximity of the vasal defect to the epididymis may require the surgeon perform a convoluted vasovasostomy (CVV). CVV is considered more technically demanding given the thin muscular wall and discrepant luminal diameters often found in the convoluted vas deferens. De-tethering should be avoided to prevent iatrogenic injury and to preserve the native blood supply. Transection site selection is paramount to avoid creating an oblique lumen. If an oblique lumen is observed, the convoluted vas can be transected at 1 mm intervals to help ensure a more optimal transverse cut [54].

The need for crossed vasovasostomy is exceedingly rare, but should be considered in men with unilateral inguinal obstruction of the vas deferens and a contralateral atrophic testicle. It may also be performed when ipsilateral obstruction of the inguinal vas or ejaculatory duct is present with obstruction of the contralateral epididymis. The vas ipsilateral to the atrophic testis is transected at the junction of the straight and convoluted portions. The contralateral vas is freed superiorly toward the site of obstruction. An incision is made in the scrotal septum and the vas is pulled to the side of the atrophic testis. The anastomosis is performed as previously described.

Wound Closure

Following completion of the anastomosis, the wound is copiously irrigated with normal saline, and hemostasis is achieved using bipolar and monopolar cautery. All holding stitches are removed, and the testicle is returned to its appropriate location within the hemiscrotum. The dartos layer is closed with 4-0 chromic suture in a locked, running fashion. The scrotal skin can be closed with a 4-0 monocryl suture using a running horizontal mattress suture. Bacitracin ointment, sterile fluff dressings, and a scrotal support are then used to dress the wound.

Outcomes

A wide range of reported patency and pregnancy rates for microsurgical vasectomy reversal have been reported. These numbers can be challenging to interpret because they are often derived from small single surgeon series (Table 4.2). However, in 1991 a large (1,469 patients) multicenter study of microsurgical vasectomy reversal outcomes was published by The VVSG, with patency and pregnancy rates of 86 and 52% respectively [32]. Though these rates are lower than those reported in many of the single surgeon series, it is remains the largest multi-surgeon study to date.

The VVSG also confirmed the interval of obstruction as the most important preoperative predictor of success [32]. A progressive decline in patency and pregnancy rates were observed with increased obstructive interval: <3 years (97, 76%), 3–8 years (88, 53%), 9–14 (79, 44%), to >15 years (71, 31%) [32]. Sperm grade, vasal length, and type of microsurgical reconstruction (VV or VE) also have a significant impact on the return of sperm to the ejaculate following the procedure [32, 40, 55, 56]. Interestingly, men with the same female partner have also been shown to have superior outcomes following microsurgical vasal repair [57, 58].

The sperm grading scale established by the VVSG is based on the presence or absence of sperm and sperm parts (Table 4.1) [32]. A score of 1–5 is assigned to the sample after microscopic observation. The authors summarized the sperm grade descriptions and their corresponding patency and pregnancy rates following vasovasostomy [32]. The semen appearance and sperm grade guide the surgeon's decision to proceed with vasovasostomy or perform a more technically challenging epididymovasostomy. Compared to vasovasostomy, epididymovasostomy is associated with significantly lower patency and pregnancy rates [59]. A separate chapter in this text thoroughly addressed the issue of epididymovasostomy, including operative techniques and outcomes.

Table 4.2 Comparison of studies reporting vasovasostomy outcomes

Authors	Year	*N*	Mean obstructive interval (year)	Vasal patency (%)	Pregnancy (%)	Notes
Grober et al. [70]	2011	164		85/89 (96)		Mini-incision vasectomy reversal
Jee and Hong [71]	2010	50	7.1 (microsurgical) 6.9 (loupe)	Microsurgical 24/25 (96) versus loupe 18/25 (72)	Microsurgical 10/25 (40) versus loupe 7/25 (28)	Microsurgical versus loupe-assisted results
Patel [61]	2008	106	8.6 (convoluted vas), 7.7 (straight vas)	Convoluted 52/53 (98), straight 36/37 (97)		Comparing convoluted versus straight vas deferens
Bolduc et al. [41]	2007	605	6.8	Primary 491/559 (88), secondary 27/46 (59)	Primary 53% at 2 years, secondary 30% at 2 years	
Hsieh et al. [72]	2005	74	Microsurgery 8.1, loupe 9.2	Microsurgical 32/35 (91), loupe 25/28 (89)	Microsurgical 15/35 (43), loupe 11/28 (39)	Compared microsurgical to loupe-assisted VV
Sandlow and Kolettis [54]	2005	48	10	38/43 (88)	15/31 (48)	VV in convoluted vas deferens
Silber and Grotjan [73]	2004	3,904		3,022 (89.5)	1,559/1,738 (89.7)	
Boorjian et al. [42]	2004	213	All patients <15 years	196 (92)	174 (82)	Evaluated obstructive interval on vasectomy reversal outcomes
Kolettis et al. [74]	2003	46	10	22/27 (81)	14/40 (33)	Outcomes with female partners 35 years or older
Kolettis et al. [57]	2003	34	5	27/29 (93)	15/25 (60)	Outcomes of men with vasectomy reversal with same female partner
Kolettis et al. [75]	2002	70	14.5	57/74 (77)	23/62 (37)	Outcomes in patients with obstruction at least 10 years
Holman et al. [76]	2000	1,817			59% (includes repeat VV)	Population-based outcomes
Fischer and Grantmyre [51]	2000	40	One layer 4.7, two layers 2.9	One layer 14/17 (82), two layers 20/23 (87)	Not reported	Compared one versus two layer VV
Feber and Ruiz [77]	1999	160		87%	50% (among patients <5 years from vasectomy)	
Belker et al. [32]	1991	1,469		865/1,012 (86)	421/810 (52)	

VV Vasovasostomy

Table 4.3 Variables which may affect outcomes of vasovasotomy/epididymovasostomy

Clinical variables	
	Age of female partner
	Interval since vasectomy
	Need for repeat vasovasostomy
	Presence of anti-sperm antibodies
	Prior pregnancy in female partner
Operative variables	
	Clips versus suture utilized at vasectomy
	Convoluted versus straight vas
	Microsurgical versus loupe anastomosis
	Need for epididymovasostomy
	One versus two layer anastomosis
	Presence and quality of vasal fluid
	Presence and quality of sperm in vasal fluid
	Presence of alpha glucosidase in epididymal secretions
	Presence of a sperm granuloma
	Unilateral versus bilateral vasovasostomy

A fairly recent study also reported an association between the length of the testicular vasal remnant and the presence of whole sperm intraoperatively [60]. Whole sperm were found in the vasal fluid of 94% of units with a testicular vasal remnant length of greater than 2.7 cm, but only 85% of units with a testicular vasal remnant length less than 2.7 cm [60]. Proximity of the vasal defect to the epididymis appears to increase the chance of intravasal azoospermia. Based on these findings, one might expect poorer outcomes associated with CVV. However, patency and pregnancy rates following CVV are comparable to vasovasostomy performed in the straight portion of the vas [54, 61]. Crossed vasovasostomy patency rates are similar; however, pregnancy rates are significantly lower [62, 63]. Factors which have been linked to vasectomy reversal outcomes are presented in Table 4.3.

Obstruction at the anastomotic site is responsible for the majority of failed reconstructions. Given the fairly good outcomes associated with repeat vasovasostomy (57–78% patency, 32–44% pregnancy rate), the initial failure is likely a consequence of the surgical technique [64]. Although repeat vasovasostomy is more cost effective, IVF with ICSI is also an appropriate option and should be discussed with patients who do not wish to pursue a repeat procedure [64–66].

Follow-Up Care

Patients are advised to wear briefs or a scrotal supporter for 2 weeks postoperatively to reduce movement and swelling. Some patients report positive results with ice intermittently applied to the affected area. Postoperative prophylactic antibiotics are used at the surgeon's discretion. There are no prospective randomized control trials comparing postoperative antibiotic prophylaxis in the setting of vasovasostomy. Oral analgesics, initially narcotics and then NSAIDS, are typically adequate for pain control. Patients are instructed to return to work when they feel well enough to do so, and this is generally on postoperative day 3–5. In order to facilitate healing, most urological microsurgeons recommend that the patient should refrain from sexual activity and strenuous lifting for at least 2 weeks postoperatively.

The first semen analysis is typically checked at 4–8 weeks postoperatively, and then approximately every 2–3 months until the sperm concentration and motility are within normal limits or until a plateau has been demonstrated. Following normalization, semen analysis should be performed every 4 months until pregnancy. Close monitoring of semen parameters enables early detection of treatment failures and/or re-obstruction at the anastomotic site. If the semen analysis reveals declining parameters over consecutive tests, this may be a sign of early anastomotic stenosis. Some clinicians will initiate therapy with anti-inflammatory agents or oral corticosteroids in an effort mitigate this process and preserve anastomotic patency. To date, no prospective studies assessing the use of these agents in the postoperative period have been published.

Complications

Complications following vasovasostomy are rare. The most common complications are wound infection and scrotal hematoma. Wound infections should be treated with antibiotics and drainage as required. Careful maintenance of hemostasis intraoperatively, particularly at the level of the dartos, is paramount to avoid hematoma formation. In order to prevent breakdown and fibrosis at the anastomotic site, the threshold for hematoma drainage should be low.

The Future of Vasovasostomy

The field of urology has been welcoming to technological advancements, with one recent successful example being Da Vinci robotic system. Some have argued that robotic surgery could also be used to achieve better patency and pregnancy outcomes during vasectomy reversal by improving visualization, increasing the number of degrees of freedom, and reducing tremor while using microsurgical instruments with fine suture. Parekattil et al. performed the first prospective randomized control trial in humans, comparing robotic and microscopic vasovasostomy in a group of 90 patients. They showed significantly improved patency, and increased postoperative sperm recovery rate as compared to the same surgeon's microsurgical series [67]. Though these early results are promising, further evaluation is necessary to determine the true clinical benefit and costs associated with robotic vasovasostomy.

There have been a number of attempts to improve patency and pregnancy outcomes, particularly with techniques aimed to facilitate securing the vasal anastomosis such as fibrin glue or laser soldering. However, these procedures continue to require sutured anastomosis and current published data reveal inferior or similar outcomes to traditional microsurgical techniques [46, 68].

Techniques aimed at reducing postoperative morbidity have also been investigated. Using principles similar to the "no scalpel vasectomy," Grober et al. developed the "mini-incision vasectomy reversal" (MIVR). In a retrospective analysis, the group showed similar patency and pregnancy rates when comparing traditional incision size microsurgical reversal with their MIVR (<1 cm) [69]. Patient's also reported significantly diminished postoperative pain and quicker return to normal daily function [69]. The authors acknowledge that postoperative complications are rare, and the MIVR technique may not be appropriate in all patients (i.e., significant scrotal or vasal fibrosis, wide vasal gaps, large sperm granulomas). However, they argue that an initial attempt with the MIVR procedure should be made given the ease of conversion to a traditional scrotal incision.

References

1. Barone MA, Hutchinson PL, Johnson CH, Hsia J, Wheeler J. Vasectomy in the United States, 2002. J Urol. 2006;176(1):232–6. discussion 236.
2. Potts JM, Pasqualotto FF, Nelson D, Thomas Jr AJ, Agarwal A. Patient characteristics associated with vasectomy reversal. J Urol. 1999;161(6):1835–9.
3. Cos LR, Valvo JR, Davis RS, Cockett AT. Vasovasostomy: current state of the art. Urology. 1983;22(6):567–75.
4. Martin E, Carnett JB, Levi JV, Pennington ME. The surgical treatment of sterility due to obstruction at the epididymis; together with a study of the morphology of human spermatozoa. Univ Pa Med Bull. 1902;15(1):2–15.
5. Jequier AM. Edward Martin (1859–1938). The founding father of modern clinical andrology. Int J Androl. 1991;14(1):1–10.
6. O'Conor VJ. Anastomosis of the vas deferens after purposeful division for sterility. J Urol. 1948;59(2):229–33.
7. Mosher WD, Pratt WF. Contraceptive use in the United States, 1973–88. Patient Educ Couns. 1990;16(2):163–72.
8. Howard G. Who asks for vasectomy reversal and why? Br Med J (Clin Res Ed). 1982;285(6340):490–2.
9. Amelar RD, Dubin L. Vasectomy reversal. J Urol. 1979;121(5):547–50.
10. Schmidt SS. Vas anastomosis: a return to simplicity. Br J Urol. 1975;47(3):309–14.
11. Dorsey JW. Surgical correction of post-vasectomy sterility. J Urol. 1973;110(5):554–5.
12. Roland SI. Splinted and non-splinted vasovasostomy. A review of the literature and a report of nine new cases. Fertil Steril. 1961;12:191–5.
13. Derrick Jr FC, Yarbrough W, D'Agostino J. Vasovasostomy: results of questionnaire of members of the American Urological Association. J Urol. 1973;110(5):556–7.
14. Shessel FS, Lynne CM, Politano VA. Use of exteriorized stents in vasovasostomy. Urology. 1981;17(2):163–5.
15. Owen ER. Microsurgical vasovasostomy: a reliable vasectomy reversal. Aust N Z J Surg. 1977;47(3):305–9.

16. Silber SJ. Microscopic vasectomy reversal. Fertil Steril. 1977;28(11):1191–202.
17. Silber SJ. Microsurgery in clinical urology. Urology. 1975;6(2):150–3.
18. Silber SJ. Vasectomy and vasectomy reversal. Fertil Steril. 1978;29(2):125–40.
19. Phadke GM, Phadke AG. Experiences in the re-anastomosis of the vas deferens. J Urol. 1967;97(5):888–90.
20. Mehta KC, Ramani PS. A simple technique of re-anastomosis after vasectomy. Br J Urol. 1970;42(3):340–3.
21. Lee L, McLoughlin MG. Vasovasostomy: a comparison of macroscopic and microscopic techniques at one institution. Fertil Steril. 1980;33(1):54–5.
22. Lee HY. A 20-year experience with vasovasostomy. J Urol. 1986;136(2):413–5.
23. Silber SJ, Cohen R. Microsurgical reversal of tubal sterilization: factors affecting pregnancy rate, with long-term follow-up. Obstet Gynecol. 1984;64(5):679–82.
24. Belker AM. Urologic microsurgery–current perspectives: I. Vasovasostomy. Urology. 1979;14(4):325–9.
25. Robb P, Sandlow JI. Cost-effectiveness of vasectomy reversal. Urol Clin North Am. 2009;36(3):391–6.
26. Garceau L, Henderson J, Davis LJ, et al. Economic implications of assisted reproductive techniques: a systematic review. Hum Reprod. 2002;17(12):3090–109.
27. Hsieh MH, Meng MV, Turek PJ. Markov modeling of vasectomy reversal and ART for infertility: how do obstructive interval and female partner age influence cost effectiveness? Fertil Steril. 2007;88(4):840–6.
28. Meng MV, Greene KL, Turek PJ. Surgery or assisted reproduction? A decision analysis of treatment costs in male infertility. J Urol. 2005;174(5):1926–31. discussion 1931.
29. Shridharani A, Sandlow JI. Vasectomy reversal versus IVF with sperm retrieval: which is better? Curr Opin Urol. 2010;20(6):503–9.
30. Jarow JP, Sigman M, Kolettis PN, Lipshultz LR, McClure RD, Nangia AK, Naughton CK, Prins GS, Sandlow JL, Schlegel PN, Hubbard H, Janus C, Folmer M, Kadiatu K, Hurley J. The management of obstructive azoospermia: AUA best practice statement. Linthicum: American Urological Association Education and Research Inc; 2010.
31. Hull MG, Fleming CF, Hughes AO, McDermott A. The age-related decline in female fecundity: a quantitative controlled study of implanting capacity and survival of individual embryos after in vitro fertilization. Fertil Steril. 1996;65(4):783–90.
32. Belker AM, Thomas Jr AJ, Fuchs EF, Konnak JW, Sharlip ID. Results of 1,469 microsurgical vasectomy reversals by the Vasovasostomy Study Group. J Urol. 1991;145(3):505–11.
33. Malizia BA, Hacker MR, Penzias AS. Cumulative live-birth rates after in vitro fertilization. N Engl J Med. 2009;360(3):236–43.
34. Wright VC, Schieve LA, Reynolds MA, Jeng G. Assisted reproductive technology surveillance–United States, 2000. MMWR Surveill Summ. 2003;52(9):1–16.
35. Clarke L, Gregson S. Who has a vasectomy reversal? J Biosoc Sci. 1986;18(3):253–9.
36. Parekattil SJ, Kuang W, Agarwal A, Thomas AJ. Model to predict if a vasoepididymostomy will be required for vasectomy reversal. J Urol. 2005;173(5):1681–4.
37. Parekattil SJ, Kuang W, Kolettis PN, et al. Multi-institutional validation of vasectomy reversal predictor. J Urol. 2006;175(1):247–9.
38. Hsiao W, Sultan R, Goldstein M. Increased follicle-stimulating hormone is associated with higher assisted reproduction use after vasectomy reversal. J Urol. 2011;185(6):2266–71.
39. Mulhall JP, Stokes S, Andrawis R, Buch JP. Simultaneous microsurgical vasal reconstruction and varicocele ligation: safety profile and outcomes. Urology. 1997;50(3):438–42.
40. Witt MA, Heron S, Lipshultz LI. The post-vasectomy length of the testicular vasal remnant: a predictor of surgical outcome in microscopic vasectomy reversal. J Urol. 1994;151(4): 892–4.
41. Bolduc S, Fischer MA, Deceuninck G, Thabet M. Factors predicting overall success: a review of 747 microsurgical vasovasostomies. Can Urol Assoc J. 2007;1(4):388–94.
42. Boorjian S, Lipkin M, Goldstein M. The impact of obstructive interval and sperm granuloma on outcome of vasectomy reversal. J Urol. 2004;171(1):304–6.

43. Flickinger CJ, Yarbro ES, Howards SS, et al. The incidence of spermatic granulomas and their relation to testis weight after vasectomy and vasovasostomy in Lewis rats. J Androl. 1986;7(5):285–91.
44. Amarin ZO, Obeidat BR. Patency following vasectomy reversal. Temporal and immunological considerations. Saudi Med J. 2005;26(8):1208–11.
45. Paick J, Kim SH, Kim SW. Ejaculatory duct obstruction in infertile men. BJU Int. 2000;85(6):720–4.
46. Kolettis PN. Restructuring reconstructive techniques–advances in reconstructive techniques. Urol Clin North Am. 2008;35(2):229–34. Viii–ix.
47. Boyle KE, Thomas Jr AJ, Marmar JL, Hirshberg S, Belker AM, Jarow JP. Sperm harvesting and cryopreservation during vasectomy reversal is not cost effective. Fertil Steril. 2006;85(4): 961–4.
48. Schrepferman CG, Carson MR, Sparks AM, Sandlow JI. Need for sperm retrieval and cryopreservation at vasectomy reversal. J Urol. 2001;166(5):1787–9.
49. Sheynkin YR, Starr C, Li PS, Goldstein M. Effect of methylene blue, indigo carmine, and Renografin on human sperm motility. Urology. 1999;53(1):214–7.
50. Busato Jr WF. Vasectomy reversal: a seven-year experience. Urol Int. 2009;82(2):170–4.
51. Fischer MA, Grantmyre JE. Comparison of modified one- and two-layer microsurgical vasovasostomy. BJU Int. 2000;85(9):1085–8.
52. Goldstein M, Li PS, Matthews GJ. Microsurgical vasovasostomy: the microdot technique of precision suture placement. J Urol. 1998;159(1):188–90.
53. Buch JP, Woods T. Retroperitoneal mobilization of the vas deferens in the complex vasovasostomy. Fertil Steril. 1990;54(5):931–3.
54. Sandlow JI, Kolettis PN. Vasovasostomy in the convoluted vas deferens: indications and outcomes. J Urol. 2005;173(2):540–2.
55. Kolettis PN, Thomas Jr AJ. Vasoepididymostomy for vasectomy reversal: a critical assessment in the era of intracytoplasmic sperm injection. J Urol. 1997;158(2):467–70.
56. Ho KL, Wong MH, Tam PC. Microsurgical vasoepididymostomy for obstructive azoospermia. Hong Kong Med J. 2009;15(6):452–7.
57. Kolettis PN, Woo L, Sandlow JI. Outcomes of vasectomy reversal performed for men with the same female partners. Urology. 2003;61(6):1221–3.
58. Chan PT, Goldstein M. Superior outcomes of microsurgical vasectomy reversal in men with the same female partners. Fertil Steril. 2004;81(5):1371–4.
59. Matsuda T, Horii Y, Muguruma K, Komatz Y, Yoshida O. Microsurgical epididymovasostomy for obstructive azoospermia: factors affecting postoperative fertility. Eur Urol. 1994;26(4):322–6.
60. Jarow JP, Sigman M, Kolettis PN, Lipshultz LR, McClure RD, Nangia AK, Naughton CK, Prins GS, Sandlow JL, Schlegel PN, Hubbard H, Janus C, Folmer M, Kadiatu K, Hurley J. The evaluation of the azoospermic male: AUA best practice statement. Linthicum: American Urological Association Education and Research Inc; 2010.
61. Patel SR, Sigman M. Comparison of outcomes of vasovasostomy performed in the convoluted and straight vas deferens. J. Urol. 2008;179(1):256–9.
62. Lizza EF, Marmar JL, Schmidt SS, et al. Transseptal crossed vasovasostomy. J Urol. 1985;134(6):1131–2.
63. Sabanegh Jr E, Thomas Jr AJ. Effectiveness of crossover transseptal vasoepididymostomy in treating complex obstructive azoospermia. Fertil Steril. 1995;63(2):392–5.
64. Hollingsworth MR, Sandlow JI, Schrepferman CG, Brannigan RE, Kolettis PN. Repeat vasectomy reversal yields high success rates. Fertil Steril. 2007;88(1):217–9.
65. Paick JS, Park JY, Park DW, Park K, Son H, Kim SW. Microsurgical vasovasostomy after failed vasovasostomy. J Urol. 2003;169(3):1052–5.
66. Donovan Jr JF, DiBaise M, Sparks AE, Kessler J, Sandlow JI. Comparison of microscopic epididymal sperm aspiration and intracytoplasmic sperm injection/in-vitro fertilization with repeat microscopic reconstruction following vasectomy: is second attempt vas reversal worth the effort? Hum Reprod. 1998;13(2):387–93.

67. Parekattil SJ, Atalah HN, Cohen MS. Video technique for human robot-assisted microsurgical vasovasostomy. J Endourol. 2010;24(4):511–4.
68. Seaman EK. The application of laser techniques to vasectomy reversal surgery. J Clin Laser Med Surg. 1998;16(1):45–8.
69. Jarvi K, Grober ED, Lo KC, Patry G. Mini-incision microsurgical vasectomy reversal using no-scalpel vasectomy principles and instruments. Urology. 2008;72(4):913–5.
70. Grober ED, Jarvi K, Lo KC, Shin EJ. Mini-incision vasectomy reversal using no-scalpel vasectomy principles: efficacy and postoperative pain compared with traditional approaches to vasectomy reversal. Urology. 2011;77(3):602–6.
71. Jee SH, Hong YK. One-layer vasovasostomy: microsurgical versus loupe-assisted. Fertil Steril. 2010;94(6):2308–11.
72. Hsieh ML, Huang HC, Chen Y, Huang ST, Chang PL. Loupe-assisted vs. microsurgical technique for modified one-layer vasovasostomy: is the microsurgery really better? BJU Int. 2005;96(6):864–6.
73. Silber SJ, Grotjan HE. Microscopic vasectomy reversal 30 years later: a summary of 4010 cases by the same surgeon. J Androl. 2004;25(6):845–59.
74. Kolettis PN, Sabanegh ES, Nalesnik JG, D'Amico AM, Box LC, Burns JR. Pregnancy outcomes after vasectomy reversal for female partners 35 years old or older. J Urol. 2003;169(6):2250–2.
75. Kolettis PN, Sabanegh ES, D'Amico AM, Box L, Sebesta M, Burns JR. Outcomes for vasectomy reversal performed after obstructive intervals of at least 10 years. Urology. 2002;60(5):885–8.
76. Holman CD, Wisniewski ZS, Semmens JB, Rouse IL, Bass AJ. Population-based outcomes after 28,246 in-hospital vasectomies and 1,902 vasovasostomies in Western Australia. BJU Int. 2000;86(9):1043–9.
77. Feber KM, Ruiz HE. Vasovasostomy: macroscopic approach and retrospective review. Tech Urol. 1999;5(1):8–11.

Chapter 5
Epididymovasostomy: Tips and Tricks of the Trade

James F. Smith and Ajay K. Nangia

Abstract The first reported successful vas deferens to epididymis bypass was reported by Martin (Univ Pa Med Bull 15:2–15, 1902). His side–side technique brought together the cut edge of epididymal tunica vaginalis to the longitudinally incised seromuscular layer of the vas deferens, relying upon the creation of a fistula between opened epididymal tubules and vas deferens. Reports by Martin and later, Hagner, demonstrated patency rates of 43 and 64%; however, low patency rates and frequent late failures among other surgeons led to further technical advances in the latter part of the twentieth century. Silber's microsurgical end–end approach in 1978 [Silber (Fertil Steril 30:565–71, 1978)] and the development of the end–side approach in the mid-to-late 1980s formed the basis for modern epididymovasostomy (EV).

Keywords Epididymovasostomy • Vasectomy reversal • Microsurgery • Male infertility • Vasectomy • Reconstruction • Vasal obstruction • Epididymal obstruction

J.F. Smith, M.D., M.S. (✉)
Departments of Urology, Obstetrics, Gynecology, and Reproductive Sciences, UCSF, 1600 Divisadero, Box 1695, San Francisco, CA 94143, USA

A.K. Nangia, M.B.B.S.
Department of Urology, University of Kansas Medical Center, 3901 Rainbow Blvd, Kansas City, KS 66160, USA

J.I. Sandlow (ed.), *Microsurgery for Fertility Specialists: A Practical Text*,
DOI 10.1007/978-1-4614-4196-0_5, © Springer Science+Business Media New York 2013

Introduction

The first reported successful vas deferens to epididymis bypass was reported by Martin in 1902 [1]. His side–side technique brought together the cut edge of epididymal tunica vaginalis to the longitudinally incised seromuscular layer of the vas deferens, relying upon the creation of a fistula between opened epididymal tubules and vas deferens. Reports by Martin and later, Hagner, demonstrated patency rates of 43 and 64%; however, low patency rates and frequent late failures among other surgeons led to further technical advances in the latter part of the twentieth century. Silber's microsurgical end–end approach in 1978 [2] and the development of the end–side approach in the mid-to-late 1980s formed the basis for modern epididymovasostomy (EV).

Epididymal obstruction is suspected for men presenting with azoospermia, normal follicle-stimulating hormone levels, palpably normal vasa deferentia, semen volume greater than 1.5 ml, normal-sized testicles, and a full epididymis. In men with idiopathic or infectious epididymal obstruction, fullness of the epididymis was associated with epididymal obstruction 100% of the time [3]. For men undergoing vasectomy reversal, a palpably normal epididymis on preoperative clinical examination required EV only 6% of the time. However, preoperative epididymal fullness in these men was less helpful and associated with need for EV only 20% of the time (positive predictive value 20%) [3]. Epididymal obstruction can be caused by epididymitis, trauma, congenital abnormalities, and, most commonly, prior vasectomy [4]. In the latter group, epididymal obstruction is determined by examination of fluid from the testicular vas segment at the time of vasectomy reversal. The presence of thick, pasty fluid, absence of vasal fluid, or absence of sperm or sperm parts strongly suggests epididymal obstruction [5].

Three techniques have been described to perform a modern, microsurgical epididymis single tubule to vas deferens anastomosis.

End–End Epididymovasostomy

Indication for Surgery

First described by Silber in 1978 [2], this technique begins with careful mobilization of the vas deferens and delivery of the epididymis and testicle through the parietal tunica vaginalis. This technique is not often used currently, but can be a useful option if the obstruction is found at the vasoepididymal junction. The epididymal diameter at this junction more closely matches the vasal lumen. There is also more of a muscular layer around the epididymal tubule for an end-to-end anastomosis. This technique is potentially useful when the vasal length is compromised for mobilization or when epididymal tubules are not dilated. Goldstein and Schlegel have suggested that the end–end technique may also be indicated when the level of obstruction is not clearly demarcated [6].

Surgical Technique

Vas Deferens Exposure and Division

Obtaining sufficient length on the vas deferens is a critical portion of the early stages of the operation. Vas deferens exposure is generally accomplished by making parallel paramedian incisions in the scrotum. Midline incisions have been used successfully for this technique but limit the surgeon's ability to extend the incision cephalad for increased vas exposure. The testicle can be used as a backing to facilitate this incision. Alternatively, incision through the skin and blunt dissection through the Dartos muscle can mobilize the cord adequately to deliver the testicle. The vas deferens is isolated and transected near the level of the convoluted vas or at the site of the prior vasectomy, preserving as much length and perivasal tissue as possible. Blunt dissection with the tip of a finger, the use of a Penfield osteal elevator, or Peanut is often helpful to push away loose connective tissue [5]. Extending the incision to the level of the inguinal canal is occasionally necessary to achieve adequate vasal length. A useful tool for transection of the vas deferens and the epididymis is the slotted nerve clamp (Accurate Surgical and Scientific Instruments, ASSI NHF2-ASSI NHF6 for sizes ranging from 2.0 to 6.0 mm) [7]. An ultrasharp blade (Accurate Surgical and Scientific Instruments, ASSI-CBS-35) fits through the slot in this nerve holder and makes excellent 90° cuts. The blade dulls quickly after 2–3 cuts.

The vas deferens is mobilized sufficiently to achieve a tension-free length that will easily meet the epididymis. Preserving perivasal adventia and sheath is important to preserve blood supply and assist in subsequent closure [7]. After verifying abdominal vasal patency with a 2-0 nylon suture, saline vasogram, methylene blue vasogram, or contrast vasography, the abdominal vas deferens is sutured to the posterior edge of the epididymal tunic with 2–3 interrupted 9-0 nylon sutures. Some surgeons prefer using the Microspike approximator (ASSI, Westbury, New York) to align the vas deferens and epididymis at this step [7]. The vas deferens should be transected cleanly after control of the vasal vessels. One of the authors uses 6-0 prolene suture to control the vessels, other surgeons use 6-0 nylon or bipolar cautery.

Epididymal Evaluation and Surgical Approach

The epididymis is inspected for signs of obstruction. The most distal portion of unobstructed appearing epididymis is transected leaving multiple tubules exposed (Fig. 5.1). Gentle irrigation of these tubules by the surgical assistant will expose the single tubule effluxing fluid. Only the tubules above the level of obstruction will efflux sperm. Examination of the fluid under 200–400× light microscopy will reveal motile or nonmotile sperm from this tubule. If no fluid is identified, repeat sectioning of the epididymis at a higher level will ultimately lead to identification of an unobstructed

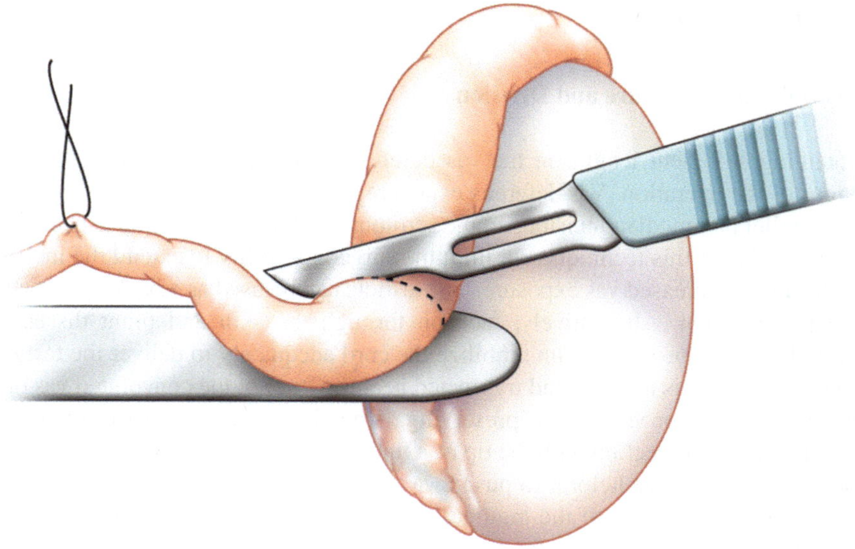

Fig. 5.1 Transection of the distal epididymis during epididymovasostomy

tubule. This process should be continued until many normal-appearing, motile sperm are identified in the epididymal fluid. The presence of only sperm parts suggests an additional obstruction above that level with an associated lower rate of patency [2]. Aspiration of sperm for cryopreservation is an option at this point.

Using the end–end EV technique, it is often necessary to mobilize the epididymis free from the testis by incising the tunical plane between the testis and epididymis distally. Care must be taken not to injure epididymal blood supply. This is usually less evident in the cauda epididymis. Occasionally, the medial and inferior epididymal arteries may need to be ligated, often at the corpus or cauda epididymis level. The superior epididymal vessels need to be preserved at the caput epididymis. Once the epididymis is transected at the correct level the cut tubule edges may be outlined by applying methylene blue to the cut end.

Vas to Epididymis Anastomosis

Anastomosis to a single cut tubule is recommended. If fluid effluxes from more than one site, reevaluation of the tubules under high magnification should be performed. Further transection to isolate a single tubule may be needed. The lumen of the epididymal tubule is anastomosed to the vasal mucosal lumen with equally spaced, inside-out, double-arm 10-0 Nylon sutures [5]. Facilitating the placement of all three stitches, the first stitch is placed at 6 o'clock and tied, but the other three stitches are

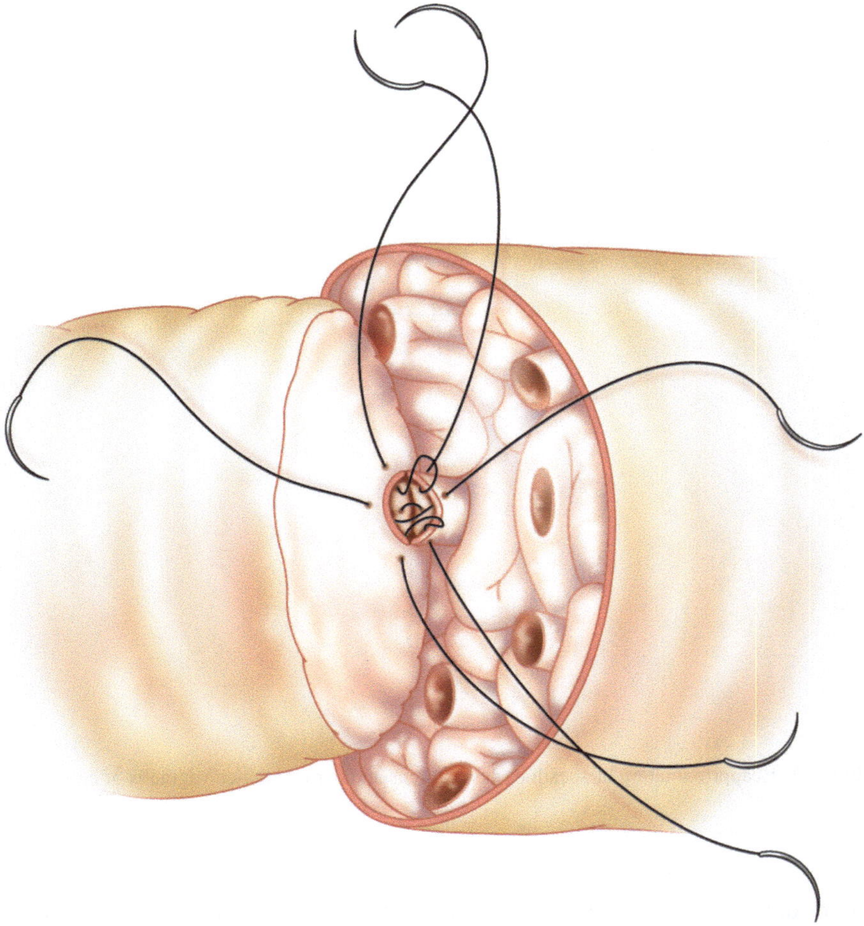

Fig. 5.2 Placement of mucosal sutures for end-to-end epididymovasostomy

placed prior to tying (Fig. 5.2). Care must be taken not to tangle these sutures. Wide bites for the mucosal sutures should be avoided. Wide bites have the risk of occluding an adjacent convoluted epididymal tubule. The seromuscular layer of the vas and visceral tunica vaginalis overlying the epididymal tubules are approximated with interrupted 9-0 Nylon sutures (Fig. 5.3). Meticulous hemostasis is essential to ensure the maximal chance for patency. The parietal tunica vaginalis is approximated with absorbable suture and the testicle is replaced within the scrotum.

Needles and suture choices are important to the success of this operation (Table 5.1). For the thick seromuscular layer of the vas deferens, the Ethicon 9-0 nylon (6 in. length) on a vas100-4 cutting needle (Ethicon, Johnson and Johnson) is sturdy and very effective. For mucosal vas surface to epididymal tubule, a

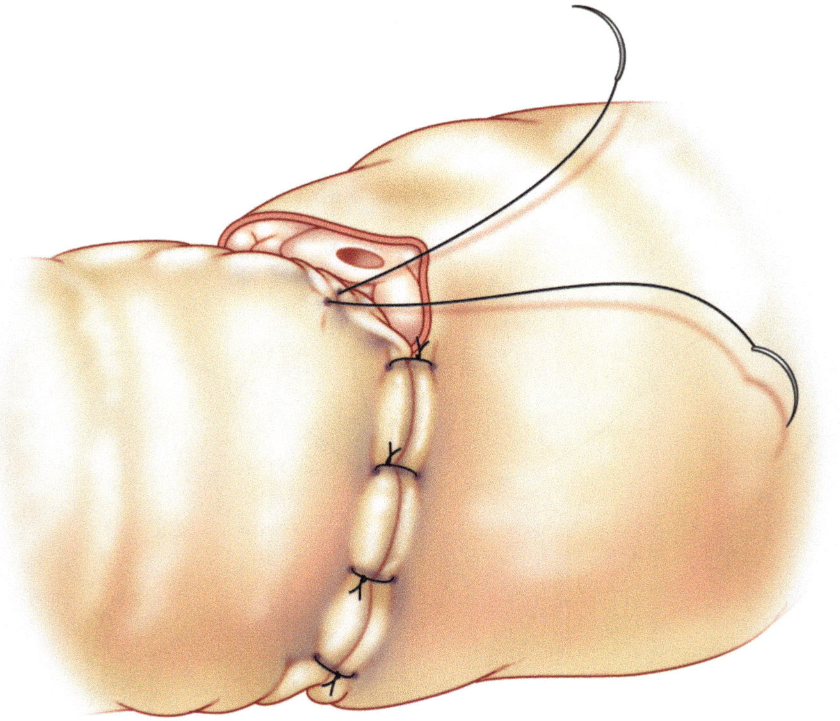

Fig. 5.3 Reapproximation of sheath of vas deferens and parietal tunica vaginalis of epididymis

more delicate needle is required. The Sharpoint 10-0 nylon (1 in.) double-arm suture with a 70 μm needle is very effective for the mucosal anastomosis (Surgical Specialties Corporation, Reading Pennsylvania, USA). The Ethicon 10-0 nylon (single arm, 6 in.) on a BV100-3 taper needle (Ethicon, Johnson and Johnson) can be a good choice; however, the shape of the needle is not as ideal as the Sharpoint 3/8 circle needle described above. Careful needle handling is necessary to minimize bending of the needle and dulling of the point for many of these needles.

In a recent review, this technique demonstrated a mean patency rate of 61%, ranging from 35 to 81% [5]. In these studies, the mean pregnancy rate was 31%, ranging from 10 to 56%. Pregnancy rates may be higher the more distal the anastomosis on the epididymis occurs [8].

Problems with this approach include troublesome bleeding at the site of epididymal transection leading to poor visualization of the epididymal tubule [4]. Identifying the patent tubule with this technique can be time-consuming and require repeat division of the epididymis [6]. Subsequent techniques developed in 1983 and 1989 sought to overcome these limitations.

Table 5.1 Suture and needles used for epididymovasostomy

Suture/manufacturer	Purpose	Needle characteristics	Description	Cost/suture	Manufacturer
5-0 PDS	Traction		Sturdy		
5-0 Maxon	Traction				
6-0 Nylon	Ligate vasal vessels				
7-0 Prolene	Traction, closure of tunic, reinforce anastomosis	Large, sturdy, taper	Packaged as double-armed suture. Memory, sturdy		
9-0 Nylon with VAS100-3	Muscular layer vas to epid tunic	Poor thru vas. Dulls quickly	Single arm		
Ethilon 9-0 Nylon with VAS100-4	Muscular layer vas to epid tunic	Relatively sturdy, circle taper. Easy thru muscle of vas			Ethicon company, Summerville, NY
Ethilon 10-0 Nylon with VAS100-3		Too large for mucosa			
Sharpoint, 9-0 nylon black monofilament HSV 6 100 μm vas cutting needle	Muscular layer vas to epid tunic	Silber			
Sharppoint 10-0 Nylon with DRM 4 needle black monofilament nylon, 70 μm, 135° curve	Mucosal stitch	Good size for mucosal suture—Silber	Single or double arm		Sharp Point
Ethicon monofilament black nylon 10-0 V75-3 taper cut needle	Mucosal stitch	Silber (2004)	Single arm		

End-to-Side Epididymovasostomy

Described first by Fogdestam and Fall in 1983 [9] and Thomas in 1989 [4], this approach attaches the cut end of the abdominal vas deferens to the side of a epididymal tubule. The end-to-side anastomosis has some advantages over the end-to-end EV: less dissection; no transection of any part of the epididymis with less associated bleeding; only one epididymal tubule is deliberately exposed and opened; and identification of a single tubule is more straightforward. Determination of the level of epididymal obstruction is necessary by inspection. A demarcation between dilated and non-dilated tubules may be seen, otherwise incision of tubules under high magnification may be needed from cauda to caput until intact sperm are seen. Controversy regarding the requirement for motility still exists.

Surgical Technique

As for all EV approaches, adequate mobilization of the vas deferens leaving intact its blood supply is necessary for a tension-free anastomosis as described above. The vas deferens is passed through a small window in the parietal tunica vaginalis from medial to lateral aspect of the cord. A small incision is made in the epididymal tunic (visceral tunica vaginalis) above the level of obstruction to expose intact epididymal tubules. Often, one or two interrupted 6-0 or 7-0 non-absorbable sutures are placed between vas deferens and visceral tunica vaginalis on the epididymis to reduce tension on the anastomosis. These sutures are placed in the perivasal tissue 1–2 cm away from the cut edge of the vas deferens and in the visceral tunica vaginalis 1–2 cm away from the epididymal anastomosis.

Epididymal Tubule Exposure and Division

Epididymal exposure is achieved by opening the parietal tunica vaginalis and delivering the testicle and epididymis into the operating field. A 5 mm opening is made in the most distal portion of the visceral tunica vaginalis overlying epididymal tubules that appears to have dilated tubules. Gentle compression of the proximal epididymis using the nondominant fingers of the surgeon's hand will cause tubules to bulge into view, allowing for dissection of a single tubule [4]. The tubule of interest can be mobilized by gently dissecting it free from the overlying tunica vaginalis and surrounding loose connective tissue. Blunt dissection with a fine non-locking

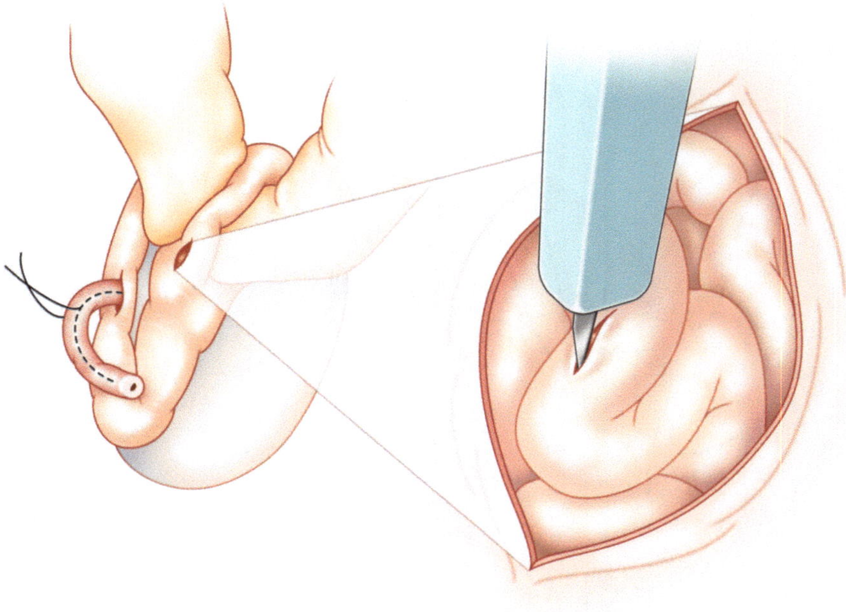

Fig. 5.4 Incision for end–side epididymovasostomy

Castroviejo needle holder is one effective technique. Incising subtunical connective tissue sharply is sometimes necessary.

After identification of the obstructed epididymal segment, a single epididymal tubule is opened longitudinally for approximately 0.5 mm (Fig. 5.4). Some surgeons may remove an elliptical segment from the convexity of the tubule exposed. This is either done directly with fine curved epididymal scissors, by placing a 10-0 suture through the apex of the convexity with incision of the epididymal tubule underneath the suture to create a lumen, or by incision of the tubule with the cutting surface of a 9-0 nylon needle. Fluid from this incision is examined with the side-table microscope. Sperm can be cryopreserved at this stage if desired. If no sperm is identified, additional more proximal epididymal tubules are opened until normal-appearing motile sperm are identified.

Vas to Epididymis Anastomosis

After setting up the anastomosis, with two or three 9-0 nylon sutures placed between the posterior seromuscular layer of the vas deferens and visceral tunica vaginalis, 3–4 double-armed 10-0 nylon sutures are placed inside-out at the cut edge of the

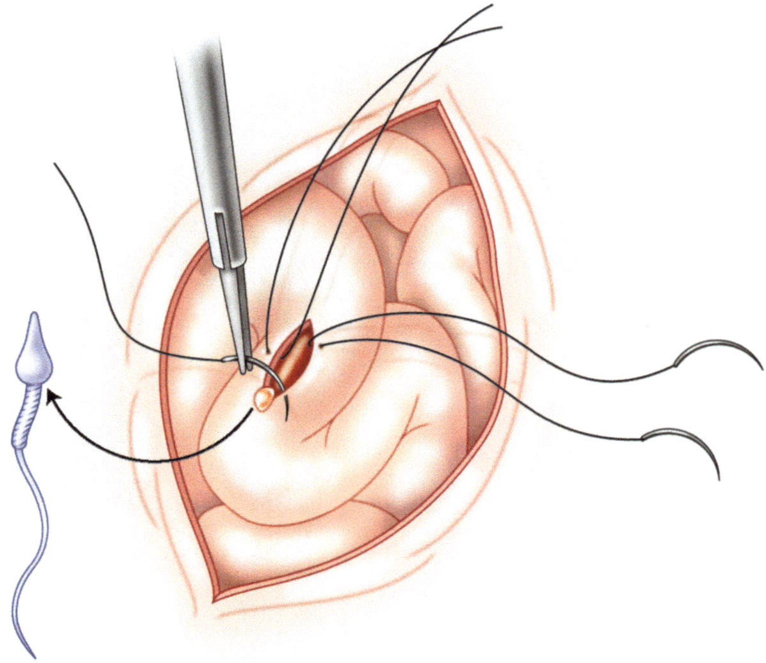

Fig. 5.5 Initial mucosal suture placement for end–side epididymovasostomy

epididymal tubule in a triangular or rectangular pattern (Fig. 5.5). The second arm is placed inside-out on the mucosal surface of the vasal segment and tied (Fig. 5.6). Some surgeons prefer to use a single-arm 10-0 suture passing from outside-in on the epididymal tubule and inside-out on the vasal mucosa. Approximately 4–6 interrupted stitches are placed to complete the leakproof anastomosis. After completing the mucosal anastomosis, the anterior seromuscular surface of the vas deferens is sutured to the epididymal tunic with interrupted 9-0 nylon sutures in the same fashion described for the end–end EV approach.

A recent summary of the patency rate for the end-to-side EV technique demonstrated very similar results to that of the end-to-end EV approach (mean patency 64%, range 31–85%) [5]. Mean pregnancy rate among these studies was approximately 35%, ranging from 13 to 50%.

Although this technique does overcome some of the difficulties inherent in the end-to-end EV and has a similar probability of successful anastomosis, it introduces new difficulties. The primary difficulty is the challenge of placing sutures on a 0.2 mm collapsed epididymal tubule. The small size of the tubule makes "backwalling" of the epididymis a significant danger. Subsequent modification of this technique by Berger in 1998 and Marmar in 2000, sought to overcome these challenges.

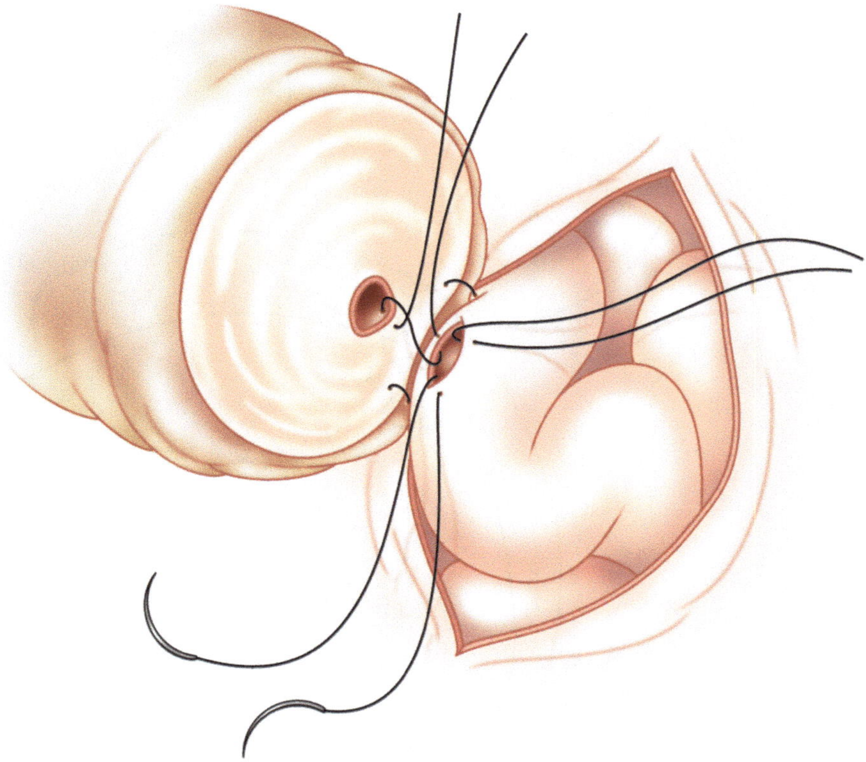

Fig. 5.6 Mucosal suture placement for end–side epididymovasostomy

Intussusception End-to-Side Epididymovasostomy

In 1998, Berger [10] reported a triangular stitch, and Marmar in 2000 [11] a parallel stitch intussusception technique. These approaches extended the modifications of the end-to-side EV by preplacing two or three stitches in the epididymal tubule prior to epididymal tubule incision. The first report of a similar approach on a single patient was by Lespinasse in 1918 [12]. These techniques allow the surgeon to avoid the difficulty of placing sutures across the cut edge of a collapsed epididymal tubule that can be obscured by leakage of epididymal fluid.

Surgical Technique

Isolation of the vas deferens and preparation of the epididymis is identical to that described above for the end-to-side EV. As emphasized above, adequate vasal

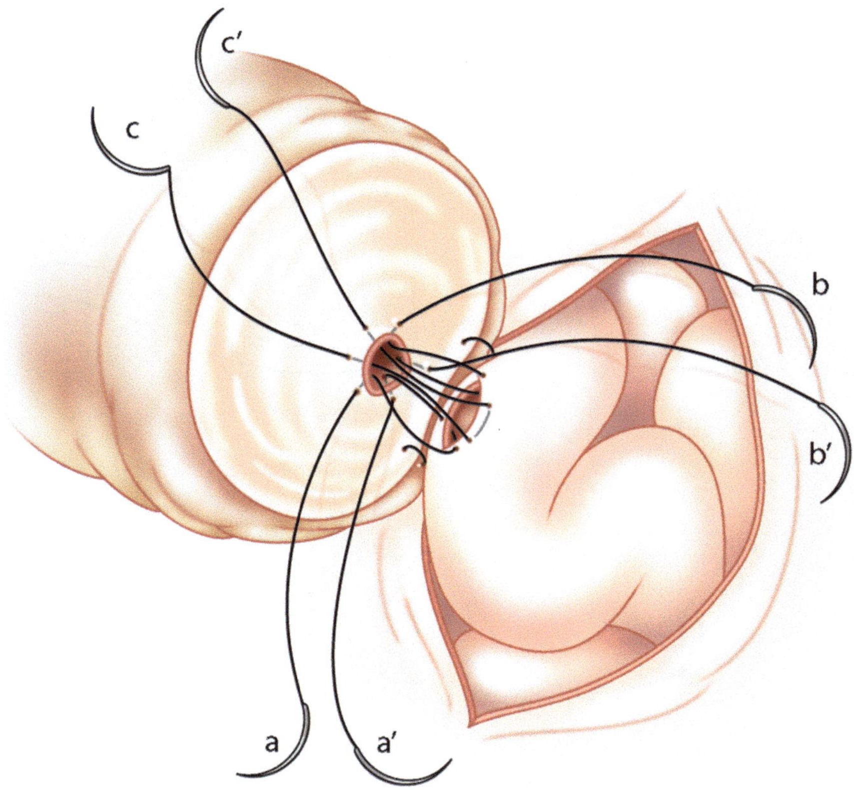

Fig. 5.7 Three-stitch intussusception technique

length is of critical importance. After identification of the unobstructed tubule, the posterior aspect of the vasal seromuscular layer is sewn to the cut edge of the epididymal tunic with 2–3 interrupted 9-0 Nylon sutures. The primary difference between the standard end-to-side EV and the intussusception end-to-side EV technique lies is in the preplacement of two or three 10-0 nylon needles in the tubule before opening the tubule. In the Berger technique, three 10-0 nylon needles are placed in a triangular fashion in the epididymal tubule prior to opening the epididymal tubule (Fig. 5.7) [10]. For the Marmar technique [11], two double-armed 1 in. 10-0 nylon needles (e.g., Sharpoint, Ethicon) are placed across the epididymal tubule through the tubule wall prior to opening the tubule (Fig. 5.8). A further subtle modification of the Marmar technique described by Chan and Goldstein in 2005 places these two stitches in a longitudinal fashion and may simplify this technique even further [13] (Fig. 5.9). With the needles still in place, the epididymal tubule is opened by one of the methods described above. Caution must be taken to not cut out the previously placed sutures. Each needle is then passed through the rest of the tubule. The closer 10-0 needle to the vasal mucosa is placed

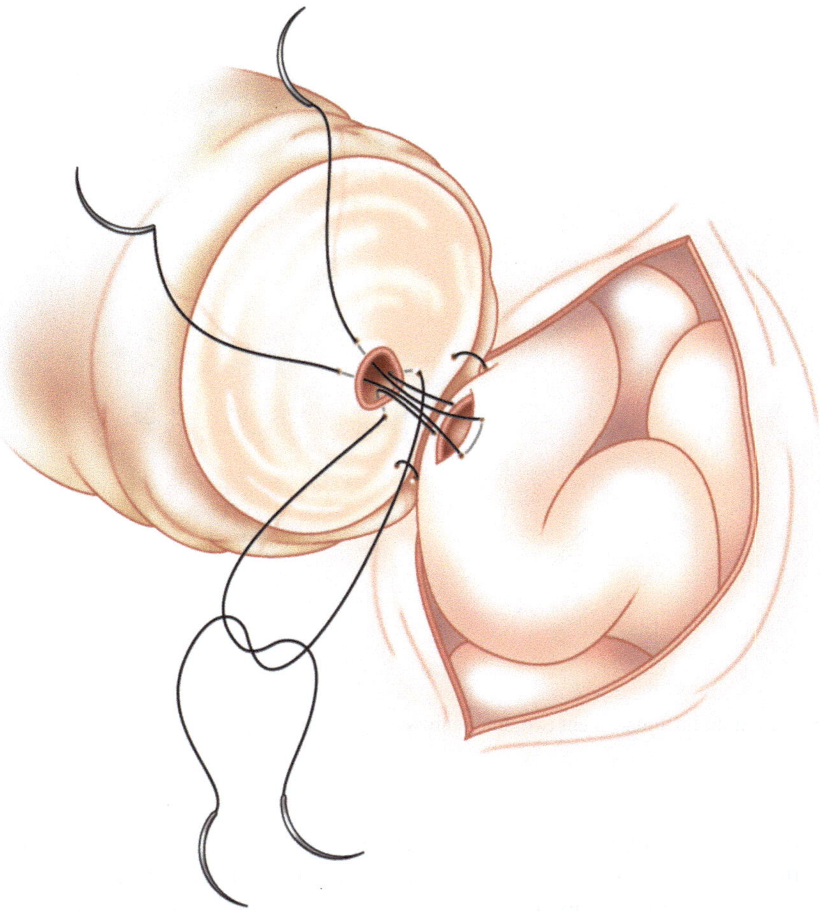

Fig. 5.8 Two-stitch intussusception mucosal needle placement

first, followed by the 10-0 needle furthest away to the vasal mucosa that sits higher up on the same side. Placement of sutures in this manner avoids crossing or having to pass needles behind previously placed mucosal suture (see Fig. 5.8). Depending on the orientation of the epididymal tubule to the vas, using the longitudinal suture placement technique described by Chan and Goldstein [13] may serve an alternative method to place these 10-0 sutures without having to cross/pass needles. It is essential to spend a minute or two to analyze the orientation of the vasal mucosa to the epididymal tubule after placement of the back wall muscular 9-0 sutures. The 10-0 suture orientation should be such to allow the intussuscepting vasal mucosal sutures to come out at 90° to the back 9-0 sutures, so that as the vas lays down on the tubule the 10-0 sutures can be tied. Also before tying the 10-0 sutures on each side, it is often necessary to place a single 9-0 suture at the apex of the vasal muscular layer and sutured to the opposite epididymal tunical layer

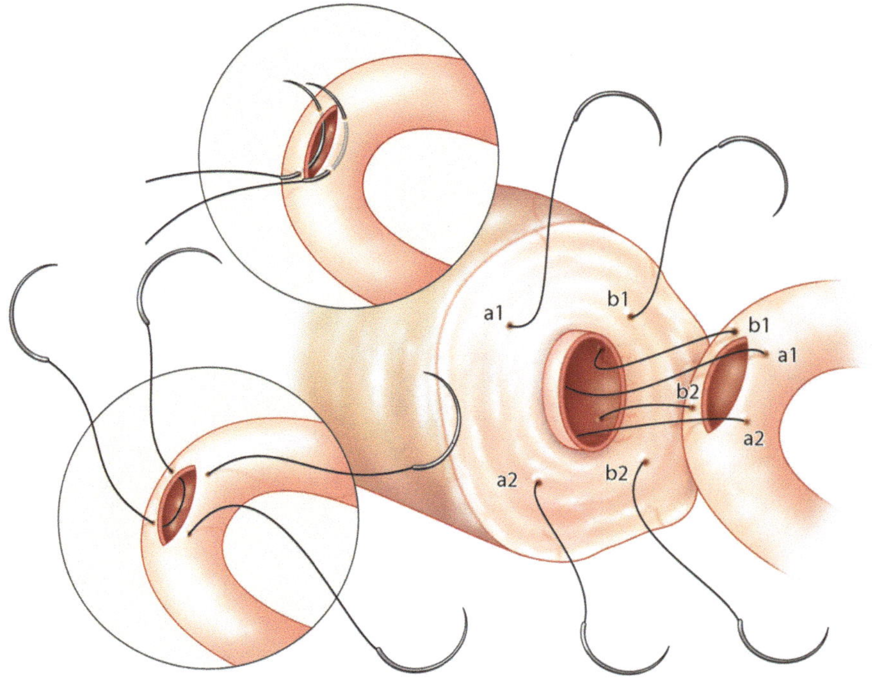

Fig. 5.9 Longitudinal placement two-stitch intussusception technique

(i.e., directly opposite [180°] from the previously placed back wall 9-0 suture)—thus allowing a tension-free environment for the 10-0 sutures to be tied. Care must be taken if this is done to pivot the vas from side to side as the 10-0 suture is being tied to watch that the slack of suture is removed and ensure that the intussusception approximation occurs without an air knot or gap at the mucosal level. This is repeated on the other side. The outer anastomosis of the muscularis layer of the vas to tunical layer of the epididymis is completed with two or three interrupted 9-0 sutures. To minimize the problem of overlapping untied sutures, keeping the surgical field moist uses the power of water surface tension to keep sutures in place and untangled.

Although the intussusception technique is relatively new, it has been adopted by many microsurgeons because of its relative simplicity in needle placement and good success rates. Patency was reported in 92% in the initial series [10] and was approximately 80% in two other series [5, 11]. Limited pregnancy data have been reported as yet. Even in the hands of an experienced surgeon, intussusception end-to-side EV appears to provide better results. In one single surgeon study, higher patency rates and fewer late failures were observed for the intussusception technique compared to the end-to-end EV and classic end–side EV [14].

Postoperative Care

Scrotal support and fluffed gauze dressings are placed at the time of surgery. An ice pack should be applied to the scrotum for the first 24–36 h. Men should utilize scrotal support night and day for 3–4 weeks. After 2 days, men can begin showers. Immersion bathing should not occur for at least 7 days after surgery. Men should abstain from sexual activity and ejaculation for 3–4 weeks. Standard narcotic pain medications are prescribed. Semen analyses are obtained postoperatively at 1 month and every 2–3 months afterward until stable sperm concentrations are achieved or the couple achieves a pregnancy. Patency can be delayed 6–12 months or more for some men after EV.

Acknowledgments This research was supported by Male Reproductive Health Research (K12, NIH/NICHD) (J.F.S.). There is no conflict of interest to be declared.

References

1. Martin E, Carnett JB, Levi JV, Pennington ME. The surgical treatment of sterility due to obstruction at the epididymis; together with a study of the morphology of human spermatozoa. Univ Pa Med Bull. 1902;15:2–15.
2. Silber SJ. Microscopic vasoepididymostomy: specific microanastomosis to the epididymal tubule. Fertil Steril. 1978;30:565–71.
3. Kolettis PN. Is physical examination useful in predicting epididymal obstruction? Urology. 2001;57:1138–40.
4. Thomas Jr AJ. Vasoepididymostomy. Urol Clin North Am. 1987;14:527–38.
5. Lipshultz L, Thomas A, Khera M. Surgical management of male infertility. In: Wein A, Kavoussi L, Novick A, Partin A, Peters C, editors. Campbell-Walsh urology. Philadelphia, PA: Saunders Elsevier; 2002. p. 654–705.
6. Schlegel PN, Goldstein M. Surgery of the epididymis. In: Marshall D, Gunter A, editors. Surgical management of urologic disease: an anatomic approach. St. Louis, MO: Mosby Year Book; 1992. p. 949–58.
7. Schlegel PN, Goldstein M. Microsurgical vasoepididymostomy: refinements and results. J Urol. 1993;150:1165–8.
8. Goldstein M. Surgery of male infertility. Philadelphia, PA: W.B. Saunders and Co; 1995. p. 120–7.
9. Fogdestam I, Fall M. Microsurgical end-to-end and end-to-side epididymovasostomy to correct occlusive azoospermia. Scand J Plast Reconstr Surg. 1983;17:137–40.
10. Berger RE. Triangulation end-to-side vasoepididymostomy. J Urol. 1998;159:1951–3.
11. Marmar JL. Modified vasoepididymostomy with simultaneous double needle placement, tubulotomy and tubular invagination. J Urol. 2000;163:483–6.
12. Lespinasse V. Obstructive sterility in the male. Treatment by direct vaso-epididymostomy. JAMA. 1918;70:448–50.
13. Chan PT, Brandell RA, Goldstein M. Prospective analysis of outcomes after microsurgical intussusception vasoepididymostomy. BJU Int. 2005;96:598–601.
14. Schiff J, Chan P, Li PS, Finkelberg S, Goldstein M. Outcome and late failures compared in 4 techniques of microsurgical vasoepididymostomy in 153 consecutive men. J Urol. 2005;174: 651–5 [quiz 801].

Chapter 6
Sperm Retrieval Techniques in Obstructive Azoospermia: MESA, PESA, and TESA

Anand Shridharani and Jay I. Sandlow

Abstract Advances in assisted reproductive technologies (ART), specifically intracytoplasmic sperm injection (ICSI) and sperm retrieval (SR) techniques, allow azoospermic men to father biologic offspring. High success rates have been demonstrated in the cohort of men with obstructive azoospermia. Sperm may be retrieved from the testis or epididymis, for immediate use or cryopreservation in conjunction with ICSI. The choice of SR modality, source of sperm, and the decision to use fresh versus cryopreserved sperm depends largely upon the reproductive surgeon, the reproductive lab personnel, facility in which the sperm is retrieved and patient preferences. Currently there is no expert consensus on which SR modality or sperm source is superior, and it is recommended that decisions be made on a case-by-case basis. The following chapter will review the technical aspects of several SR modalities. In addition, a review of the pros and cons as well as the success rates of each procedure will be discussed.

Keywords Sperm retrieval • Azoospermia • Testicular • Epididymal

A. Shridharani, M.D. (✉) • J.I. Sandlow, M.D.
Department of Urology, Medical College of Wisconsin, 9200 W. Wisconsin Avenue, CLCC Bldg., 4th Floor, Milwaukee, WI 53226, USA
e-mail: ashridha@mcw.edu; jsandlow@mcw.edu

J.I. Sandlow (ed.), *Microsurgery for Fertility Specialists: A Practical Text*,
DOI 10.1007/978-1-4614-4196-0_6, © Springer Science+Business Media New York 2013

Introduction

One of every five couples in the United States will experience difficulty achieving pregnancy. The male factor is involved in approximately 50% of cases [1]. Of these male factor-involvement couples, 5–10% will experience difficulty due to azoospermia, which can be classified as obstructive azoospermia (OA) or non-obstructive azoospermia (NOA) [2]. OA accounts for approximately one-third of azoospermic individuals and may be due to either acquired or congenital etiologies. Acquired OA causes include previous vasectomy, previous inguinal or abdominal surgery, trauma, or infection. Congenital OA causes include cystic fibrosis, congenital absence of the vas deferens (CAVD), prostatic/ejaculatory duct cysts, or syndromes of poor ciliary motility, such as Kartagener's or Young's Syndrome.

In the past, artificial insemination by donor (AID) has been the only option available to these couples with azoospermia. However, due to the advent of intracytoplasmic sperm injection (ICSI), very small numbers of live sperm can be used in conjunction with in vitro fertilization (IVF). This has allowed many men who are azoospermic, either due to obstruction or lack of production, the ability to father a child. For these men, sperm acquisition in conjunction with IVF is a highly successful option [3, 4].

Sperm can be retrieved either from the testis, epididymis or vas deferens. The goal of sperm retrieval is to obtain the maximum amount of viable sperm with minimal damage to the reproductive tract. Multiple techniques of sperm acquisition have been described, each with their own inherent risks and success rates. For OA there is evidence that the sperm source, testicular or epididymal, or retrieval modality does not significantly impact the outcome of IVF [5–8]. Additionally, there is no conclusive evidence on whether fresh versus cryopreserved sperm achieves better fertilization and/or live pregnancies [9, 10]. The decision to use a specific retrieval modality depends largely upon the surgeon retrieving the specimen, the embryologist, and the lab utilized to manipulate and store the specimen. It is strongly recommended that a trained surgeon perform the sperm retrieval given the potential complications requiring management, including but not limited to bleeding and infection [11].

Preoperative Patient Evaluation

Patients are evaluated for the etiology of azoospermia preoperatively. In addition to a thorough history and physical, a semen analysis, post-ejaculate urine, and hormonal studies, including FSH and testosterone are obtained. Genetic testing, including CFTR and poly T analysis, is obtained when appropriate. Once spermatogenesis is confirmed, the patient is counseled regarding treatment options, including ductal bypass (if applicable), sperm acquisition, or donor insemination. Female factors may also be present, and a focused evaluation should be included in the work-up of all men with obstructive azoospermia.

If genetic testing reveals an abnormality, a discussion regarding the possibility of passing the abnormality to their offspring needs to take place. Genetic testing of the partner and genetic specialist counseling should be sought when appropriate.

Patients with CBAVD are tested for mutations associated with cystic fibrosis owing to the high prevalence of CFTR mutations in this population [12]. Again, those that test positive should seek genetic counseling and have their partners undergo testing as well in order to better counsel the couple regarding the chances of having a child with cystic fibrosis.

Techniques

MESA

Microsurgical epididymal sperm aspiration (MESA), first described by Temple-Smith and Silber in the 1980s, involves microsurgical puncture or incision of an epididymal tubule and aspiration of its contents [13, 14]. The procedure is indicated in men who have obstructive azoospermia due to failed vasectomy reversal, bilateral congenital absence of the vas deferens [15], post-infectious obstruction [16], or idiopathic causes. Men who are anejaculatory are functionally obstructed, and may be suitable candidates as well. The procedure is not indicated in men who have non-obstructive causes of azoospermia, such as varicoceles, maturation arrest, or testicular failure. The procedure requires microscopic magnification and a trained microsurgeon experienced in accessing the epididymis for sperm and reconstruction. Epididymal aspiration may be performed in conjunction with a vasoepididymostomy or as a primary retrieval method. In the author's current practice, MESA is rarely performed due to the increased cost and morbidity; however, some practices still find it useful when using a less experienced lab person who requires epididymal sperm for IVF.

Technique

Under adequate anesthesia, the testis is delivered through a midline scrotal incision. The tunica vaginalis is opened sharply and the epididymis is inspected. Alternatively, a small 1–2 cm incision may be used to perform "mini-MESA," in which the epididymis is brought anteriorly [17]. The epididymis is examined using the operating microscope, and dilated epididymal tubules are identified. Typically, the most distal tubules are grossly yellow and dilated, and tend to contain many white cells and degenerating sperm. As one proceeds proximally, the tubules contain clearer

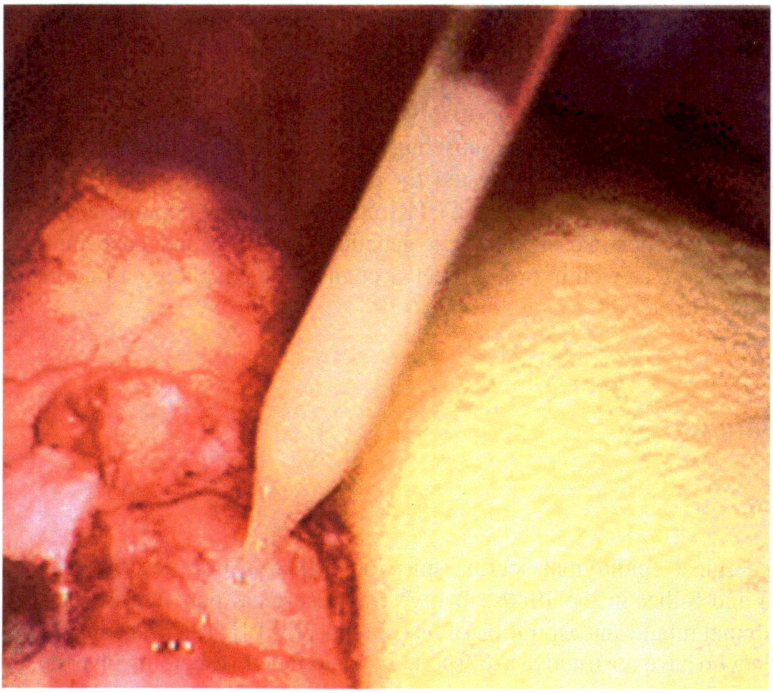

Fig. 6.1 Micropipette aspirating thin, milky fluid containing numerous motile sperm

fluid, and the sperm is found to be motile (Fig. 6.1). Unlike vasoepididymostomy, where only intact sperm need be identified, it is extremely important that motile sperm are present. The tunica of the epididymis is incised to expose the dilated tubule, and a glass micropipette is used to puncture the tubule. We have found that direct micro puncture yields the cleanest specimen, as opposed to opening the tubule and aspirating the fluid. Gentle aspiration from within the tubule is performed until fluid can no longer be obtained. Manual compression of the testis and/or epididymis may enhance fluid retrieval. Retrieval of the fluid without aspiration, by micropipette capillary action, has also been described to prevent tubular mucosal disruption [18]. This is then placed in media, and passed to the IVF lab personnel, where an aliquot is examined for motile sperm. Repeat aspirations are performed until no more fluid can be obtained. In some cases the efferent ductules have been exposed and aspirated, yielding sperm of comparable quality to the epididymis. The procedure may be repeated on the contralateral side to obtain the most sperm possible. The authors close the epididymal tubules with 10-O nylon sutures to minimize scarring in order to facilitate subsequent MESA procedures if necessary. If adequate amounts of motile sperm are not retrieved, a testicular FNA or TESE may be performed under the same anesthetic. Finally, the testis is replaced within the scrotum, which is then closed with absorbable sutures.

Percutaneous Epididymal Sperm Aspiration

This procedure was first described by Craft and Shrivastav, and called for percutaneous aspiration of semen from the epididymis under local anesthesia by skin infiltration and cord block [19, 20]. This procedure can be performed in the office, is less invasive than MESA/TESE and does not require microscopic magnification [21]. There has been concern regarding unreliable sperm acquisition/DNA damage compared to testicular aspiration or microsurgical epididymal aspiration [22]. Nevertheless, if adequate numbers of sperm are not retrieved, a testicular aspiration (TESA) can be performed at the same procedure, or more invasive MESA, or TESE may be performed at a later date after sufficient counseling. PESA is not indicated in patients with NOA.

Technique

The scrotum is cleaned with antiseptic and then thoroughly washed with saline to eliminate any residual antiseptic. Under local anesthesia the head of the epididymis is palpated and stabilized between thumb and forefinger. It is then punctured directly through the scrotal skin, with a 22–26 G needle attached to a tuberculin needle containing 0.1 ml of sperm-washing medium. An air bubble is kept between the medium and the rubber stopper of the plunger to prevent direct contact between the rubber and medium. The assistant pulls the plunger all the way to the top of the syringe thus creating a suction force. The needle is gently and slowly advanced through the epididymal tubule. The needle is rotated 180° and then withdrawn partially, staying within the epididymis. It is then advanced in a different direction, all the while maintaining suction. The suction is partially released and the needle is withdrawn from the epididymis. Sometimes droplets of fluid can be seen entering the syringe, but on other occasions the epididymal aspirate may be so thin and scanty that there is no visible aspirate. Some authors have described using a larger butterfly needle on a 20-ml syringe whereby the aspirated droplets may be visualized easier in the butterfly tubing. One can expect no more than 0.3–1 ml of fluid to be obtained per aspirate [23]. The contents of the syringe are gently flushed into a dish and examined for the presence of sperm. If motile sperm are not seen, the procedure is repeated at a slightly different location moving towards the epididymal head from the tail. Since this is a blind procedure sometimes several attempts are required before good quality sperm are found. Only one paper describes the effect of PESA on subsequent reconstruction. The authors found that it did not disrupt the ability to perform reconstructive surgery [24].

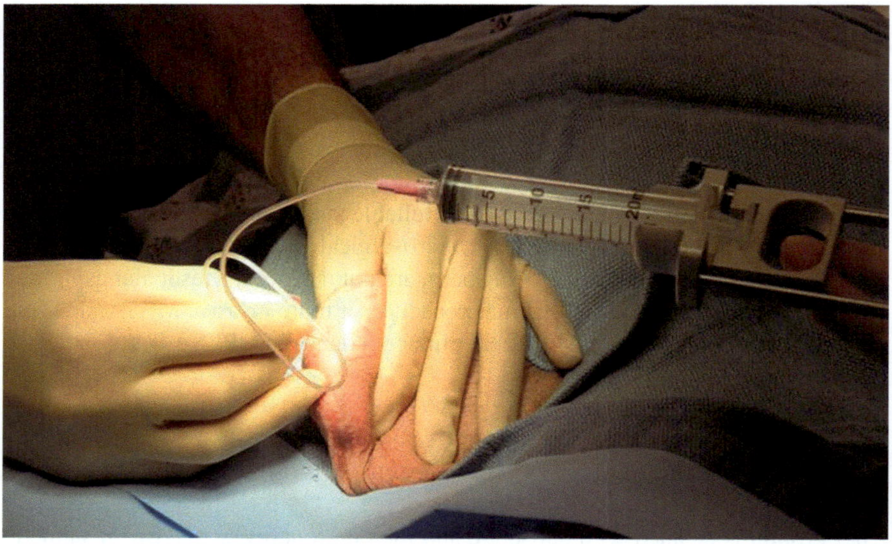

Fig. 6.2 Photo of TESA procedure, with Cameco piston syringe handle creating negative pressure while 19 G butterfly needle is inserted into testis

TESA

Testicular sperm aspiration (TESA) is a minimally invasive method of sperm retrieval. First described by Belker in 1998, it has proven to be a safe and effective means of sperm retrieval and is the first line modality at our institution for patients not undergoing microsurgical reconstruction [25]. Pregnancy rates of up to 62%, and live delivery rates up to 50% have been in reported [26]. Adequate amounts of sperm retrieved, a concern associated with percutaneous retrievals, is optimized by having an embryologist in the vicinity for immediate analysis and assessment of the aspirated tissue for immediate use or cryopreservation. If adequate amounts are not retrieved, more invasive retrieval techniques may be pursued.

Technique

The scrotum is cleaned with antiseptic and then thoroughly washed with saline to eliminate any residual antiseptic. Anxiolytics may be offered to reduce anxiety. Local anesthesia is administered in the form of spermatic cord blockade in addition to the planned testicular aspiration sites at the skin level. After adequate anesthesia is obtained, the testis is fixed with the surgeon's hand, and a 19-G butterfly needle attached to a 20 cm^3 syringe is used to aspirate testicular tissue with the aid of a Cameco piston syringe handle (see Fig. 6.2). Multiple passes are made through the same puncture site and the aspirated tissue and fluid is sent to the reproductive lab for confirmation of mature, viable sperm. Attempts are made to obtain enough tissue for at least three fresh cycles of IVF. The contralateral side may be tried if adequate tissue is not obtained. Once adequate tissue is obtained pressure is applied to the puncture sites until adequate hemostasis is achieved. Sterile dressings, Kerlix fluffs, and an athletic supporter are applied, and the patient is instructed in routine post-procedural care.

The testicular tissue may be cryopreserved. The planned cryopreservation specimens are mixed with an equal volume of test yolk buffer (TYB) and glycerol and incubated at room temperature. The specimens are transferred to cryopreservation vials in aliquots of 1 ml. The filled vials are incubated at 2–6 °C for 60–90 min. After incubation, the vials are suspended in liquid nitrogen vapor for 30 min. Then the vials are submerged in liquid nitrogen for 2 h and a post-thaw analysis was also performed.

TESE

Testicular sperm extraction (TESE) or open biopsy of the testicular tissue may be utilized in cases of obstructive azoospermia; however, its use is more commonplace for the diagnosis and treatment of non-obstructive azoospermia (NOA). Other SR techniques have proven more efficacious and reliable and less invasive with decreased complications and therefore has led to its decreased utilization as a primary SR modality [20]. It is also more costly than the previously mentioned percutaneous forms of sperm retrieval.

Technique

Under adequate anesthesia (local, regional, or general), after sterile preparation of the genitalia, the testis is either delivered through a midline or transverse scrotal incision between the skin lines, if being done in conjunction with surgical exploration. Alternatively, the procedure may also be performed using the “window” technique not requiring delivery of the testis. The tunica vaginalis is opened sharply and the testis is inspected. A transverse incision along the anterior aspect of the testis between the blood vessels is made. Blood vessels may be encountered underneath the tunica are managed with bipolar electrocautery. The tubules are examined and are gently removed with a fine forceps or micro needle holder. Manual compression of the testis aids in extrusion of the testicular tissue. Once adequate tissue is delivered out of the testis it is excised sharply at its base, placed in tubal fluid media and handed off to the laboratory technician. This is repeated until adequate amounts of sperm are harvested. Hemostasis is achieved with bipolar electrocautery. The tunica albuginea is closed with 5-0 absorbable sutures. The tunica vaginalis and subsequently skin are closed with fine absorbable suture.

Postoperative Care

Postoperative care recommendations are relatively common between SR techniques; however, may differ between practitioners. All retrieval techniques are performed on an outpatient basis, either in a hospital, ambulatory surgical care center or office setting. Patients often resume their normal activities on the following day after percutaneous retrievals, and after 2–3 days following open surgical retrievals. A scrotal support should be worn for several days following the procedure to prevent scrotal edema and pain. No strenuous activity is recommended for 3–5 days. Patients should refrain from sexual activity for the same interval. All patients are discharged with prn oral narcotics and scheduled a scheduled anti-inflammatory medication unless contraindicated.

Summary table for sperm retrieval techniques

Sperm retrieval techniques for obstructive azoospermia		
	Pros	Cons
MESA	Higher likelihood to obtain ample sperm in one procedure compared to percutaneous SR	Higher cost associated with OR time/anesthetic
	May perform reconstruction under same anesthetic	Requires microscope
	Decreased risk of hematoma	More invasive/recovery
PESA	Fast, may be performed in clinic	May not retrieve adequate amounts of sperm
	Microscope not required	Hematoma formation
	Minimal recovery	May obstruct epididymis at puncture site
TESA	Fast, may be performed in clinic	May not retrieve adequate amounts of sperm
	Microscope not required	Hematoma/hematocele formation
	Minimal recovery	Risk of testicular atrophy
	Repeatable	
TESE	Fast, and repeatable	Requires exploration
	Microscope not required	More invasive/recovery
		Testicular atrophy

Complications

Complications that may occur at varying degrees, depending on SR technique, include persistent pain, infection, hydrocele, bleeding/hematoma, epididymal obstruction, testicular fibrosis, and testicular atrophy. Contemporary series utilizing MESA, PESA, and TESA report very minor complications if at all [17, 26, 27]. Minor complications such as these are typical of all sperm retrieval techniques. Nevertheless, sperm retrieval from the proximal epididymis may lead to fibrosis and obstruction complicating or precluding later microsurgical reconstruction. Testicular atrophy and fibrosis increase as the amount of percutaneous or open testicular retrieval attempts increase [28]. The use of operative magnification will aid in avoiding vascular injuries.

SR Outcomes for OA

The success rates for surgical retrieval of sperm in patients with OA are generally good and ranges from 90 to 100% [29]. However, when comparing SR techniques to one another, each has its own inherent advantages and disadvantages. A recent Cochrane meta-analysis of various techniques found "insufficient evidence to recommend any specific sperm retrieval technique" [8]. The choice of SR technique ultimately depends on the experience and preferences of the surgeon, and within the constraints of the facility in which the procedure is performed. The safest and most effective technique specific to the practitioner and specific lab utilizing the sperm should be performed.

References

1. Jarow JP, Espeland MA, Lipshultz LI. Evaluation of the azoospermic patient. J Urol. 1989;142:62–5.
2. Irvine DS. Epidemiology and aetiology of male infertility. Hum Reprod. 1998;13 Suppl 1:33–44.
3. Silber SJ, Nagy Z, Van Steirteghem A, et al. Andrology: conventional in-vitro fertilization versus intracytoplasmic sperm injection for patients requiring microsurgical sperm aspiration. Hum Reprod. 1994;9:1705.
4. Schlegel PN, Palermo GD, Rosewaks Z, et al. Micropuncture retrieval of epididymal sperm with in vitro fertilization: importance of in vitro micromanipulation techniques. Urology. 1995;241:238–41.
5. Kamal A, Fahmy I, Mansour R, et al. Does the outcome of ICSI in cases of obstructive azoospermia depend on the origin of the retrieved spermatozoa or the cause of obstruction? A comparative analysis. Fertil Steril. 2010;94:2135–40.
6. Nicopoullos JDM, Gilling Smith C, Ramsay JW, et al. The results of 154 ICSI cycles using surgically retrieved sperm from azoospermic men. Hum Reprod. 2004;19:579–85.
7. Schwarzer JU, Fiedler K, Lochner-Ernst D, et al. Sperm retrieval procedures and intracytoplasmatic spermatozoa injection with epididymal and testicular sperms. Urol Int. 2003;70: 119–23.
8. Proctor M, Johnson N, Phillipson G, et al. Techniques for surgical retrieval of sperm prior to intra-cytoplasmic sperm injection (ICSI) for azoospermia. Cochrane Database Syst Rev. 2008;2:CD002807.
9. Janzen N, Goldstein M, Schlegel PN, et al. Use of electively cryopreserved microsurgically aspirated epididymal sperm with IVF and intracytoplasmic sperm injection for obstructive azoospermia. Fertil Steril. 2000;74:696–701.
10. Nagy Z, Liu J, Van Steirteghem A, et al. Using ejaculated, fresh, and frozen-thawed epididymal and testicular spermatozoa gives rise to comparable results after intracytoplasmic sperm injection. Fertil Steril. 1995;63:808–15.
11. AUA Staff. The management of obstructive azoospermia: AUA best practice statement; 2010.
12. Yu J, Chen Z, Li Z, et al. CFTR mutations in men with congenital bilateral absence of the vas deferens (CBAVD): a systemic review and meta-analysis. Hum Reprod. 2012;27:25–35.
13. Silber SJ, Balmaceda J, Borrero C, et al. Pregnancy with sperm aspiration from the proximal head of the epididymis: a new treatment for congenital absence of the vas deferens. Fertil Steril. 1998;50:525–8.
14. Temple-Smith PD, Southwick GJ, de Kretser DM, et al. Human pregnancy by in vitro fertilization (IVF) using sperm aspirated from the epididymis. J Assist Reprod Gen. 1985;3:119–22.

15. Tournaye H, Devroey P, Van Steirteghem A, et al. Microsurgical epididymal sperm aspiration and intracytoplasmic sperm injection: a new effective approach to infertility as a result of congenital bilateral absence of the vas deferens. Fertil Steril. 1994;61:1045.
16. Tournaye H, Clasen K, Devroey P, et al. Fine needle aspiration versus open biopsy for testicular sperm recovery: a controlled study in azoospermic patients with normal spermatogenesis. Hum Reprod. 1998;13:901.
17. Nudell DM, Conaghan J, Turek PJ, et al. The mini-micro-epididymal sperm aspiration for sperm retrieval: a study of urological outcomes. Hum Reprod. 1998;13:1260.
18. Goldstein M. Surgical management of the infertile male. In: Campbell-Walsh urology. 10th ed.; 2012 pp 675–6.
19. Shrivastav P, Nadkarni P, Craft I, et al. Andrology: percutaneous epididymal sperm aspiration for obstructive azoospermia. Hum Reprod. 1994;9:2058.
20. Craft I, Tsirigotis M, Nicholson N, et al. Percutaneous epididymal sperm aspiration and intracytoplasmic sperm injection in the management of infertility due to obstructive azoospermia. Fertil Steril. 1995;63:1038–42.
21. Sheynkin YR, Ye Z, Schlegel PN, et al. Controlled comparison of percutaneous and microsurgical sperm retrieval in men with obstructive azoospermia. Hum Reprod. 1998;13:3086–9.
22. O'Connell M, McClure N, Lewis SEM. Mitochondrial DNA deletions and nuclear DNA fragmentation in testicular and epididymal human sperm. Hum Reprod. 2002;17:1565.
23. Esteves SC, Miyaoka R, Agarwal A. Sperm retrieval techniques for assisted reproduction. Int Braz J Urol. 2011;37:570–83.
24. Marmar JL, Sharlip I, Goldstein M. Results of vasovasostomy or vasoepididymostomy after failed percutaneous epididymal sperm aspirations. J Urol. 2008;179:1506–9.
25. Belker AM, Sherins RJ, Schulman JD, et al. Percutaneous testicular sperm aspiration: a convenient and effective office procedure to retrieve sperm for in vitro fertilization with intracytoplasmic sperm injection. J Urol. 1998;160:2058–62.
26. Garg T, Strawn E, Sandlow JI, et al. Outcomes after testicular aspiration and testicular tissue cryopreservation for obstructive azoospermia and ejaculatory dysfunction. J Urol. 2008;180:2577–80.
27. Wood S, Thomas K, Lewis-Jones I, et al. Postoperative pain, complications, and satisfaction rates in patients who undergo surgical sperm retrieval. Fertil Steril. 2003;79:56–62.
28. Schlegel PN, Su LM. Physiological consequences of testicular sperm extraction. Hum Reprod. 1997;12:1688–92.
29. Nicopoullos JDM, Gilling Smith C, Ramsay JWA, et al. Use of surgical sperm retrieval in azoospermic men: a meta-analysis. Fertil Steril. 2004;82:691–701.

Chapter 7
Microsurgical Testicular Sperm Extraction: Technical Considerations

Peter N. Schlegel

Abstract Treatment of nonobstructive azoospermia (NOA) has changed radically over the past 15 years, evolving from a clinical diagnosis with no direct treatment options to a highly treatable entity. The condition of NOA is typically characterized by a man who has small volume testes and elevated FSH. Therefore, the condition is often diagnosed clinically without extensive laboratory evaluation or invasive tests. Up to 1% of all men may have this condition, but it has represented a substantial therapeutic challenge for urologists. Up until recently, the only therapies that would allow a man with NOA to father a child was to provide donor insemination or adoption. Obviously, these "replacement" therapies do not directly treat the condition. Several steps allowed us the opportunity to consider treatment of men with NOA, so these men could have their own biological children. In the early mid-1990s, recognition of the potential presence of sperm in some of these men occurred (Jow et al., J Androl 14(3):194–8, 1993). Subsequent refinements in our ability to use these sperm for assisted reproduction were advanced in the late 1990s to optimize treatment for men with NOA. In this chapter, we will overview the development of a technique referred to as microdissection TESE (testicular sperm extraction) (Schlegel, Hum Reprod 14(1):131–5, 1999). This surgical technique appears to optimize the ability of treating physicians to localize small regions of sperm production within the testis. Micro-TESE's utility, in comparison to other techniques of sperm retrieval, safety, and efficacy will be discussed.

Keywords Testicular failure • Azoospermia • Microsurgery • Nonobstructive • TESE

P.N. Schlegel, M.D. (✉)
Department of Urology, Weill Cornell Medical College, 525 East 68th St., New York, NY 10021, USA

New York Presbyterian Hospital, Weill Cornell Medical Center, 525 East 68th St., New York, NY 10021, USA
e-mail: pnschleg@med.cornell.edu

J.I. Sandlow (ed.), *Microsurgery for Fertility Specialists: A Practical Text*, DOI 10.1007/978-1-4614-4196-0_7, © Springer Science+Business Media New York 2013

Introduction

Treatment of nonobstructive azoospermia (NOA) has changed radically over the past 15 years, evolving from a clinical diagnosis with no direct treatment options to a highly treatable entity. The condition of NOA is typically characterized by a man who has small volume testes and elevated FSH. Therefore, the condition is often diagnosed clinically without extensive laboratory evaluation or invasive tests. Up to 1% of all men may have this condition, but it has represented a substantial therapeutic challenge for urologists. Up until recently, the only therapies that would allow a man with NOA to father a child was to provide donor insemination or adoption. Obviously, these "replacement" therapies do not directly treat the condition. Several steps allowed us the opportunity to consider treatment of men with NOA, so these men could have their own biological children. In the early mid-1990s, recognition of the potential presence of sperm in some of these men occurred [1]. Subsequent refinements in our ability to use these sperm for assisted reproduction were advanced in the late 1990s to optimize treatment for men with NOA. In this chapter, we will overview the development of a technique referred to as microdissection TESE (testicular sperm extraction) [2]. This surgical technique appears to optimize the ability of treating physicians to localize small regions of sperm production within the testis. Micro-TESE's utility, in comparison to other techniques of sperm retrieval, safety, and efficacy will be discussed.

Men with NOA have severely deficient spermatogenesis, with inadequate sperm production within the testis for sperm to reach the ejaculate. Despite this defective sperm production, recent studies have suggested that at least 60% of men with NOA will actually have sperm production within the testes [2]. Histological evaluation of the testes of men with NOA is always abnormal and demonstrates Sertoli cell-only pattern within the seminiferous tubules, maturation arrest, or hypospermatogenesis. Commonly, a combination of different patterns of spermatogenesis is seen within the seminiferous tubules. Since a diagnostic biopsy samples very little (typically less than 5% of seminiferous tubules) within the testis, the ability of a diagnostic biopsy to identify limited, small sites of sperm production is very poor. Even if the most advanced pattern of spermatogenesis is used as a predictive factor (rather than the overall pattern of spermatogenesis), then the prediction of sperm retrieval with micro-TESE is very limited. Not surprisingly, the correlation between findings on diagnostic biopsy and sperm retrieval is unreliable. In an early study by Tournaye et al., sperm retrieval rates in men who had a predominant pattern of Sertoli cell-only was 50%, with maturation arrest and hypospermatogenesis on diagnostic biopsy having little effect on the chance of subsequent sperm retrieval [3].

One of the most misunderstood paradigms of NOA is that testicular histology is uniform. Fortunately, testicular histology is not typically uniform, especially for men who have impaired spermatogenesis. Even men with normal spermatogenesis will often have small areas of the testicle that show Sertoli cell-only or sclerosis. Similarly, men with NOA will commonly have small areas with spermatogenesis, so one area of the testis may have predominantly Sertoli cell-only whereas another region of the testis may have rare sperm being produced. This heterogeneity helps to explain why diagnostic testis biopsies are poorly predictive of sperm retrieval. It also helps to explain why men with NOA may have no sperm in the ejaculate but substantive sperm production within the testicle. An understanding of the heterogeneity of the testis (structurally and functionally) is critical to recognition of how NOA can be treated.

Preoperative Preparation

Genetic testing to identify the cause of low sperm production may provide important prognostic and diagnostic information for men with NOA. Y chromosome microdeletion testing and karyotype analysis will typically identify the cause of low sperm production in 15–20% of men with NOA. Favorable prognostic information is provided for men with Klinefelter syndrome (47, XXY) or AZFc deletions (70%), whereas a very poor prognosis (near 0) exists for men with complete deletions of AZFa or AZFb (or AZFb+c). Karyotypic abnormalities are an indication to consider embryo biopsy to detect known genetic anomalies that may be transmitted to the fetus.

Men with NOA may have very limited pockets of sperm production. This limited production should be optimized before undergoing an invasive procedure. If sperm production is marginal to begin with and impaired by other/external conditions, then it is possible that sperm may not be found despite application of effective surgical techniques. Several interventions may enhance sperm production in these men. Since sperm production takes 3 months and it can be adversely affected by inflammation or hematoma formation after prior surgery, at least 6 months should be allowed to pass after a prior biopsy or other scrotal surgical procedure before proceeding with attempted TESE [4].

In the presence of a varicocele, men with NOA may be considered for varicocelectomy to optimize sperm production prior to testicular sperm extraction. The benefit of optimizing sperm production or allowing sperm to return to the ejaculate is attractive. Unfortunately, benefits from varicocelectomy may take 6 months or longer to be realized. In a series of men with well-documented azoospermia and varicoceles treated at Cornell, <10% of men had adequate sperm return to the ejaculate after varicocelectomy to avoid TESE [5]. Furthermore, performance of varicocelectomy prior to TESE did not appear to affect sperm retrieval rates for men with clinical varicoceles, based on retrospective review of treated patients. Therefore, I usually restrict varicocele repair to men who have had documented sperm in the ejaculate or who have a number of years to benefit from sperm in the ejaculate, if they have a beneficial result (i.e., female partner less than 30–32 years old).

Many men with NOA have compromised serum testosterone levels and could have low intratesticular testosterone. These patients will typically have relatively increased estrogen levels in association with low testosterone, suggesting that increased aromatase activity from the testis is responsible for the low circulating (serum) testosterone levels [6]. Enhancement of intratesticular (endogenous) testosterone levels could result from treatment of men with low serum testosterone levels and elevated testosterone/estradiol ratios with an aromatase inhibitor such as anastrazole (Arimidex). This off-label use of anastrazole reliably increases circulating testosterone and decreases estradiol with an associated increase in sperm production for affected men with oligospermia [7]. We usually treat men with low serum testosterone and relatively elevated estradiol (e.g., T <300 mg/dL and estradiol >30 pg/mL) with 1 mg p.o. per day of anastrazole, obtaining a repeat testosterone and estradiol in 1 month to evaluate success of treatment. It is not expected that testosterone levels will increase enough to allow sperm to return to the ejaculate, but it could optimize intratesticular T levels and spermatogenesis.

Treatment Approach and IVF/ICSI

If spermatozoa are present within the testes of men with NOA, then the sperm have limited viability. Indeed, these sperm are incapable of surviving epididymal transit, as they are not detectable within the ejaculate. Therefore, the ability of sperm to survive other insults such as cryopreservation may be limited. We have found that only 33% of testicular samples from men with NOA will reliably survive freeze–thaw and have documentable viability, that is considered a requirement for optimal ICSI results [8]. For this reason, we perform sperm extraction procedures during a programmed IVF cycles, to allow sperm to be used fresh after sperm extraction. For cases where no sperm are found and the couple has not elected to have donor sperm available for use, the remaining segment of the IVF cycle is cancelled.

Sperm retrieval is usually timed to occur on the day before oocyte retrieval. In cases where sperm retrieval cannot logistically occur before oocyte retrieval, or if ovarian stimulation has not reliably allowed good follicular development, or if rare sperm have previously been seen in the ejaculate, then sperm retrieval is done on the same day as oocyte retrieval during the IVF cycle. There appears to be no difference in pregnancy rates whether sperm are retrieved on the day before or the same day as oocyte retrieval. Testicular sperm (from men with NOA) often acquire at least twitching motility after they are retrieved and incubated overnight.

Surgical Approaches

Approaches for sperm retrieval have included fine needle aspiration, percutaneous testis biopsy, open testicular biopsy, multiple testicular biopsy (testicular sperm extraction) and microdissection TESE. Fine needle aspiration has the advantage of being a minimally invasive procedure. However, the adverse consequences of fine needle aspiration on testicular function may be greater than that seen after simple biopsies. In a systematic review of the literature on surgical sperm retrieval for NOA, Tournaye et al. described surgical sperm retrieval as the most effective approach for sperm retrieval in NOA, at least for patients who have predominant Sertoli cell-only pattern [9]. They also reported that microdissection had the lowest rate of complications with fine needle aspiration next in risk of intratesticular complications, and multiple biopsies as the highest risk procedure. The FNA approach had a lower chance of sperm retrieval than multiple biopsy. Overall, microdissection TESE carried the highest chance of sperm retrieval with the lowest risk of complications.

Fine needle aspiration of the testis involves making multiple blind entries into the testicular parenchyma with a 19–22 gauge needle that is passed in and out through testicular parenchyma with strong negative force applied by syringe attached to the needle. Small sections of seminiferous tubules are thereby aspirated into the needle that is discharged into sperm medium. The presence of spermatozoa can be analyzed for each aspiration site. In a modification of this technique, Dr. Paul Turek has described FNA mapping, a technique to identify the site of sperm production within the testis to guide future biopsies [10]. Significant cytologic experience is required to analyze these testicular specimens, and the results of FNA are used to guide subsequent sperm retrieval attempts. An open biopsy is subsequently used for sperm retrieval. Although they report a high success rate of FNA mapping, the only patients who undergo sperm retrieval procedures are those that are demonstrated to have sperm production by FNA to begin with.

In an early study that documented the heterogeneity of sperm production, Jow et al. identified sperm within the testes of approximately one-third of men with NOA [1]. This was based on a single biopsy, done for diagnostic purposes. Substantial confusion has developed between the techniques for sperm retrieval and sperm retrieval rates. Subsequent techniques of multiple biopsy testicular sperm extraction have shown up to 50% sperm retrieval rates in a variety of different clinical series. Unfortunately, the testicular blood supply runs immediately underneath the surface of the tunica albuginea so multiple biopsies carries a risk of damage to the testicular blood supply which, in case reports, has led to complete testicular devascularization and testicular loss. A technique of identification of the subtunical blood vessels was described by Goldstein [11]. This approach helps to minimize the risk of damage to the testicular blood supply. A lower complication rate was reported in diagnostic testis biopsies done with this approach. The use of an operating microscope can also be applied during testicular exploration to identify sites within the testis that have sperm production. This approach is referred to as testicular microdissection [2]. In brief, the testis is opened widely in an equatorial plane along the midportion of the testis. This allows wide exposure of seminiferous tubules in a physiological approach that follows the blood supply of the testis and preserves intratesticular blood flow (see Fig. 7.1). The use of the operating microscope at 15–20× power allows identification the seminiferous tubules that are most likely to contain sperm. If sperm production is present within a seminiferous tubule then it contains more cells than seminiferous tubules without sperm. Seminiferous tubules with complete spermatogenesis are therefore larger and more opaque than tubules without spermatogenesis. Microdissection TESE allows identification of the seminiferous tubules that contain sperm, improving the yield of sperm retrieval and limiting the amount of testicular tissue that needs to be removed.

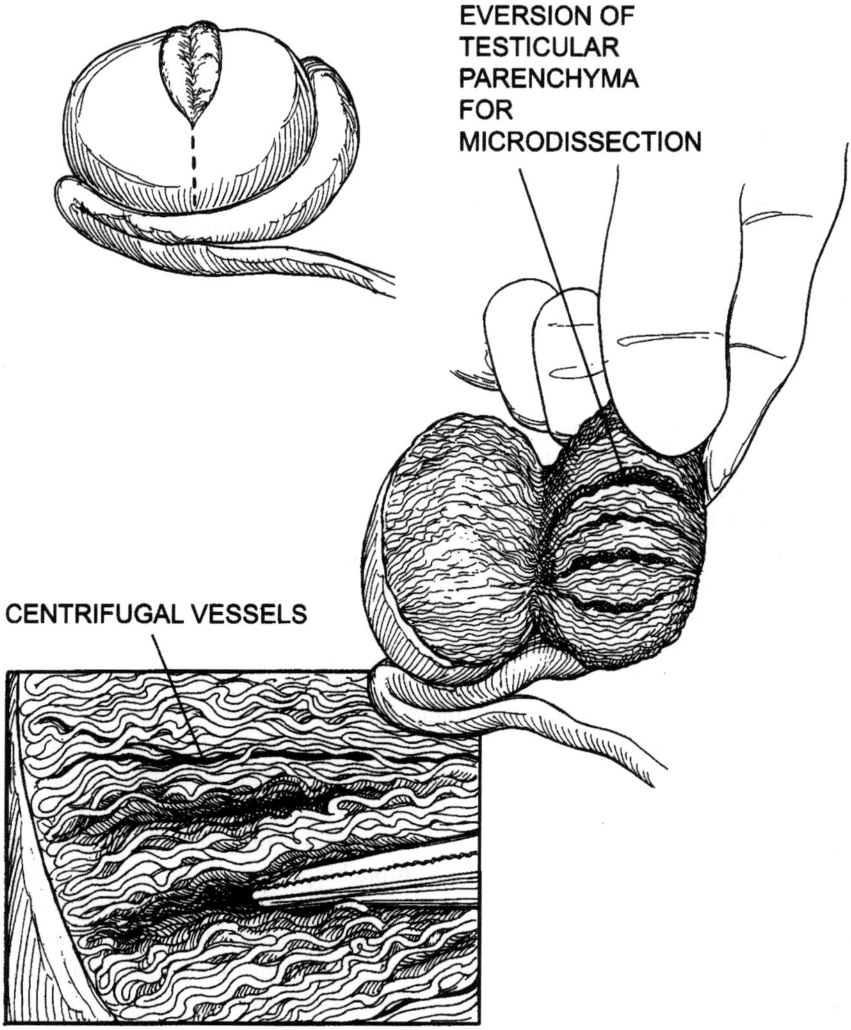

Fig. 7.1 Schematic illustration of testicular microdissection technique, demonstrating initial incision with wide exposure of seminiferous tubules, digital pressure exerted on the tunica albuginea to evert tissue, allowing the ability to dissect deep within testicular parenchyma

Microdissection TESE

In order for all areas of potential sperm production to be identified, microdissection must allow examination of all seminiferous tubules within the testis. Seminiferous tubules are highly convoluted and exist within very fine septae, with centrifugal vessels running in parallel to the tubules and septae (Fig. 7.1.) Dissection between the tubules allows access to deeper sections of the seminiferous tubules, down to the level of the tunica albuginea. It is critical to maintain blood supply along the tubules during the dissection and to avoid separation of tubules from the tunica albuginea. The space between the tubules and tunica has an extensive array of subtunical vessels that are prone to excessive bleeding and very difficult to control if this space is entered during microdissection. The higher the power of magnification used during microdissection, the easier it is to determine which of the tubules is larger/more normal. The sperm retrieval procedure can be tedious, especially in larger testes, and may take several hours to adequately and safely examine all areas of the testis, even for microsurgeons experienced in this technique.

Critical Points of Surgical Technique

- Wide incision along an equatorial plane allows complete exposure of seminiferous tubules.
- Exposure of the initially exposed tubules is inadequate to find many sites of sperm production.
- Dissection parallel to the centrifugal vessels allows dissection deep within testicular parenchyma.
- Gentle pressure across the tubules being dissected is important to allow blunt separation of tissue.
- Pressure under the tunica albuginea to evert the testicular tissue for microdissection.
- A vertical incision in the tunica albuginea is an alternative, but carries a greater risk of injury to testicular vessels and does not allow organized dissection of seminiferous tubules.

The original description of microdissection TESE was published in 1999. In the study, Schlegel reported that historical rate of sperm retrieval using multibiopsy TESE was 45%. Sperm retrieval increased to 63% with application of micro-TESE. In a controlled study, where testicular sperm extraction was performed on one side with TESE on the other, sperm retrieval using TESE with multiple biopsies alone would miss sperm in nearly a third of the men who could have sperm found by micro-TESE. Another study by Amer et al. in 2000 documented higher sperm retrieval rates with micro-TESE (47%) compared to standard, multibiopsy TESE (30%). In addition, the rate of acute and chronic complications including testicular atrophy and devascularization was markedly lower for patients who had micro-TESE [12]. A further study by Okada et al. documented improved sperm retrieval rates using microdissection TESE compared to standard TESE, with differences most pronounced in those patients who had predominant Sertoli cell-only pattern (where the difference in size of seminiferous tubules is more dramatic.). In an update of results of this technique, with experience in 460 patients who underwent microdissection for NOA, sperm retrieval was accomplished with micro-TESE in 62% of cases whereas the sperm retrieval rate with standard multibiopsy TESE was only 32% [13]. The safety of micro-TESE was also demonstrated in a retrospective review by Ramasamy et al. from Cornell. In this study, effects of testicular sperm extraction using a multibiopsy technique or microdissection were compared by following patients with serial scrotal ultrasound as well as serial testosterone levels after TESE. Patients had earlier and more complete recovery of testosterone production after microdissection TESE, with return of serum testosterone to 95% of baseline after 18 months, whereas patients after standard TESE had recovery only to 85% of baseline levels. Similarly, acute and chronic changes as detected on scrotal ultrasound were less common in patients who had microdissection TESE. The lower complication rate after microdissection TESE is likely related to the ease and complete achievement of hemostasis during this procedure.

Sperm Processing

If sperm production is present within testicular parenchyma for men with NOA, then the sperm are within the seminiferous tubules. The efficiency of finding sperm is enhanced by aggressively mincing the testicular tissue to allow sperm to be released from the tubules and identified. The amount of tissue that is removed during microdissection TESE is typically much less obtained from multibiopsy TESE procedures (50-fold less tissue excised). To assure that the testicular tissue suspension has been adequately disrupted and sperm can be most easily identified on wet-prep in the operating room, the testicular suspension is passed sequentially through a 24-guage angiocatheter to confirm adequate suspension. This approach can increase sperm yield up to 300-fold [14]. Each specimen with enlarged seminiferous tubules should be sequentially examined for the presence of sperm in the operating room, since the procedure can be terminated once sperm are found. Since sperm do not survive freeze–thaw very efficiently, intentional removal of additional testicular tissue may waste the sperm production that is present and create additional scar tissue within the testis, potentially compromising future attempts at fertility treatment.

Overall Results with micro-TESE at Cornell

Encouraging experience has been obtained at Weill Cornell with TESE-ICSI in the past 1,357 attempted treatment cycles for couples in whom the man had NOA. The mean age of patients entering treatment was 36.1 years for men and 31.8 years for women. In men, the initial mean serum FSH level was 21.6 IU/L (normal 1–8 IU/L), and average testis volume 9.6 cm^3. During the past 1,357 attempted TESE-ICSI cycles, sperm were retrieved for injection in 763 cycles (56.1% retrieval rate). For those cycles in which sperm were retrieved, the fertilization rate per injected oocyte was 51.1% (4,272/8,365), and embryo transfer occurred in 92% of cycles. Clinical pregnancies (fetal heartbeat on ultrasound) were established in 49.1% (375/763) of evaluable cycles and live deliveries occurred in 40% of cycles with retrieved sperm for which sufficient time had passed for completed gestation. Over 320 children have been born from our center. Twin deliveries occurred in 11% of cases, triplets in <1%, and singleton deliveries for the remainder.

No etiology of azoospermia provided an absolute predictor for the presence or absence of sperm within the testes, except for complete deletions of the AZFa and AZFb regions of the Y chromosome, that was associated with a 0% retrieval rate.

Micro-TESE After Failed Standard TESE

The superiority of microdissection TESE as an approach for sperm retrieval in NOA is also suggested by a recent publication by Ramasamy et al. where patients who had previous failed biopsy or TESE procedures subsequently underwent microdissection TESE [15]. In this report, patients who had no prior biopsy had a 52% rate of sperm retrieval with micro-TESE. Patients who had one or two biopsies per testis for an attempt at testicular sperm extraction had a sperm retrieval rate of 50% as well. If three or four or more biopsies per testis were done in an attempt to extract sperm, the subsequent sperm retrieval rate with microdissection TESE was 22%. These data strongly suggest that blind, random biopsies of the testis will commonly miss areas of sperm production. Indeed, one or two biopsies per testis provide inadequate evaluation of testicular parenchyma and provides information that is little better than proceeding with micro-TESE with no prior biopsies whatsoever. Even if TESE is done with three or more biopsies per testis, the chance of sperm identification using the micro-TESE approach was still 22%. So, failure of sperm retrieval with standard TESE still leaves open the opportunity of sperm retrieval with micro-TESE.

Predictors of micro-TESE Success

FSH

In another study performed at Cornell, the relationship between serum FSH and sperm retrieval results were analyzed for men who underwent microdissection TESE. Patients who had serum FSH of 15–30, 30–45, or greater than 45 all had similar sperm retrieval results (average of 63%). Even men with FSH levels over 90 IU/L can have sperm retrieved with micro-TESE. These observations suggest that small areas of spermatogenesis, inadequate to affect serum FSH (or testicular volume) may be present and will commonly be found using microdissection TESE [16]. Indeed, the only patients with NOA who had a different rate of sperm retrieval was for men with an FSH <15, where sperm retrieval rate is 51%. This subgroup of patients has an increased risk of uniform maturation arrest, where genetic abnormalities are common and the chance of sperm retrieval is adversely affected [17]. Previous studies have suggested that serum FSH is a good predictor of the chance of sperm retrieval. These studies were done predominantly with single or multiple random biopsies of the testis for sperm retrieval. These observations suggest that random biopsies of the testis may identify the predominant pattern of sperm production but do not necessarily identify the best area of sperm production within the testis. The observation from this retrospective review that microdissection TESE is superior in finding sperm for men with the most severe defects in sperm production further supports micro-TESE as the optimal approach for sperm retrieval in men with NOA.

Klinefelter Syndrome

One paradigm for the most severe cases of NOA is those men with Klinefelter syndrome. These patients typically have a testicular volume of 2.5 cm^3's with markedly elevated FSH. In an initial report, the chance of sperm retrieval for men with Klinefelter syndrome who underwent microdissection TESE was 71%. These excellent results were obtained despite the very small testicular volume present in these patients, likely because the micro-TESE technique is effective at finding small, limited areas of sperm production within the testis.

We update here the results of treatment for 68 men with classic, nonmosaic Klinefelter syndrome (47, XXY, or mosaic patterns that do not include 46, XY) who underwent attempted sperm retrieval during simultaneous 88 ICSI cycles at our institution. An additional three IVF cycles were done in which cryopreserved sperm from previous TESE procedures were used. Sperm were found in 68% (62/91) of the fresh retrieval attempts. Of the cycles in which sperm were retrieved by TESE, the fertilization rate per injected oocyte was 55%, embryo transfer occurred in 51/62 (83%) cases, and clinical pregnancy was achieved in 53% (33/62), with 44 children born to date. All children have been healthy (all 46, XX girls and 46, XY boys). Pretreatment testicular biopsy histology was not helpful in distinguishing who would succeed with microdissection TESE for patients with Klinefelter syndrome. Although a majority of men had Sertoli cell-only on diagnostic biopsy, 70% of these patients had sperm found on subsequent microdissection TESE. Even though two of the patients treated had previously undergone multiple random biopsy TESE with no sperm found, sperm were retrieved in a subsequent procedure using the microdissection TESE technique. These findings illustrate the potential for TESE-ICSI to provide fertility despite underlying genetic abnormalities [18].

History of Cryptorchidism

Men with a history of prior cryptorchidism, corrected by orchiopexy, account for up to 7–10% of all men with NOA. These men may have had surgery for correction of the position of the testes after the age currently recommended for such intervention (before age 1). In some cases, the testes were inguinal or intraabdominal until adulthood. Anecdotal observations at Cornell demonstrate that neovascularity of the testes is common, with positional abnormalities such as an anterior epididymis in many cases. These observations make surgical exploration difficult, although it may reflect the underlying difference that made these men azoospermic. Since most men with a history of cryptorchidism are fertile, for a man to be azoospermic after orchiopexy, something must be different for these individuals. We suspect that the abnormality is vascular compromise, perhaps by using a suture at the inferior pole of the testis—limiting arterial inflow where the artery exists under the tunica albuginea.

Fortunately, the sperm retrieval rate is favorable for azoospermic men with a history of cryptorchidism, 74% overall. Men who underwent orchiopexy before age 10, but were azoospermic, had better sperm retrieval rates than men who underwent the procedure later in life. However, sperm retrieval has been successful in several adult males who had testes that were inguinal, even after attempted orchiopexy. We have not yet retrieved sperm from intraabdominal testes, so attempts at orchiopexy may be reasonable for these adolescents or young adults prior to attempts at sperm retrieval [19].

History of Prior Chemotherapy

Another treated subset of men with NOA includes the cohort of 73 men with a history of chemotherapy administered for a variety of diagnoses who underwent 84 sperm retrieval attempts with TESE for persistent NOA. All men were azoospermic and at least 6 years post-chemotherapy at the time of treatment. The mean interval from chemotherapy to TESE was 19.0 years. Sperm were successfully retrieved in 43% (36/84) of attempts, with clinical pregnancy occurring in 50% (14/42) couples. Men treated for lymphoma had a sperm retrieval rate per attempt of 33% (14/42), whereas after treatment for germ cell tumor, the retrieval rate was 85%. Diagnostic biopsy was not helpful in determining the prognosis for sperm retrieval. Most patients had predominantly Sertoli cell-only pattern, even if germ cells were present in some seminiferous tubules. Males previously treated with alkylating agents had a lower chance of sperm retrieval (21%) relative to patients treated with other agents [20].

Y Chromosome Microdeletions

Genetic testing for Y chromosome microdeletions is of prognostic significance for TESE procedures. For men with complete deletions of the AZFb region the chance of sperm retrieval during TESE is severely impaired. In our experience, 0 of 23 men with Y chromosome partial deletions involving all of AZFb had sperm retrieved with TESE, whereas the sperm retrieval rate in a contemporary series of men with NOA but no AZFb deletions was 67% (85/126). The presence of a complete deletion of AZFa appears consistently associated with Sertoli cell-only and a poor chance of sperm retrieval. Of the men with complete deletions of the AZFa region, who had diagnostic biopsies or TESE at our institution, zero out of ten had sperm found. Therefore, for men with complete AZFa or AZFb deletions, we do not recommend proceeding with TESE [21].

Pregnancy rates for ICSI using sperm from men with Y microdeletions appear to be very similar to those obtained for couples with similar sperm production. For men with AZFc deletions alone (the only Y-deleted patients who have had sperm in our experience), most (75%) men will have at least rare sperm in the ejaculate. For those men who are AZFc-deleted and azoospermic, most (50–75%) will have sperm found with biopsy or micro-TESE [20]. We reported a series of 27 IVF cycles involving men with AZFc microdeletions who were azoospermic (12 cycles) or severely oligospermic (15 cycles.) The clinical pregnancy rates per cycle were comparable to that obtained for nonaffected men from azoospermic (TESE cycles) and oligospermic men (ejaculated sperm). All children born were phenotypically normal, but we expect all boys to have deletions involving the AZFc region, with resulting impairments in spermatogenesis [22].

Summary

Sperm retrieval from the testis is possible in a majority of men with NOA. Despite severely abnormal testicular function, limited regions of sperm production can be found in these men. The technique of microdissection TESE is an effective approach to treatment of these patients. The procedure may be somewhat tedious, but it allows successful treatment of men despite markedly elevated FSH, limited testicular volume, and conditions previously associated with sterility (e.g., Klinefelter syndrome).

References

1. Jow WW, Steckel J, Schlegel PN, Magid MS, Goldstein M. Motile sperm in human testis biopsy specimens. J Androl. 1993;14(3):194–8.
2. Schlegel PN. Testicular sperm extraction: microdissection improves sperm yield with minimal tissue excision. Hum Reprod. 1999;14(1):131–5.
3. Tournaye H, Liu J, Nagy PZ, Camus M, Goossens A, Silber S, Van Steirteghem AC, Devroey P. Correlation between testicular histology and outcome after intracytoplasmic sperm injection using testicular spermatozoa. Hum Reprod. 1996;11(1):127–32.
4. Schlegel PN, Su LM. Physiological consequences of testicular sperm extraction. Hum Reprod. 1997;12(8):1688–92.
5. Schlegel PN, Kaufmann J. Role of varicocelectomy in men with nonobstructive azoospermia. Fertil Steril. 2004;81(6):1585–8.
6. Pavlovich CP, King P, Goldstein M, Schlegel PN. Evidence of a treatable endocrinopathy in infertile men. J Urol. 2001;165(3):837–41.

7. Raman JD, Schlegel PN. Aromatase inhibitors for male infertility. J Urol. 2002;167(2 Pt 1): 624–9.
8. Schlegel PN, Liotta D, Hariprashad J, Veeck LL. Fresh testicular sperm from men with nonobstructive azoospermia works best for ICSI. Urology. 2004;64(6):1069–71.
9. Donoso P, Tournaye H, Devroey P. Which is the best sperm retrieval technique for NOA? A systematic review. Hum Reprod Update. 2007;13(6):539–49.
10. Turek PJ, Cha I, Ljung BM. Systematic fine-needle aspiration of the testis: correlation to biopsy and results of organ "mapping" for mature sperm in azoospermic men. Urology. 1997;49(5):743–8.
11. Dardashti K, Williams RH, Goldstein M. Microsurgical testis biopsy: a novel technique for retrieval of testicular tissue. J Urol. 2000;163(4):1206–7.
12. Amer M, Ateyah A, Hany R, Zohdy W. Prospective comparative study between microsurgical and conventional testicular sperm extraction in NOA: follow-up by serial ultrasound examinations. Hum Reprod. 2000;15(3):653–6.
13. Okada H, Dobashi M, Yamazaki T, Hara I, Fujisawa M, Arakawa S, Kamidono S. Conventional versus microdissection testicular sperm extraction for nonobstructive azoospermia. J Urol. 2002;168(3):1063–7.
14. Ostad M, Liotta D, Ye Z, Schlegel PN. Testicular sperm extraction for nonobstructive azoospermia: results of a multibiopsy approach with optimized tissue dispersion. Urology. 1998;52(4):692–6.
15. Ramasamy R, Schlegel PN. Microdissection testicular sperm extraction: effect of prior biopsy on success of sperm retrieval. J Urol. 2007;177(4):1447–9.
16. Ramasamy R, Lin K, Gosden LV, Rosenwaks Z, Palermo GD, Schlegel PN. High serum FSH levels in men with nonobstructive azoospermia does not affect success of microdissection testicular sperm extraction. Fertil Steril. 2009;92(2):590–3.
17. Hung AJ, King P, Schlegel PN. Uniform testicular maturation arrest: a unique subset of men with nonobstructive azoospermia. J Urol. 2007;178(2):608–12.
18. Ramasamy R, Ricci JA, Palermo GD, Gosden LV, Rosenwaks Z, Schlegel PN. Successful fertility treatment for Klinefelter's syndrome. J Urol. 2009;182(3):1108–13.
19. Raman JD, Schlegel PN. Testicular sperm extraction with intracytoplasmic sperm injection is successful for the treatment of nonobstructive azoospermia associated with cryptorchidism. J Urol. 2003;170(4 Pt 1):1287–90.
20. Hsiao W, Stahl PJ, Osterberg EC, Nejat E, Palermo GD, Rosenwaks Z, Schlegel PN. Successful treatment of postchemotherapy azoospermia with microsurgical testicular sperm extraction: the Weill Cornell experience. J Clin Oncol. 2011;29(12):1607–11.
21. Hopps CV, Mielnik A, Goldstein M, Palermo GD, Rosenwaks Z, Schlegel PN. Detection of sperm in men with Y chromosome microdeletions of the AZFa, AZFb and AZFc regions. Hum Reprod. 2003;18(8):1660–5.
22. Choi JM, Chung P, Veeck L, Mielnik A, Palermo GD, Schlegel PN. AZF microdeletions of the Y chromosome and in vitro fertilization outcome. Fertil Steril. 2004;81(2):337–41.

Chapter 8
Noninfertility Scrotal Microsurgery

Akanksha Mehta and Marc Goldstein

Abstract The use of microsurgical techniques for noninfertility urologic surgery is growing. Urologic literature published over the past three decades describes the use of microsurgery for a variety of penile, scrotal, and upper urinary tract reconstructive procedures, testicular autotransplantation for cryptorchidism, testis-sparing surgery for testis tumors, spermatic cord denervation for chronic pain, as well as routine urologic procedures such as hernia repair, hydrocelectomy, spermatocelectomy. In the hands of skilled microsurgeons, superior outcomes have been reported following these procedures. With further improvements in microsurgical technology, and training of dedicated microsurgeons, the role for microsurgery will only continue to grow.

Keywords Cryptorchidism • Denervation • Epididymal cyst • Hydrocelectomy Hernia repair • Ilioinguinal nerve • Lymphedema • Lymphovenous anastomosis • Microsurgery • Orchalgia • Orchidopexy • Spermatocele • Spermatocelectomy • Testis autotransplantation • Testis reimplantation • Undescended testes • Vascular anastomosis

A. Mehta, M.D. (✉)
Department of Urology, Weill Cornell Medical College, Cornell University, 525 East 68th St., Starr 900, New York, NY 10065, USA
e-mail: akm9009@med.cornell.edu

M. Goldstein, M.D.
Department of Urology, Center for Male Reproductive Medicine and Microsurgery, Weill Cornell Medical College, Cornell University, 525 East 68th St., Box 580, New York, NY 10065, USA
e-mail: mgoldst@mail.med.cornell.edu

J.I. Sandlow (ed.), *Microsurgery for Fertility Specialists: A Practical Text*,
DOI 10.1007/978-1-4614-4196-0_8, © Springer Science+Business Media New York 2013

Introduction

Since the introduction of microsurgery for vasal reanastomosis by Silber [1] and Owen [2] in the 1970s, microsurgery has evolved to become a urologic subspecialty. Significant technical advances in optical magnification, illumination, microsurgical instrumentation, and sutures have allowed for improvement in microsurgical techniques, and expanded the use of microsurgical methodologies for a variety of urologic procedures.

In addition to surgery of the male reproductive tract, such as vasovasostomy and vasoepididymostomy, and testicular and epididymal sperm extraction for the treatment of obstructive and nonobstructive azoospermia, respectively, microsurgery has been used for penile, scrotal, and upper urinary tract reconstruction. Microsurgical penile revascularization for the treatment of arteriogenic erectile dysfunction has been successfully described in several series [3, 4]; its utility has also been considered for improving graft outcomes in posterior urethral reconstructive surgery [5]. In the pediatric population, hypospadias repair using the operating microscope has been shown to have equivalent or better outcomes compared to using 3.5× loupe magnification [6]. Microvascular testis autotransplantation for the treatment of cryptorchidism has also been described in the pediatric population, with reasonable success [7]. More recently, testis-sparing surgery for testis cancer has been shown to provide safe and effective oncologic control in the German testicular Cancer Study Group [8]. In such settings, microsurgical testis exploration allows for accurate identification and excision of the target lesion, with appropriate margins, while minimizing trauma to the surrounding parenchyma [9, 10]. Microsurgery plays a role in surgery of the upper urinary tract as well. Brannen et al. [11] have described microsurgical renovascular repair in the organ-transplant setting, with the goal of maximizing renal function. Likewise, microsurgical ureteroureteral anastomosis has led to excellent long-term outcomes while averting the need for urinary diversion [12–14].

Microsurgical varicocelectomy has become the gold standard for varicocele repair, with contemporary series showing negligible complication and recurrence rates. While indications for varicocelectomy have traditionally been impaired semen parameters or pain, evidence of improvement in serum testosterone levels following varicocelectomy has led some authors to advocate for microsurgical varicocelectomy for the treatment of hypoandrogenism in the appropriate clinical setting [15, 16].

While the application of microsurgery in urology has traditionally been for the treatment of male infertility, the advantages offered by the microsurgical approach are evident for noninfertility surgery as well. This chapter discusses the use of microsurgical techniques for noninfertility surgery, focusing on spermatocelectomy, hydrocelectomy, herniorrhaphy, denervation, and vascular and lymphatic reconstructive surgery. Readers are referred to Chaps. 3, 9 and 13 for further discussion on the role of microsurgery for varicocelectomy, testis-sparing surgery, and penile revascularization, respectively.

Advantages and Limitations of Microsurgery

An operating microscope allows for 6–25× magnification of the operating field, thereby considerably enhancing the surgeon's visual acuity and ability for precision. This magnification also allows for meticulous hemostasis and avoidance of inadvertent iatrogenic injuries. Microsurgery is ideally suited for the execution of any procedure that involves fine dissection or anastomoses, and which aims to limit manipulation of tissues surrounding the operative field. However, costs associated with an operating microscope and microsurgical instruments can be substantial. Training in microsurgical techniques also demands time and patience. Case selection for microsurgery should, therefore, should be carefully performed by the operating surgeon, and be guided by surgical outcomes.

Denervation of the Spermatic Cord

Chronic orchalgia, defined as unexplained, intermittent or constant unilateral or bilateral testicular pain lasting for more than 3 months [17], presents a challenging management dilemma for urologists. Although surgical intervention is considered the last line of treatment, by the time of presentation to a urologist, most patients have experienced the condition for years, and have tried and failed multiple other therapies such as anti-inflammatory agents, antibiotics, and antidepressants.

Surgical therapy for idiopathic chronic orchalgia includes epididymectomy, orchiectomy, and microsurgical denervation of the spermatic cord (MDSC). Variable success rates have been reported in the literature with each of these procedures, ranging from as low as 20% [18] to as high as 96% [19]. Recent series of microsurgical denervation, however, show more consistent and promising results. The largest of these series comprised 95 testicular units, and resulted in complete, durable pain relief in 71%, partial relief in 17%, and no change from baseline in 11% of testicular units, at a mean follow-up of 20.3 months [17]. The most severe complication was testicular atrophy, seen in 2 of 79 patients. No complications were noted in a smaller series of 35 patients followed for 31.5 months after MDSC [19].

Appropriate patient selection is important. Candidates for MDSC should have no identifiable reversible pathology, and should demonstrate a partial or complete response to spermatic cord nerve block with local anesthetic. Following an inguinal incision, the spermatic cord is delivered over a penrose drain, as shown in Fig. 8.1. The ilioinguinal nerve is identified and divided, and a section of the nerve is removed to prevent reunion of the cut ends. The external and internal spermatic fascia are then opened. Testicular, cremasteric, and vasal arteries, as well as lymphatics of the spermatic cord, are identified and spared. The vas deferens is also identified and spared. The remaining cremasteric fibers, veins, and perivasal fascia are ligated and divided.

Chronic orchalgia is thought to result from persistently upregulated central- and peripheral-nervous system pain pathways. MDSC was first described by Devine and Schellhammer [20], and has been popularized over the past decade as a testis-preserving surgical approach for the treatment of chronic orchalgia.

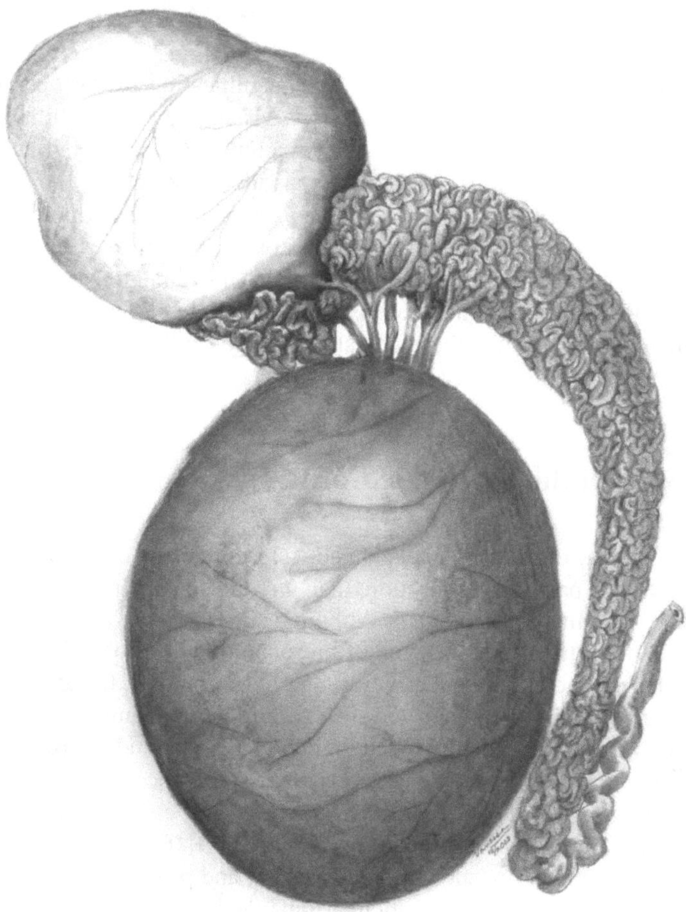

Fig. 8.1 Microsurgical spermatocelectomy

The use of microsurgical techniques certainly contributes to the high success rate and low complication rate associated with this procedure.

Hydrocelectomy

Hydrocelectomy, along with inguinal herniorrhaphy, spermatocelectomy, renal transplantation, and appendectomy, is a recognized cause of iatrogenic injury to the vas deferens. Adherence of the epididymis or spermatic cord to the tunica vaginalis places these structures at risk of unintentional resection or injury by suture ligation, at the time of resection or posterior deflection of the tunica vaginalis during a bottleneck repair [21]. Zahalsky et al. reported a 5.62% rate of injury to the epididymis alone during hydrocelectomy [22].

Prior to surgery, a scrotal ultrasound should be performed to confirm absence of testis tumor. Following transverse scrotal skin-fold incision, the testicle is delivered, and the spermatic cord and vas are identified and surrounded with a Penrose drain. An opening is made in the tunica vaginalis under the microscope, the hydrocele fluid drained, and the testis and epididymis delivered. Use of the operating microscope at the time of hydrocelectomy provides a detailed view of the vas deferens, vasal vessels, and the epididymis, minimizing the possibility of iatrogenic injury. Transillumination of the opened hydrocele sac using the operating room lights can help identify the vas and epididymis, which may be splayed out within the walls of a thick and long-standing hydrocele sac, and be difficult to otherwise identify. The vas should be traced from the cord to the vasoepididymal junction. In cases where the margins of the epididymis are indistinct, the operating microscope is indispensable to assure that epididymal tubules are not transected during hydrocele sac excision. Redundant tunica vaginalis is resected, leaving a fingerbreadth margin of tunic around the epididymis. The edges of the tunic are then oversewn for control of hemostasis. A bipolar cautery is used to control small bleeding vessels. Although there is no published data available comparing the outcomes of microsurgical or nonmicrosurgical hydrocelectomy, in our experience, the microsurgical technique minimizes iatrogenic complications without significantly extending the operative time.

Spermatocelectomy

Spermatoceles are extratesticular, sperm-containing cystic structures emanating from the caput epididymis. They are caused by aneurysmal dilatation of an efferent duct, usually due to distal obstruction of the involved efferent duct. As such, spermatoceles are distinct from epididymal cysts, which do not contain sperm. Surgical indications for spermatocelectomy are pain or discomfort secondary to large size; sperm aspirated from spermatoceles are often of poor quality and cannot be used for intrauterine insemination, but in men with vasoepididymal obstructive azoospermia, they can serve as an easily accessible reservoir for sperm adequate for in vitro fertilization and intracytoplasmic sperm injection.

Following transverse scrotal skin-fold incision and delivery of the testis, the tunica vaginalis is opened and the testis, epididymis, and spermatocele are inspected. The spermatocele is microsurgically dissected off the epididymis down to its origin from a single efferent duct, as shown in Fig. 8.2. Care is taken to avoid puncturing the spermatocele. The isolated efferent duct is then ligated with 5-0 absorbable suture and the spermatocele is removed intact. In the only reported series of microsurgical spermatocelectomy, 23 men underwent a total of 36 microsurgical spermatocelectomy procedures, with no postoperative complications or recurrences at a mean follow-up of 17.3 months [23]. In contrast, the reported incidence of complications after nonmicrosurgical spermatocelectomy is 10–30%, with injuries to the epididymis occurring in 17.12% of cases [22].

The optical magnification provided by an operating microscope facilitates dissection of the spermatocele of the epididymis and allows clear identification of the

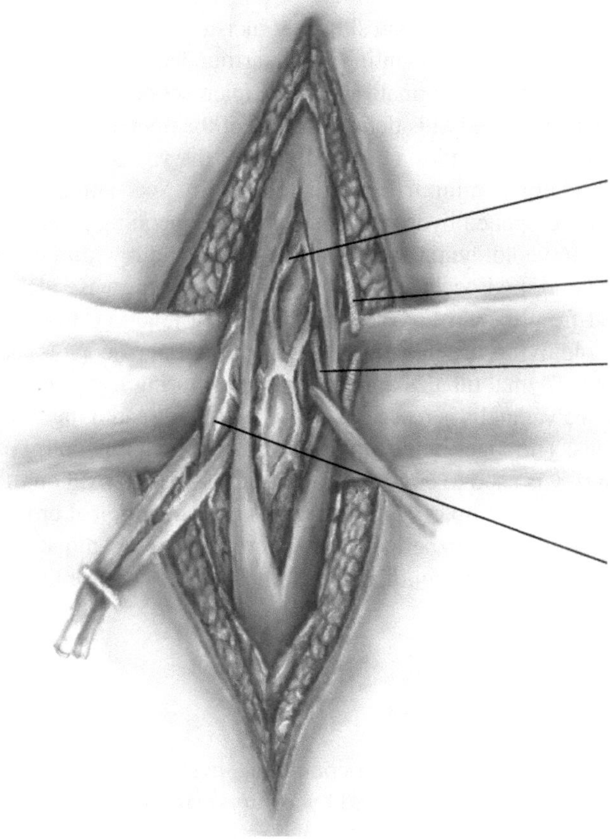

Fig. 8.2 Microsurgical denervation of the spermatic cord

spermatocele neck for ligation, and prevents injury to adjacent epididymal tubules. Outcomes and recurrence rates are significantly improved after microsurgical compared to nonmicrosurgical intervention. The described technique can also be applied for management of epididymal cysts, albeit the lack of communication with an efferent ductule obviates the need to ligate an efferent duct.

Herniorrhaphy

Inguinal herniorrhaphy is the most common cause of iatrogenic injury to the vas deferens, causing obstructive azoospermia, as well as injury to the testicular arterial supply, resulting in ischemic orchitis and testis atrophy [24]. The repair of indirect inguinal hernias, which requires the hernia sac to be dissected off the contents of the spermatic cord and ligated, can be particularly challenging, as indirect hernia sacs are often adherent to the vas deferens. Additionally, placement of surgical mesh at the time of herniorrhaphy can be associated with entrapment of the ilioinguinal or genitofemoral nerves, leading to postoperative neuropathic pain.

A skin incision is made in the inguinal crease between the internal and external rings. The superficial epigastric artery and vein are identified, ligated, and divided. The external oblique aponeurosis is opened in the direction of its fibers, and held open using a Scott retractor. Under 10× magnification, the ilioinguinal nerve is identified and retracted out of the operative field. The hernia sac is identified on the anteromedial aspect of the spermatic cord, and dissected off the surrounding cord structures to the level of the internal ring, where is twisted, suture ligated, and divided. The vas deferens, vasal vessels, and internal spermatic artery are preserved. Surgical mesh with a preformed opening for the spermatic cord is then placed around the cord, and seated in a flat position along the floor of the inguinal canal. The ilioinguinal nerve is revisualized to ensure it is not entrapped by the mesh. The mesh is then sewn to itself around the spermatic cord, and secured to the pubic tubercle using interrupted 2-0 monofilament absorbable suture. The external oblique fascia is closed over the mesh using absorbable suture. Use of long-lasting but absorbable sutures minimizes the risk of nerve entrapment syndrome, even if a nerve is inadvertently included under the suture.

Microsurgically assisted hernia repair may be performed as an independent procedure, or concurrently at the time of ipsilateral or contralateral varicocelectomy. Use of the operating microscope minimizes iatrogenic injuries and urologic complications, and should certainly be considered for recurrent or otherwise challenging indirect inguinal hernia repairs.

Scrotal Vascular and Lymphatic Surgery

Lymphedema of the scrotum may be idiopathic, or secondary to parasitic infection, radiation, or radical pelvic surgery. The traditional approach for treatment of lymphedema has been excision of the involved tissue, but this approach is invasive, and still carries a risk of recurrence [25]. The use of microsurgery for the treatment of genital lymphedema was first described by Huang et al. in 1981, based on the technique previously developed for treatment of lymphedema in the upper and lower extremities [26].

In their original approach, the authors used bilateral curved scrotal incisions, and outlined the scrotal lymphatics by subcutaneous, intradermal injection of methylene blue. Under the operating microscope, the stained lymphatics were then anastomosed to superficial scrotal veins [27]. The maximum number of possible anastomoses was performed, averaging about two per side. In three patients treated by this technique, scrotal size returned to nearly normal, and was maintained at 18-month follow-up. The authors noted that appropriate patient selection was important. Long-standing excess lymphatic fluid accumulated in the intercellular space leads to chronic inflammation, and compression of the lymphatic channels, making surgical reconstruction challenging [27]. Therefore, lymphovenous anastomosis is ideally performed prior to the onset of fibrosis.

Mukenge et al. described a modification of the above technique in which lymphovenous anastomoses were performed between the lymphatics of the spermatic cord and the veins of the pampiniform plexus, thereby allowing testicular lymphatic drainage [28]. In their series of five patients, progressive improvement was noted in terms of visual improvement in scrotal size, consistency and color, decrease in patient-reported discomfort, and by scrotal lymphangiography, in all cases. 90–100% resolution of edema was noted at 3 years of follow-up [28].

The advantages of microsurgical lymphovenous anastomoses over traditional scrotoplasty for treatment of scrotal lymphedema include a limited dissection, either in the superficial scrotum, or in the spermatic cord, with minimal tissue trauma and bleeding, and significantly fewer complications, such as cellulitis and scrotal hematoma. The experience with microsurgical lymphovenous anastomoses is certainly limited, given the infrequent presentation of scrotal lymphedema. One drawback of the procedure is its lengthy duration, with Mukenge et al. reporting an operative time of over 7 h in some patients with long-standing scrotal edema and fibrosis [28].

Testis Autotransplantation and Reimplantation

The incidence of undescended testes in full term infants is approximately 3% at birth. The majority of cryptorchid testes descend spontaneously during the first year of life, with 0.8% of male infants having undescended testes at 1 year of age. For intra-abdominal testes, a staged orchidopexy procedure consisting of division of the spermatic vessels, followed by testicular mobilization and scrotal orchidopexy, has been the mainstay of operative approaches since its description by Fowler and Stephens [29]. The facility of this procedure has been increased by the introduction of laparoscopy and minimally invasive techniques.

As an alternative to the Fowler–Stephens technique, Silber and Kelly described using a microvascular anastomosis to bring extra blood supply to the testicle after mobilization of a high intra-abdominal testicle into the scrotum [30]. Slight modifications have been made to the original technique over the years [7]. A high inguinal incision is made to avoid injury to the epigastric vessels. The retroperitoneum is entered and the testicle is identified. High ligation of the testicular arteries and veins is performed to provide maximal length for vascular anastomosis following scrotal transplantation. The testicle is mobilized, taking a wide strip of peritoneum with the vas deferens. A subdartos pouch is created in the scrotum to accommodate the testicle in a dependent position, without tension on the vas. The inferior epigastric vessels are then isolated and distally ligated, leaving an intact 8–9 cm intact length from their origin at the external iliac vessels. Small vascular branches along this length are also ligated. Under the microscope, the vessels are cleaned of excess adventitial tissue and flushed with heparinized saline. An end-to-end or end-to-side anastomosis using 10-0 nylon may be performed between the testicular and inferior epigastric arteries, based on the discrepancy in their sizes, while an end-to-end anastomosis between the testicular and inferior epigastric vein usually suffices. The testicle is then secured within the dartos pouch.

Several groups have reported excellent long-term results with microsurgical testicular autotransplantation. In the largest series by Bukowski et al., over 95% of the 30 autotransplants performed over a 17-year period were successful [7]. Combined with the results of other small series, there is an aggregate success rate of over 88–95% [31–33]. Despite these promising results, microsurgical testicular autotransplantation has not been widely adopted, due to the need of an operating microscope, microsurgical skill, and the long duration of cases. Recently, the combination of laparoscopic surgery for testicular harvesting with minimal morbidity and maximal vascular pedicle length, and microsurgery for execution of the vascular reanastomosis has been described [34, 35], with comparable success rates, even in patients who had failed previous Fowler–Stephens orchidopexy [34]. The use of microsurgery for orchidopexy of high intra-abdominal testis may, therefore, again increase.

Since the introduction of the operating microscope, various experimental protocols to evaluate testicular transplantation between individuals have also been performed, using similar surgical techniques as described above. In some cases, functional transplants have been successfully executed [36]. However, at present, the risks associated with testicular transplantation between individuals, such as immunosuppression, far outweigh its benefits, and this procedure is not recommended.

Microsurgical technique has also been used for reimplantation of the traumatically avulsed testis [37–39], with or without concomitant avulsion of the penis. While there is no large series of this experience, and reporting bias is possible, a review of the case reports demonstrates reasonable outcomes. Transplanted testes remained viable, with preserved histologic architecture and steroidogenic function in all reported cases [37–39]. Spermatogenesis was not noted in any report. Interestingly, one case report describes temporary ectopic replantation of a traumatically avulsed testis on the forearm with refabrication and subsequent successful orthotopic microsurgical transfer to the perineum [38]. In the case of a unilateral testis injury, with a normal contralateral testis, fertility and hormonal function are not expected to be severely affected. Testicular reimplantation may be considered in the setting on a unilateral testis or an atrophic contralateral testis.

Summary

Microsurgical techniques can be applied to a variety of urologic procedures outside the field of male infertility surgery. However, the advantages of microsurgery, including optical magnification, minimal tissue trauma and meticulous hemostasis, must be balanced with its limitations, such as operative cost and time, and the microsurgical skills of the operating surgeon. As discussed in this chapter, the use of microsurgical techniques leads superior outcomes in the appropriately selected case and patient population. The ability to successfully perform detailed procedures such as denervation of the spermatic cord, and the execution of fine vascular of lymphovascular anastomoses, is clearly enhanced with the use of the operating microscope. Equally importantly, postoperative complications in procedures such as varicocelectomy, hydrocelectomy, and spermatocelectomy are minimized under the microscope. With technical advances in microsurgery, and training of dedicated microsurgeons, the application of microsurgical techniques in urology will likely continue to expand.

References

1. Silber JS. Microsurgery in clinical urology. Urology. 1975;6(2):150–3.
2. Owen ER. Microsurgical vasovasostomy. A reliable vasectomy reversal. Aust N Z J Surg. 1977;47(3):305–9.
3. Melman A, Riccardi R. The success of microsurgical penile revascularization in treating arteriogenic impotence. Int J Impot Res. 1993;5(1):47–52.
4. Janssen T, Sarramon JP, et al. Microsurgical arterio-arterial and arterio-venous penile revascularization in patients with pure arteriogenic impotence. Br J Urol. 1994;73(5):561–5.
5. Nelson AK, Wessells H, Friedrich JB. Review of microsurgical posterior urethral reconstruction. J Reconstr Microsurg. 2011;27(3):179–86.
6. Shapiro SR. Hypospadias repair: optical magnification versus Zeiss reconstruction microscope. Urology. 1989;33(1):43–6.
7. Bukowski TP, Wacksman J, et al. Testicular autotransplantation for the intra-abdominal testis. Microsurgery. 1995;16:290–5.
8. Heidenreich A, Weissbach L, et al. Organ sparing surgery for malignant germ cell tumor of the testis. J Urol. 2001;166:2161–5.
9. Hopps CV, Goldstein M. Ultrasound guided needle localization and microsurgical exploration for incidental non-palpable testicular tumors. J Urol. 2002;168:1084–7.
10. Rolle L, Tamagnone A, et al. Microsurgical "testis-sparing" surgery for nonpalpable hypoechoic testicular lesions. Urology. 2006;68:381–5.
11. Brannen GE, Bush WH, et al. Microvascular management of multiple renal injuries in transplantation. J Urol. 1982;128:112–5.
12. Oesterwitz H, Metz L, Weber H. Microsurgical end-to-end anastomosis in ureteral injuries. Eur Urol. 1988;14(3):251–2.
13. Oesterwitz H, Bick C, et al. Reconstructive microsurgery of the upper urinary tract. Int Urol Nephrol. 1988;20(5):453–9.
14. Ponig BF. Microsurgical ureteroureterostomy in ureteral injuries. J Urol. 1982;128(3):594–5.
15. Tanrikut C, Goldstein M. Varicocele repair for the treatment of androgen deficiency. Curr Opin Urol. 2010;20:500–2.
16. Zohdy W, Ghazi S, Arafa M. Impact of varicocelectomy on gonadal and erectile functions in men with hypogonadism and infertility. J Sex Med. 2011;8:885–93.
17. Strom KH, Levine LA. Microsurgical denervation of the spermatic cord for chronic orchalgia: long-term results from a single center. J Urol. 2008;180:949–53.
18. Costabile RA, Hahn M, McLeod DG. Chronic orchalgia in the pain prone patient: the clinical perspective. J Urol. 1991;146:1571–4.
19. Heidenreich A, Olbert P, Engelmann UH. Management of chronic testalgia by microsurgical testicular denervation. Eur Urol. 2002;41(4):392–7.
20. Devine CJ, Schellhammer PF. The use of microsurgical denervation of the spermatic cord for orchalgia. Trans Am Assoc Genitourin Surg. 1978;70:149–51.
21. Hopps CV, Goldstein M. Microsurgical reconstruction of iatrogenic injuries to the epididymis from hydroceletomy. J Urol. 2006;176:2077–80.

22. Zahalsky MP, Berman AJ, Nagler HM. Evaluating the risk of epididymal injury during hydroceletomy and spermatocelectomy. J Urol. 2004;171(6 Pt 1):2291–2.
23. Kauffman EC, Kim HH, et al. Microsurgical spermatocelectomy: technique and outcomes of a novel surgical approach. J Urol. 2011;185:238–42.
24. Sheynkin YR, Hendin B, et al. Microsurgical repair of iatrogenic injury to the vas deferens. J Urol. 1998;159:139–41.
25. Mukenge SM, Pulitano C, et al. Secondary scrotal lymphedema: a novel microsurgical approach. Microsurgery. 2007;27:655–6.
26. Huang GK, Hu RQ, et al. Microlymphaticovenous anastomosis for treating lymphedema of the extremities and external genitalia. J Microsurg. 1981;3(1):32–9.
27. Huang GK, Hu RQ, Liu ZZ. Microlymphaticovenous anastomosis for treating scrotal elephantiasis. Microsurgery. 1985;6:36–9.
28. Mukenge SM, Catena M, et al. Assessment of follow-up of patency after lymphovenous microsurgery for treatment of secondary lymphedema in external male genital organs. Eur Urol. 2011;60:1114–9.
29. Fowler R, Stephens FD. The role of testicular vascular anatomy in the salvage of high undescended testes. Aust N Z J Surg. 1959;29:92–106.
30. Silber SJ, Kelly J. Successful autotransplantation of an intra-abdominal testicle to the scrotum by microvascular technique. J Urol. 1976;115:452–4.
31. Giuliani L, Carmignani G. Microsurgical testis autotransplantation. A critical review. Eur Urol. 1983;9:129–32.
32. Boeckx W, Vereecken R, Depuydt K. Microsurgery for intra-abdominal testicular retention. Eur J Obstet Gynecol Reprod Biol. 1998;81(2):191–6.
33. Wacksman J, Dinner M, Handler M. Results of testicular autotransplantation using the microvascular technique: experience with 8 intra-abdominal testes. J Urol. 1982;128(6):1319–21.
34. Tackett LD, Wacksman J, et al. The high intra-abdominal testis: technique and long-term success of laparoscopic testicular autotransplantation. J Endourol. 2002;16(6):359–61.
35. Kelley BP, Higuera S, et al. Combined laparoscopic and microsurgical techniques for testicular autotransplantation: is this still an evolving technique? J Reconstr Microsurg. 2010;26(8): 555–8.
36. Silber SJ. Transplantation of a human testis for anorchia. Fertil Steril. 1978;30:181–7.
37. Lin SD, Lai CS, Su PY. Replantation of the testis by microsurgical technique. Plast Reconstr Surg. 1985;76(4):620–5.
38. Ramdas S, Thomas A, Thomas A, Arun Kumar S. Temporary ectopic testicular replantation, refabrication and orthotopic transfer. J Plast Reconstr Aesthet Surg. 2007;60(7):700–3.
39. Altarac S. A case of testicle replantation. J Urol. 1993;150(5 Pt 1):1507–8.

Chapter 9
Testis-Sparing Surgery for Testicular Masses

Oleksandr Stakhovskyi and Michael A.S. Jewett

Abstract Patients with palpable and nonpalpable testicular lesions may have benign rather than malignant tumors. The organ-sparing approach with partial orchiectomy is an option to preserve testicular function. The role for partial orchiectomy (PO) is less well established for malignant tumors but can be safely performed for solitary tumors, <2 cm in diameter when the blood supply to the remaining testis can be preserved. Residual androgen and fertility function is usually worth the risk of recurrence, which is low. Careful monitoring of the residual testis is required. The presence of carcinoma in situ (CIS) in the testis can complicate further management, but adjuvant radiation is effective and can be delayed to allow for fertility.

Keywords Testis-sparing surgery • Partial orchiectomy • Testis cancer

Radical orchiectomy is the standard treatment for a primary germ cell tumor (GCT) of the testis. It provides diagnostic tissue and is curative in most stage I tumors. There is however functional, physical, and psychological morbidity [1]. For many years, the testis-sparing alternative of partial orchiectomy has been available but it has not been widely adopted [2]. The attractions of partial orchiectomy are cosmetic and the potential for preservation of function, both fertility and hormonal.

Testicular GCT represents 2% of male malignancies but is the most common solid tumor in men between the ages of 15 and 35 years. Worldwide, the incidence has more than doubled in the past 40 years with an estimated 8,290 new cases diagnosed in the United States in 2011 [3–5]. Cure rates of almost 100% are expected with early stage testicular GCT. Even with metastatic disease, stratified by the International Germ Cell Cancer Collaborative Group (IGCCCG) classification into

O. Stakhovskyi, M.D. • M.A.S. Jewett, M.D., F.R.C.S.C., F.A.C.S. (✉)
Division of Urology, Departments of Surgery and Surgical Oncology,
Princess Margaret Hospital and the University Health Network, University of Toronto,
610 University Ave, 3-130, Toronto, ON, Canada M5G 2M9
e-mail: m.jewett@utoronto.ca

J.I. Sandlow (ed.), *Microsurgery for Fertility Specialists: A Practical Text*,
DOI 10.1007/978-1-4614-4196-0_9,

good, intermediate, and poor groups. *Five-year survival rates of 90, 80, and 50% are achieved* [6]. The high cure rates, particularly in low stage GCT have focused management on minimizing morbidity while preserving the excellent oncological outcomes. Examples of changes in treatment include introducing active surveillance for stage I tumors, nerve-sparing retroperitoneal lymph node dissection (RPLND), insertion of testicular prostheses after orchiectomy and radiation of carcinoma in situ (CIS) rather than radical orchiectomy [7–10]. Partial orchiectomy (PO) represents another such strategy in GCT management to reduce morbidity. Contributing to the uptake of PO is the observation that many small testicular masses are being discovered earlier, which are benign. Orchiectomy usually represents overtreatment of these lesions.

Until the mid-1980s, all testicular masses that were suspicious for tumor were treated by radical orchiectomy because of concern for tumor seeding with transscrotal biopsy [11]. About 1% were benign at final histopathology [11]. The first report of partial orchiectomy by Richie in 1984, was for bilateral tumors to preserve fertility and androgen function and to reduce psychological stress [12]. There has been a gradual increase in PO since with expanded potential indications including a suspected metachronous GCT. More recently, PO has been performed for masses that are suspected of being benign as the number of small nonpalpable lesions detected by ultrasound has increased [13]. It is now recognized that benign lesions represent a significantly higher proportion of testicular masses [14–17]. Radical surgery is overtreatment of these benign lesions. Furthermore, tumor seeding appears to be rare when an unrecognized malignancy is biopsied or incised [18]. Therefore, a paradigm shift to organ preservation appears feasible in selected cases of testicular masses.

Indications for Partial Orchiectomy

The indications for testis-sparing PO can be considered imperative, relative, or elective.

Imperative indications include circumstances in which orchiectomy would render the patient castrate requiring hormonal replacement therapy. Suspected testicular tumors in solitary testes or bilateral testicular tumors are imperative indications. *Relative* indications include those in which the contralateral testis is compromised in some way, e.g., epididymitis, microlithiasis, hypogonadism, etc. Eberhard et al. showed that preoperative hypogonadism and microlithiasis by ultrasound are strong predictors of subsequent hypogonadism [19]. *Elective* indications include those patients with small, peripheral (polar) tumors and a normal contralateral testis.

There is an increased risk for the development of a second tumor in the contralateral testis in men who have had a GCT [20]. The incidence of contralateral testis malignancy ranges from 1 to 5% [20–22]. Bilateral metachronous tumors are seen more commonly than bilateral synchronous tumors. The interval between the first and second tumor is variable. Fossa et al. has studied the impact of lifelong hormonal replacement in these patients after bilateral orchiectomy [23]. They evaluated a cohort of 43 patients and found that psychological and sexual adjustment was satisfactory in the majority however, 20% did have severe to moderate psychological distress. Organ-sparing approaches are very likely to benefit this group of men. A number of studies report equal survival in patients with bilateral and unilateral testicular cancer after orchiectomy [20, 24, 25].

The German Testicular Cancer Group and others reported their results with PO for GCT in a small subset of carefully selected patients with a solitary testis or bilateral testicular tumors [26–32]. Selection criteria included: organ-confined disease with no infiltration of the rete testis, a mass <2 cm to preserve enough testosterone-producing parenchyma, negative postresection biopsies of the tumor bed. Intraoperative cold ischemia was employed in an attempt to preserve Sertoli and Leydig function. Using these criteria, Heidenreich et al. have reported orchiectomy results for 73 GCTs [28]. Thirty tumors were in single testis and 69 were bilateral [17 (23.3%) synchronous and 52 (71%) metachronous] and 4 (5.5%) occurred in a solitary testicle. After a median follow-up of 91 months, 98.6% patients had no evidence of disease and one died of systemic tumor progression. The presence of CIS was described in 82.3% of patients [28, 33]. Finally, 15 (20.5%) had embryonal carcinoma elements and 3 patients developed metastatic disease (with the one death).

Patient Assessment

Preoperative assessment includes history and physical examination along with imaging of the lesion, usually with ultrasound (US). Risk factors that should be recorded and which play major role in assessment include family history, Caucasian race, previous GCT, cryptorchidism, infertility, and testicular microlithiasis [34, 35]. Genetic and environmental factors contribute to GCT development. A number of studies suggest that exposure to organochlorine compounds, chlordanes, and some polychlorinated biphenyl congeners could increase the risk of development of GCT [36, 37]. Brothers of men with GCT have an eight to tenfold increased risk compared with general population, and sons of the affected have a four- to sixfold increased risk [38, 39]. Swerdlow et al. reported that dizygotic/monozygotic twin brothers of a man with GCT will have 37- and 76.5-fold elevated risks of CGT respectively [40]. Another congenital risk factor reported is cryptorchidism [41]. Several epidemiologic studies have reported the relative risk of testicular cancer in patients with cryptorchidism from 3 to 14 times higher than normal expected incidence [42–44]. Berthelsen and colleagues reported that between 5 and 10% of patients with a history of cryptorchidism develop malignancy in the contralateral, normally descended gonad [45]. An infertile man with an abnormal semen analysis has a 20-fold greater incidence of testicular cancer compared to general population [46].

Physical examination of the testis is performed by careful palpation of the testis between the thumb and the first two fingers of the examining hand. The normal testis is homogeneous in consistency, freely movable, and separable from the epididymis. Testes normally have a firm, rubbery consistency with a smooth surface.

GCTs are usually nontender and firm masses, but in many cases, lesions are not palpable or they are small and not clearly suspicious for GCT. The epididymis should be distinguished as a palpable ridge on the posterior surface of testis. Lesions in this structure are usually benign. Classically, 90–95% of palpable solid masses in the testicular were reported to be malignant GCT [47]. More recent data shows that that many will still be benign despite being palpable. Carmignan et al. reported their experience with 1,320 patients [16]. Of patients with focal testicular lesions (27), 17 (63%) had palpable nodules between 3 to 24 mm and PO was performed in 47% (8). Definitive pathological report found seven nonmalignant neoplasms and one non-Hodgkin's lymphoma. The remaining nine patients (53%) underwent radical orchiectomy based on frozen section examination (FSE) of malignancy (eight) or diffused Leydig cell hyperplasia (one). The authors surmised that a conservative surgical approach is the best option and will not expose the patient to the risk of relapse.

Bloodwork includes tumor serum markers: β-human chorionic gonadotropin (β-hCG) and α-fetoprotein (AFP). These sensitive tumor markers allow careful follow-up, with intervention earlier in the course of disease. Endocrine assessment includes serum follicle-stimulating hormone (s-FSH), serum-luteinizing hormone (s-LH), and serum free testosterone.

Fertility evaluation along with semen analysis is important. A high proportion of men with a unilateral tumor have impaired spermatogenesis in the contralateral testis [48]. Petersen et al. reported considerable impairment of semen quality before orchiectomy in patients with GCT. In their study of 83 men with testicular cancer they found that total sperm count and sperm concentration were significantly lower in the group of men affected by testicular cancer compared to healthy men. This was supported by the observation of significantly higher FSH and lower inhibin B levels in men with GCT than in controls [49]. Man with testicular cancer appears to have normal androgen levels before orchiectomy. The most likely explanation of impaired semen quality is preexisting impairment in the contralateral testis [50].

Psychological evaluation is also useful. Life-threatening illnesses and the possibility of dying are not usual life experiences of young men who are more focused on career, interpersonal relationships and starting a family [51]. Very few studies have specifically examined psychological distress symptoms and their association with GCT's in testicular cancer survivors (TCS). Moynihan et al. found a 14% prevalence rate of anxiety disorders and 9% prevalence of depression up to 5 years after primary treatment [52]. TCS's were reported to have higher scores of depression compared to normal controls [53]. Psychological distress was significantly associated with health worries, fear of relapse, unemployment, financial difficulties, whereas nonsignificant associations were observed for treatment strategies, social class, marital status at diagnosis, fertility, and sexual problems [52]. Dahl, Haaland et al. reported that anxiety disorder in TCS was associated with younger age, peripheral neuropathy, economic problems, alcohol problems, sexual problems, and previous treatment for mental problems, but evaluation of personality parameters was not done [54]. It was also reported that testicular cancer affects body image and possibly may have effects on aspects of masculine identity or self-image specifically related to gender, sexuality, and fertility [55]. The loss of a testicle, particularly if bilateral, may alter the psyche in some men, even if prostheses are provided. One study formally assessed the QOL after bilateral orchiectomy in 43 patients and concluded that most men were psychosexually well adjusted [23]. However, it was significant that 19% were categorized as "cases" according to impact of event scale. This is considerably higher than the percentage of 3.6% observed in the general population with comparable instruments. It was equivalent to that seen 1 year after radical mastectomy for breast cancer. Five patients (10%) had significant posttraumatic stress [23]. Preserving testicular tissue via organ-sparing approach could decrease this stress compared to radical orchiectomy.

Men with GCT require lifelong follow-up and very little data exists on the impact on QOL. Monitoring of serum markers, regular imaging and periodic self-examination are recommended [20]. With an organ-sparing approach to the primary tumor, additional uncertainty and scrotal imaging are necessary. Further studies to compare QOL of patients after PO versus radical orchiectomy should be conducted.

Imaging of Testicular Lesions

US remains the most widely used imaging modality for the diagnosis of testicular lesions with >95% sensitivity and specificity in identifying intratesticular lesions [56]. One of the main roles of US is to distinguish intratesticular lesions from extratesticular, since the latter are more likely to be benign. Scrotal US is performed with a linear transducer that gives adequate penetration (7–10 MHz). Images are obtained at least in two planes. The findings (size, vascularity, echogenicity) are compared to the opposite side. Power Doppler US can show increased vascularity in malignancy, but this is not specific [57]. Unfortunately benign and malignant tumors are characterized by changes in echogenicity rather than specific sonographic features [58, 59]. All GCTs demonstrate blood flow whereas benign masses will appear with limited or absent flow in most cases. Nonseminomatous GCTs generally appear heterogeneous whereas seminomas are homogenous, but overlap is significant. Sonographic markers suggestive of benign lesions do exist, such as a target appearance or onion skin sign of epidermoid cysts, but they are not 100% specific or sensitive [60, 61]. A solid hypoechogenic testicular mass (Fig. 9.1) must be considered malignant until proven otherwise, even if it is not palpable [62]. The age of the patient, history of trauma, presence of fever, and associated medical conditions are important factors that should be considered when evaluating atypical testicular lesions. Infection caused acute orchitis appears as a diffusely enlarged hypoechoic testis on US; associated focal or diffuse enlargement of the epididymis due to coexisting epididymitis should help in diagnosis.

Horstman et al. reported their experience with nine incidental nonpalpable testicular lesions in approximately 1,600 scrotal US done for other indications. Seventy-eight percent of lesions were benign and 55% were less than 1 cm. The authors concluded that incidentally discovered lesions are likely to be benign and

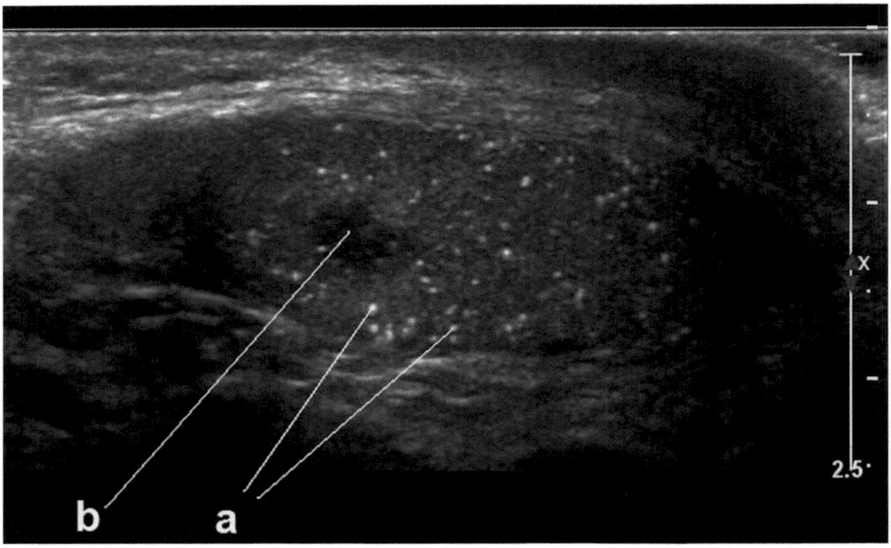

Fig. 9.1 An ultrasound of a small testicular mass ideally considered for organ sparing being located at the lower pole and palpable: (a) microcalcifications throughout the testis (b) small hypoechoic area suspicious for a focus of cancer

these patients should undergo initial excisional biopsy through an inguinal approach before proceeding to radical orchiectomy [13]. Conversely, other authors caution that impalpable lesions of the testis may be malignant [63, 64]. Furthermore, non-palpable testicular embryonal carcinoma as well as mature teratoma has been recently reported [65, 66].

Evidence of testicular microlithiasis on US was previously thought to be a risk factor for malignancy but is now known to occur in approx 5% of healthy asymptomatic men. In fact, 98.4% of men with testicular microlithiasis will not go on to develop malignancy [67]. Testicular microlithiasis is an uncommon condition in which many small nonshadowing hyperechoic foci of 1–3 mm are apparent within the testicular parenchyma, representing calcium deposits in the lumina of seminiferous tubules (Fig. 9.1). Criteria for diagnosis is the presence of ≥5 foci per US transducer field. Microlithiasis has been associated with various conditions, including Kleinfelter's syndrome, cryptorchidism, Down's syndrome, male pseudohermaphroditism, pulmonary alveolar microlithiasis, and testicular cancer [68]. Testicular microlithiasis is found in about 50% of men with GCTs so the presence of a mass and microlithiasis suggests malignancy [69].

MRI as an imaging tool for the testis is developing but is unlikely to replace US, particularly as a first line investigation [70]. It can provide additional useful information in patients with equivocal US findings. MRI can be of value when the location of a scrotal mass is uncertain or when there is difficulty in differentiating an inflammatory or vascular abnormality from a solid testicular mass [71]. Normal testis appears homogeneous with intermediate signal intensity on T1-weighted images and high signal intensity on T2-weighted images relative to skeletal muscle.

The epididymis has signal intensity characteristics similar to normal testicular parenchyma on T1-weighted images but lower signal intensity on T2-weighed images. Solid intratesticular lesions have lower signal intensity on T2-weighted images, in excellent contrast to the background high signal intensity of testicular parenchyma. At MRI, seminomas are usually homogeneous in appearance, isointense to normal testicular parenchyma on T1-weighted images and hypointense on T2-weighted images, although MRI does not allow a reliable histological diagnosis of testicular cancer subtypes. Nonseminomas, typically more heterogeneous, are usually iso- to hyperintense compared with normal testicular parenchyma on T1-weighted images, and hypointense on T2-weighted images [62].

A few nonmalignant lesions can be indistinguishable from testicular cancer, for which surgical exploration is often required. An example can be focal subacute or chronic orchitis, which can persist for months or years.

Biopsy of Testicular Lesions

Preoperative, percutaneous needle biopsy of testicular masses is not routinely recommended [11, 72]. In a meta-analysis, scrotal violation increased the risk of local recurrence from 0.4 to 2.9% [73]. The overall survival was not reduced when patients were followed with appropriate surgical management and close observation [74].

Due to concerns about seeding, excisional biopsy with FSE is more commonly undertaken as part of an organ-sparing approach. For those lesions confirmed to be benign by FSE, the remnant testis may be returned to the scrotum. If a GCT is found, CIS will occasionally be picked up on frozen section but this should not be relied upon. The concern with FSE has been misinterpretation of the mass or missing of CIS in the surrounding "normal" parenchyma when comparing to permanent sectioning and this should be discussed with patients [66, 75]. The detection of CIS is suboptimal not only because of pathological interpretation but also skip lesions amongst normal parenchyma. A FSE is generally felt to be inadequate [76]. The detection of CIS using immunohistochemistry with placental alkaline phosphatase (PLAP) is not straightforward but requires permanent section [77]. Consideration of adjuvant radiation observation or radical orchiectomy may be discussed with the patient postoperatively once the permanent sections have been examined for CIS and the GCT type determined(see below). The final stage of the primary tumor will also dictate what if any adjuvant treatment is required.

The main objective of the FSE is to confirm a GCT and confirm the lesion has a margin of normal testicular parenchyma. Some groups advocate multiple core biopsies of each sidewall and from the bottom of the tumor bed after the tumor has been excised while others (including our institution) rely on examination of the edge of the mass [78]. For detecting GCT, FSE has found to be 100% accurate for the presence of tumor in the largest study of 354 patients where there were 317 malignant patients and 37 benign patients when compared to the definitive histology [79]. A small (8%) error rate in differentiating seminoma from nonseminoma occurred in this study with no clinical consequences. A smaller study of around 30 patients also had 100% accuracy for malignancy [80]. We would suggest that equivocal results do occur and that a figure around 98% in the hands of an experienced uropathologist is probably more accurate [59].

Informed consent is a very important part of the patient evaluation and assessment for PO. The organ preserving approach is not yet established for primary GCT management, so a surgeon should very carefully select the patients after evaluating their psycho emotional status. Every patient should be informed and consented for the possibility of total testicular removal if the decision to extend the procedure is made intraoperatively or reoperation for completion orchiectomy is recommended.

Treatment

Partial Orchiectomy: Technique

PO is usually performed under general anesthesia with the patient in the supine position. In the usual sterile manner including prepping the scrotum, a 4–5 cm incision is made along the Langerhans skin line about 2 cm above and parallel to the inguinal ligament. The initial steps are the same as radical orchiectomy. The subcutaneous fat is dissected to expose Scarpa's fascia which is incised to the level of the external oblique aponeurosis which in turn is incised towards the internal inguinal ring. The ileoinguinal nerve is identified, dissected free of the cord and preserved after identification. The cord is clamped with a rubber-shod clamp or Penrose tourniquet at the level of internal ring and the testicle is delivered from the scrotum into the wound, taking care to control small vessels. The gubernaculum attachments are divided with electrocautery or ligated. Before opening tunica vaginalis, the lesion is located in the testicle by palpation or with the help of the intraoperative US [75] (Fig. 9.2). Warm or cold ischemia remains controversial but if performed, Steiner and colleagues advocate immersion of the testis in crushed ice or slush for 5 min before spermatic cord occlusion [78, 81]. If FSE is planned, the wound should be covered before opening the tunica vaginalis and incising the parenchyma. An operating microscope with 6–25× magnification can be used to help identification of testis and tumor blood supply [75]. The tumor is enucleated with an attempt to preserve surrounding normal parenchyma. There are two possible scenarios after the result of the FSE. If the lesion appears to be benign, the vessels are unclamped and after ensuring hemostasis, the tunica albuginea is closed with running 4-0 or 5-0 absorbable suture. When the FSE is positive for malignancy and a decision is made to proceed with PO, some authors recommended multiple biopsies of the remaining tumor bed to rule out other possible malignant lesions or CIS [33]. Testicle is placed back in the scrotum without twisting or tension. After returning the testis to the scrotum, the external oblique aponeurosis is closed in a running fashion with absorbable sutures after thorough hemostasis. Scarpas' fascia is also closed with absorbable sutures. Skin is closed with 4-0 subcuticular sutures. Compressive scrotal support can minimize wound edema. The patient usually goes home the same day or may stay overnight.

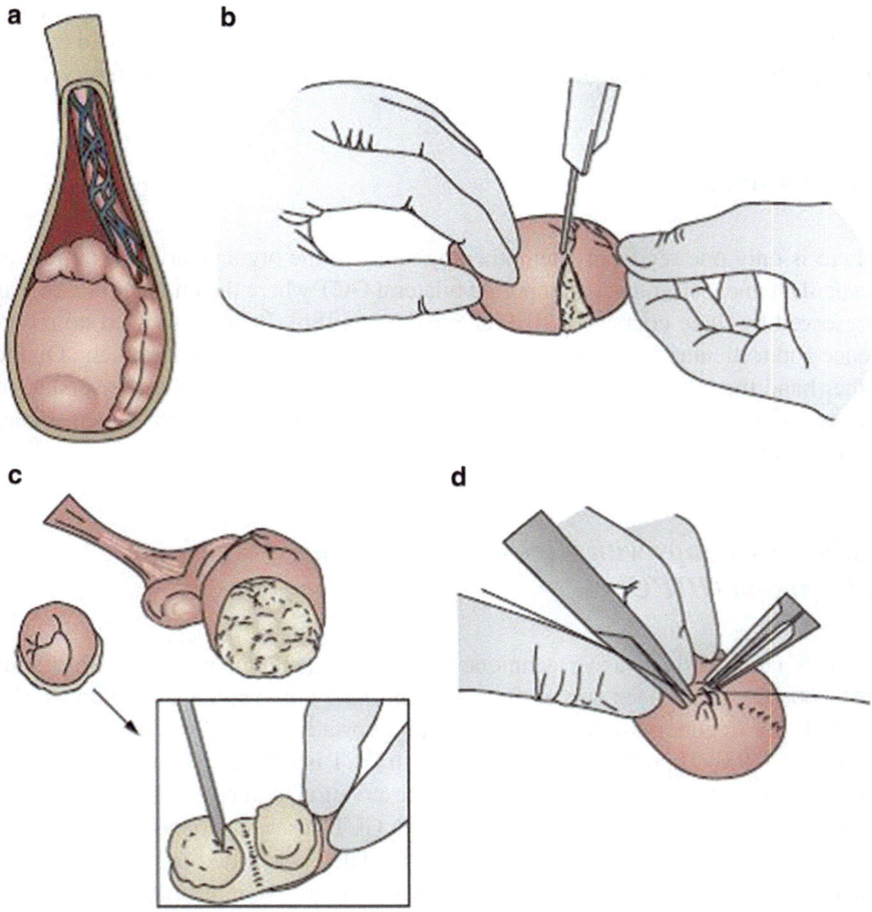

Fig. 9.2 Partial orchiectomy. After testis delivered through the inguinal incision (**a**), Penrose drain used for vascular control and incision is made of tunica albuginea (**b**), tumor is incised with up to 5 mm margin of normal testicular parenchyma (**c**). Tunica albuginea is repaired with absorbable sutures (**d**). Printed with permission of Nature Publishing Group. Alvaro Zuniga, Nathan Lawrentschuk and Michael A. S. Jewett. Organ-sparing approaches for testicular masses. Vol 7, Dec 31, 1969

Radiation

The well-known radiosensitivity of semonimas prompted several studies of treatment of primary GCT with radiation without PO [82, 83]. However, the required dose of radiation can affect hormone production and replacement therapy may be necessary. Previous studies showed that 33 Gy decrease testosterone levels in 50% of men [84]. At lower doses for CIS, there is a decline in testosterone production and 40% of men require required testosterone replacement [84, 85]. The high risk of testosterone replacement supports a surgical approach, but in selected cases radiation can be successfully used [82, 83]. Further dose-fractionation studies needed to optimize protocol of tumor eradication with acceptable hormone function preservation.

Chemotherapy

There is only one report of chemotherapy alone in the organ-sparing treatment of testicular cancer. Tomita et al. reported bilateral GCT where the unilateral testis was preserved by three courses of BEP chemotherapy [86]. Patients showed no recurrence and testicular preservation between 24 and 82 months after treatment. On the other hand the effect of chemotherapy in eradicating CIS is very controversial, so further studies with larger number of patients and longer follow-up needed to recommend chemotherapy as safe organ-sparing approach.

Ablative Therapy with High-Intensity Focused Ultrasound (HIFU)

HIFU is a minimally invasive technique to achieve coagulation necrosis of the tumor (90–100 °C). It has been successfully used in other applications in oncology, particularly for treatment of patients with rectal, prostate, breast, liver, and pancreatic tumors [87–93]. Therapeutic goal for HIFU in GCT is similar to that of local tumor excision in patients selected for organ-preservation strategy. The group from Germany have published their experience with GCT in seven patients with a solitary testis and mean follow-up of 42 months [94]. They performed transscrotal HIFU under general anesthesia with mean operative time of 31 min, followed 6 weeks later by prophylactic testicular irradiation (18–20 Gy). One patient received two cycles of chemotherapy for a single suspicious retroperitoneal lymph node diagnosed 6 months after HIFU. Other six patients remained tumor free at the mean follow-up of 42 (3–93) months. One patient who refused adjuvant radiation developed a recurrent tumor within 6 months was treated with radical orchiectomy. HIFU is a very promising treatment, producing necrosis without surgical trauma to the vascular anatomy and allows to preserve more gonadal function. But the downside of this would be lack of histological examination of the lesion.

Carcinoma In Situ Considerations

CIS is a malignant preinvasive testicular GCT [28, 33]. It is common in the nontumor part of the testis containing GCT and also seen in 5% of the contralateral testes. The cumulative probability for testicular tumor development in patients with CIS has been reported to be 50–70% after 5–7 years in Scandinavia [33, 95]. CIS has been reported to be significantly associated with poor spermatogenesis and with testicular atrophy, representing potentially impaired fertility [96]. The diagnosis of CIS at the time of PO or on permanent sections after the organ preserving procedure is challenging. Radiotherapy, chemotherapy, or surveillance are alternatives to completion radical orchiectomy [10, 97, 98].

Radiation treatment is commonly recommended, particularly in Europe. A total dose of 20 Gy (single doses of 2 Gy, five fractions per week) is recommended in the EAU guidelines [99]. Several groups have reported the results of adjuvant radiation after PO. The German Testicular Cancer Group did not observe local recurrence in 46 patients treated with adjuvant radiation but only 4 of 26 patients who did not receive radiation therapy had local recurrence [28]. This may compromise androgen production in up to 25% of men [100]. Lower doses, <20 Gy, were reported to have a variable impact on testosterone production but better preservation of Leydig cell function [10, 28, 84, 97, 100–104]. However, dose reduction may result in lower rates of complete CIS eradication. Radiotherapy may also destroy potential residual fertility, so it may be postponed in those who wish to father children as long as close surveillance is practiced [28]. The time between diagnosis of CIS and the development of a testicular tumor is usually long. This strategy was proposed by Heidenreich et al. who reported ten patients with concomitant CIS who postponed radiotherapy to father a child [28]. Five were successful with spontaneous pregnancy and five required vitro fertilization. Where radiation is undertaken, regular determination of the serum testosterone levels should be performed [97]. In case of clinical signs of androgen deficiency or subnormal testosterone levels hormone supplementation should be initiated.

Chemotherapy, particularly cisplatin-based has been reported to have some effect on CIS but the response can be variable because the cumulative risk of recurrent CIS at 10 years is 42% [105]. More recent publication from Kleinschmidt et al. reported a limited place for chemotherapy in CIS with a 63% failure rate on rebiopsy at 9 months post treatment [106].

Surveillance is the option that is frequently recommended, particularly in North America, for men who will be compliant with scheduled follow-up. Follow-up includes regular physician visits with scrotal US at yearly intervals.

Summary

Patients with palpable and nonpalpable testicular lesions may have benign rather than malignant tumors. The organ-sparing approach with partial orchiectomy is an option to preserve testicular function. The role for PO (partial orchiectomy) is less well established for malignant tumors but can be safely performed for solitary tumors, <2 cm in diameter when the blood supply to the remaining testis can be preserved. Residual androgen and fertility function is usually worth the risk of recurrence, which is low. Careful monitoring of the residual testis is required. The presence of CIS in the testis can complicate further management but adjuvant radiation is effective and can be delayed to allow for fertility.

References

1. Winter C, Albers P. Testicular germ cell tumors: pathogenesis, diagnosis and treatment. Nat Rev Endocrinol. 2011;7:43–53.
2. Lawrentschuk N, Zuniga A, Grabowksi AC, Rendon RA, Jewett MA. Partial orchiectomy for presumed malignancy in patients with a solitary testis due to a prior germ cell tumor: a large North American experience. J Urol. 2011;185:508–13.
3. Society AC. Cancer facts and figures 2011. Atlanta: American Cancer Society; 2011.
4. Pharris-Ciurej ND, Cook LS, Weiss NS. Incidence of testicular cancer in the United States: has the epidemic begun to abate? Am J Epidemiol. 1999;150:45–6.
5. Jemal A, Bray F, Center MM, Ferlay J, Ward E, Forman D. Global cancer statistics. CA Cancer J Clin. 2011;61:69–90.
6. International Germ Cell Consensus Classification: a prognostic factor-based staging system for metastatic germ cell cancers. International Germ Cell Cancer Collaborative Group. J Clin Oncol. 1997;15:594–603.
7. Zuniga A, Kakiashvili D, Jewett MA. Surveillance in stage I nonseminomatous germ cell tumours of the testis. BJU Int. 2009;104:1351–6.
8. Large MC, Sheinfeld J, Eggener SE. Retroperitoneal lymph node dissection: reassessment of modified templates. BJU Int. 2009;104:1369–75.
9. Lawrentschuk N, Webb DR. Inserting testicular prostheses: a new surgical technique for difficult cases. BJU Int. 2005;95:1111–4.
10. Bang AK, Petersen JH, Petersen PM, Andersson AM, Daugaard G, Jorgensen N. Testosterone production is better preserved after 16 than 20 Gray irradiation treatment against testicular carcinoma in situ cells. Int J Radiat Oncol Biol Phys. 2009;75:672–6.
11. Soh E, Berman LH, Grant JW, Bullock N, Williams MV. Ultrasound-guided core-needle biopsy of the testis for focal indeterminate intratesticular lesions. Eur Radiol. 2008;18:2990–6.
12. Richie J. Simultaneous bilateral tumors with unorthodox management. World J Urol. 1984;2:74–5.
13. Horstman WG, Haluszka MM, Burkhard TK. Management of testicular masses incidentally discovered by ultrasound. J Urol. 1994;151:1263–5.
14. Haas GP, Shumaker BP, Cerny JC. The high incidence of benign testicular tumors. J Urol. 1986;136:1219–20.
15. Kressel K, Schnell D, Thon WF, Heymer B, Hartmann M, Altwein JE. Benign testicular tumors: a case for testis preservation? Eur Urol. 1988;15:200–4.
16. Carmignani L, Gadda F, Gazzano G, et al. High incidence of benign testicular neoplasms diagnosed by ultrasound. J Urol. 2003;170:1783–6.
17. Carmignani L, Morabito A, Gadda F, Bozzini G, Rocco F, Colpi GM. Prognostic parameters in adult impalpable ultrasonographic lesions of the testicle. J Urol. 2005;174:1035–8.
18. Rogers DA, Rao BN, Meyer WH, et al. Indications for hemiscrotectomy in the management of genitourinary tumors in children. J Pediatr Surg. 1995;30:1437–9.
19. Eberhard J, Stahl O, Cwikiel M, et al. Risk factors for post-treatment hypogonadism in testicular cancer patients. Eur J Endocrinol. 2008;158:561–70.
20. Che M, Tamboli P, Ro JY, et al. Bilateral testicular germ cell tumors: twenty-year experience at M. D. Anderson Cancer Center. Cancer. 2002;95:1228–33.
21. Colls BM, Harvey VJ, Skelton L, Thompson PI, Frampton CM. Bilateral germ cell testicular tumors in New Zealand: experience in Auckland and Christchurch 1978–1994. J Clin Oncol. 1996;14:2061–5.

22. Osterlind A, Berthelsen JG, Abildgaard N, et al. Risk of bilateral testicular germ cell cancer in Denmark: 1960–1984. J Natl Cancer Inst. 1991;83:1391–5.
23. Fossa SD, Opjordsmoen S, Haug E. Androgen replacement and quality of life in patients treated for bilateral testicular cancer. Eur J Cancer. 1999;35:1220–5.
24. Holzbeierlein JM, Sogani PC, Sheinfeld J. Histology and clinical outcomes in patients with bilateral testicular germ cell tumors: the Memorial Sloan Kettering Cancer Center experience 1950 to 2001. J Urol. 2003;169:2122–5.
25. Tekin A, Aygun YC, Aki FT, Ozen H. Bilateral germ cell cancer of the testis: a report of 11 patients with a long-term follow-up. BJU Int. 2000;85:864–8.
26. Heidenreich A, Bonfig R, Derschum W, von Vietsch H, Wilbert DM. A conservative approach to bilateral testicular germ cell tumors. J Urol. 1995;153:10–3.
27. Heidenreich A, Holtl W, Albrecht W, Pont J, Engelmann UH. Testis-preserving surgery in bilateral testicular germ cell tumours. Br J Urol. 1997;79:253–7.
28. Heidenreich A, Weissbach L, Holtl W, et al. Organ sparing surgery for malignant germ cell tumor of the testis. J Urol. 2001;166:2161–5.
29. Houlgatte A, De La Taille A, Fournier R, Goluboff ET, Camporo P, Houdelette P. Paternity in a patient with seminoma and carcinoma in situ in a solitary testis treated by partial orchidectomy. BJU Int. 1999;84:374–5.
30. Kazem I, Danella JF. Organ preservation for the treatment of contralateral testicular seminoma. Radiother Oncol. 1999;53:45–7.
31. Sawyer EJ, Oliver RT, Tobias JS, Badenoch DF. A lesson in the management of testicular cancer in a patient with a solitary testis. Postgrad Med J. 1999;75:481–3.
32. Weissbach L. Organ preserving surgery of malignant germ cell tumors. J Urol. 1995;153:90–3.
33. Dieckmann KP, Skakkebaek NE. Carcinoma in situ of the testis: review of biological and clinical features. Int J Cancer. 1999;83:815–22.
34. McGlynn KA, Cook MB. Etiologic factors in testicular germ-cell tumors. Future Oncol. 2009;5:1389–402.
35. Greene MH, Kratz CP, Mai PL, et al. Familial testicular germ cell tumors in adults: 2010 summary of genetic risk factors and clinical phenotype. Endocr Relat Cancer. 2010;17:R109–21.
36. Purdue MP, Engel LS, Langseth H, et al. Prediagnostic serum concentrations of organochlorine compounds and risk of testicular germ cell tumors. Environ Health Perspect. 2009;117:1514–9.
37. Giannandrea F, Gandini L, Paoli D, Turci R, Figa-Talamanca I. Pesticide exposure and serum organochlorine residuals among testicular cancer patients and healthy controls. J Environ Sci Health B. 2011;46:780–7.
38. Forman D, Oliver RT, Brett AR, et al. Familial testicular cancer: a report of the UK family register, estimation of risk and an HLA class 1 sib-pair analysis. Br J Cancer. 1992;65: 255–62.
39. Heimdal K, Olsson H, Tretli S, Flodgren P, Borresen AL, Fossa SD. Risk of cancer in relatives of testicular cancer patients. Br J Cancer. 1996;73:970–3.
40. Swerdlow AJ, De Stavola BL, Swanwick MA, Maconochie NE. Risks of breast and testicular cancers in young adult twins in England and Wales: evidence on prenatal and genetic aetiology. Lancet. 1997;350:1723–8.
41. Mostofi FK. Proceedings: testicular tumors. Epidemiologic, etiologic, and pathologic features. Cancer. 1973;32:1186–201.
42. Schottenfeld D, Warshauer ME, Sherlock S, Zauber AG, Leder M, Payne R. The epidemiology of testicular cancer in young adults. Am J Epidemiol. 1980;112:232–46.
43. Henderson BE, Benton B, Jing J, Yu MC, Pike MC. Risk factors for cancer of the testis in young men. Int J Cancer. 1979;23:598–602.
44. Farrer JH, Walker AH, Rajfer J. Management of the postpubertal cryptorchid testis: a statistical review. J Urol. 1985;134:1071–6.
45. Berthelsen JG, Skakkebaek NE, von der Maase H, Sorensen BL, Mogensen P. Screening for carcinoma in situ of the contralateral testis in patients with germinal testicular cancer. Br Med J (Clin Res Ed). 1982;285:1683–6.

46. Raman JD, Nobert CF, Goldstein M. Increased incidence of testicular cancer in men presenting with infertility and abnormal semen analysis. J Urol. 2005;174:1819–22. discussion 22.
47. Richie JP. Detection and treatment of testicular cancer. CA Cancer J Clin. 1993;43:151–75.
48. Hansen PV, Trykker H, Andersen J, Helkjaer PE. Germ cell function and hormonal status in patients with testicular cancer. Cancer. 1989;64:956–61.
49. Petersen PM, Skakkebaek NE, Vistisen K, Rorth M, Giwercman A. Semen quality and reproductive hormones before orchiectomy in men with testicular cancer. J Clin Oncol. 1999;17: 941–7.
50. Dieckmann KP, Linke J, Pichlmeier U, Kulejewski M, Loy V. Spermatogenesis in the contralateral testis of patients with testicular germ cell cancer: histological evaluation of testicular biopsies and a comparison with healthy males. BJU Int. 2007;99:1079–85.
51. Jones GY, Payne S. Searching for safety signals: the experience of medical surveillance amongst men with testicular teratomas. Psychooncology. 2000;9:385–94.
52. Moynihan C. Testicular cancer: the psychosocial problems of patients and their relatives. Cancer Surv. 1987;6:477–510.
53. Arai Y, Kawakita M, Hida S, Terachi T, Okada Y, Yoshida O. Psychosocial aspects in long-term survivors of testicular cancer. J Urol. 1996;155:574–8.
54. Dahl AA, Haaland CF, Mykletun A, et al. Study of anxiety disorder and depression in long-term survivors of testicular cancer. J Clin Oncol. 2005;23:2389–95.
55. Rieker PP, Fitzgerald EM, Kalish LA, et al. Psychosocial factors, curative therapies, and behavioral outcomes. A comparison of testis cancer survivors and a control group of healthy men. Cancer. 1989;64:2399–407.
56. Rifkin MD, Kurtz AB, Pasto ME, Goldberg BB. Diagnostic capabilities of high-resolution scrotal ultrasonography: prospective evaluation. J Ultrasound Med. 1985;4:13–9.
57. Bhatt S, Jafri SZ, Wasserman N, Dogra VS. Imaging of non-neoplastic intratesticular masses. Diagn Interv Radiol. 2011;17:52–63.
58. Carkaci S, Ozkan E, Lane D, Yang WT. Scrotal sonography revisited. J Clin Ultrasound. 2010;38:21–37.
59. Kirkham AP, Kumar P, Minhas S, et al. Targeted testicular excision biopsy: when and how should we try to avoid radical orchidectomy? Clin Radiol. 2009;64:1158–65.
60. Dogra VS, Gottlieb RH, Rubens DJ, Liao L. Benign intratesticular cystic lesions: US features. Radiographics. 2001;21(Spec No):S273–81.
61. Cho JH, Chang JC, Park BH, Lee JG, Son CH. Sonographic and MR imaging findings of testicular epidermoid cysts. AJR Am J Roentgenol. 2002;178:743–8.
62. Hilton S. Contemporary radiological imaging of testicular cancer. BJU Int. 2009;104:1339–45.
63. Hindley RG, Chandra A, Saunders A, O'Brien TS. Impalpable testis cancer. BJU Int. 2003;92:572–4.
64. Comiter CV, Benson CJ, Capelouto CC, et al. Nonpalpable intratesticular masses detected sonographically. J Urol. 1995;154:1367–9.
65. Ishida M, Hasegawa M, Kanao K, Oyama M, Nakajima Y. Non-palpable testicular embryonal carcinoma diagnosed by ultrasound: a case report. Jpn J Clin Oncol. 2009;39:124–6.
66. Powell TM, Tarter TH. Management of nonpalpable incidental testicular masses. J Urol. 2006;176:96–8. discussion 9.
67. DeCastro BJ, Peterson AC, Costabile RA. A 5-year followup study of asymptomatic men with testicular microlithiasis. J Urol. 2008;179:1420–3. discussion 3.
68. Goedecker S, Teter M, Hutter J. Separable dual-space Gaussian pseudopotentials. Phys Rev B. 1996;54:1703–10.
69. Parenti GC, Zago S, Lusa M, Campioni P, Mannella P. Association between testicular microlithiasis and primary malignancy of the testis: our experience and review of the literature. Radiol Med. 2007;112:588–96.
70. Parenti GC, Feletti F, Brandini F, et al. Imaging of the scrotum: role of MRI. Radiol Med. 2009;114:414–24.
71. Kim W, Rosen MA, Langer JE, Banner MP, Siegelman ES, Ramchandani P. US MR imaging correlation in pathologic conditions of the scrotum. Radiographics. 2007;27:1239–53.

72. Shannon BA, Cohen RJ, de Bruto H, Davies RJ. The value of preoperative needle core biopsy for diagnosing benign lesions among small, incidentally detected renal masses. J Urol. 2008;180:1257–61. discussion 61.
73. Capelouto CC, Clark PE, Ransil BJ, Loughlin KR. A review of scrotal violation in testicular cancer: is adjuvant local therapy necessary? J Urol. 1995;153:981–5.
74. Giguere JK, Stablein DM, Spaulding JT, McLeod DG, Paulson DF, Weiss RB. The clinical significance of unconventional orchiectomy approaches in testicular cancer: a report from the Testicular Cancer Intergroup Study. J Urol. 1988;139:1225–8.
75. Hopps CV, Goldstein M. Ultrasound guided needle localization and microsurgical exploration for incidental nonpalpable testicular tumors. J Urol. 2002;168:1084–7.
76. Heidenreich A. Contralateral testicular biopsy in testis cancer: current concepts and controversies. BJU Int. 2009;104:1346–50.
77. Berney DM. Staging and classification of testicular tumours: pitfalls from macroscopy to diagnosis. J Clin Pathol. 2008;61:20–4.
78. Steiner H, Holtl L, Maneschg C, et al. Frozen section analysis-guided organ-sparing approach in testicular tumors: technique, feasibility, and long-term results. Urology. 2003;62:508–13.
79. Elert A, Olbert P, Hegele A, Barth P, Hofmann R, Heidenreich A. Accuracy of frozen section examination of testicular tumors of uncertain origin. Eur Urol. 2002;41:290–3.
80. Tokuc R, Sakr W, Pontes JE, Haas GP. Accuracy of frozen section examination of testicular tumors. Urology. 1992;40:512–6.
81. Billmire DF. Germ cell tumors. Surg Clin North Am. 2006;86:489–503. xi.
82. Bos SD, Ypma AF. Synchronous bilateral seminoma testis treated with unilateral orchiectomy and contralateral irradiation: a therapeutic option. Scand J Urol Nephrol. 1993;27:559–61.
83. Chung PW, Jewett MA, Warde PR. Testicular radiation for primary seminoma in a solitary testis. Can J Urol. 2006;13:2975–7.
84. Petersen PM, Giwercman A, Daugaard G, et al. Effect of graded testicular doses of radiotherapy in patients treated for carcinoma-in-situ in the testis. J Clin Oncol. 2002;20:1537–43.
85. Izard MA. Leydig cell function and radiation: a review of the literature. Radiother Oncol. 1995;34:1–8.
86. Tomita E, Kondo T, Nakazawa H, Ito F, Hashimoto Y, Tanabe K. Successful testis preservation for bilateral testicular tumors with a new chemotherapy-based protocol: initial results of three cases. Int J Urol. 2007;14:879–82.
87. Wang X, Sun J. High-intensity focused ultrasound in patients with late-stage pancreatic carcinoma. Chin Med J (Engl). 2002;115:1332–5.
88. Blana A, Walter B, Rogenhofer S, Wieland WF. High-intensity focused ultrasound for the treatment of localized prostate cancer: 5-year experience. Urology. 2004;63:297–300.
89. Jun-Qun Z, Guo-Min W, Bo Y, Gong-Xian W, Shen-Xu H. Short-term results of 89 cases of rectal carcinoma treated with high-intensity focused ultrasound and low-dose radiotherapy. Ultrasound Med Biol. 2004;30:57–60.
90. Hwang JJ, Walther MM, Pautler SE, et al. Radio frequency ablation of small renal tumors: intermediate results. J Urol. 2004;171:1814–8.
91. Uchida T, Ohkusa H, Yamashita H, et al. Five years experience of transrectal high-intensity focused ultrasound using the Sonablate device in the treatment of localized prostate cancer. Int J Urol. 2006;13:228–33.
92. Wu F, Wang ZB, Cao YD, et al. A randomised clinical trial of high-intensity focused ultrasound ablation for the treatment of patients with localised breast cancer. Br J Cancer. 2003;89:2227–33.
93. Wu F, Wang ZB, Chen WZ, et al. Extracorporeal high intensity focused ultrasound ablation in the treatment of patients with large hepatocellular carcinoma. Ann Surg Oncol. 2004;11:1061–9.
94. Kratzik C, Schatzl G, Lackner J, Marberger M. Transcutaneous high-intensity focused ultrasonography can cure testicular cancer in solitary testis. Urology. 2006;67:1269–73.

95. Hoei-Hansen CE, Rajpert-De Meyts E, Daugaard G, Skakkebaek NE. Carcinoma in situ testis, the progenitor of testicular germ cell tumours: a clinical review. Ann Oncol. 2005;16:863–8.
96. Dieckmann KP, Kulejewski M, Pichlmeier U, Loy V. Diagnosis of contralateral testicular intraepithelial neoplasia (TIN) in patients with testicular germ cell cancer: systematic two-site biopsies are more sensitive than a single random biopsy. Eur Urol. 2007;51:175–83. discussion 83–5.
97. Krege S, Beyer J, Souchon R, et al. European consensus conference on diagnosis and treatment of germ cell cancer: a report of the second meeting of the European Germ Cell Cancer Consensus group (EGCCCG): part I. Eur Urol. 2008;53:478–96.
98. Krege S, Beyer J, Souchon R, et al. European consensus conference on diagnosis and treatment of germ cell cancer: a report of the second meeting of the European Germ Cell Cancer Consensus Group (EGCCCG): part II. Eur Urol. 2008;53:497–513.
99. Albers P, Albrecht W, Algaba F, et al. EAU guidelines on testicular cancer: 2011 update. Eur Urol. 2011;60:304–19.
100. Giwercman A, von der Maase H, Berthelsen JG, Rorth M, Bertelsen A, Skakkebaek NE. Localized irradiation of testes with carcinoma in situ: effects on Leydig cell function and eradication of malignant germ cells in 20 patients. J Clin Endocrinol Metab. 1991;73:596–603.
101. Petersen PM, Daugaard G, Rorth M, Skakkebaek NE. Endocrine function in patients treated for carcinoma in situ in the testis with irradiation. APMIS. 2003;111:93–8. discussion 8–9.
102. Grigsby PW, Perez CA. The effects of external beam radiotherapy on endocrine function in patients with carcinoma of the prostate. J Urol. 1986;135:726–7.
103. Nader S, Schultz PN, Cundiff JH, Hussey DH, Samaan NA. Endocrine profiles of patients with testicular tumors treated with radiotherapy. Int J Radiat Oncol Biol Phys. 1983;9:1723–6.
104. Shalet SM, Tsatsoulis A, Whitehead E, Read G. Vulnerability of the human Leydig cell to radiation damage is dependent upon age. J Endocrinol. 1989;120:161–5.
105. Christensen TB, Daugaard G, Geertsen PF, von der Maase H. Effect of chemotherapy on carcinoma in situ of the testis. Ann Oncol. 1998;9:657–60.
106. Kleinschmidt K, Dieckmann KP, Georgiew A, Loy V, Weissbach L. Chemotherapy is of limited efficacy in the control of contralateral testicular intraepithelial neoplasia in patients with testicular germ cell cancer. Oncology. 2009;77:33–9.

Chapter 10
Robotic Microsurgery for Male Infertility

Sijo J. Parekattil, Ahmet Gudeloglu, and Jamin V. Brahmbhatt

Abstract Surgical management of male infertility began with a microsurgical approach starting in 1975 when a Zeiss operating microscope was used to fashion a two-layer vasovasostomy, achieving a higher vasal patency rate and pregnancy rate than that achieved with non-microscopic repair [1, 2]. In an attempt to further promote enhanced microsurgical efficiency, ease of performance and enhanced reproducible precision, the use of robotic-assisted microsurgery is being explored. This chapter presents a detailed description of the robotic-assisted surgical techniques that we have developed for vasovasostomy, vasoepididymostomy, varicocelectomy, and testicular sperm extraction (TESE). Preliminary outcomes from our early series of approximately 300 procedures are presented.

Keywords Robotic vasectomy reversal • Vasovasostomy • Vasoepididymostomy • Varicocelectomy • Testicular sperm extraction

S.J. Parekattil, M.D. (✉) • A. Gudeloglu, M.D.
Department of Urology, Winter Haven Hospital and University of Florida, 200 Avenue F.N.E, Winter Haven, FL 33881, USA
e-mail: sijo.parekattil@winterhavenhospital.org

J.V. Brahmbhatt, M.D.
Department of Urology, University of Tennessee Health Science Center, 910 Madison Avenue, Suite 409, Memphis, TN 38163, USA
e-mail: jaminbrahmbhatt@gmail.com

J.I. Sandlow (ed.), *Microsurgery for Fertility Specialists: A Practical Text*,
DOI 10.1007/978-1-4614-4196-0_10, © Springer Science+Business Media New York 2013

Introduction

From the very early use of the microscope for microsurgery [2], there has been an increase in its use for the operative management of male infertility [1–11]. Achieving greater fertility rates and vas patency after vasovasostomy [12] has made its use a standard for the male infertility microsurgeon. Other applications include the use of the microscope for subinguinal varicocelectomy and testicular sperm extraction (TESE). Most of these techniques require a great degree of microsurgical training and a skilled surgical assistant. Our goal was to explore the use of robotic assistance for such microsurgical procedures to assess if the use of a stable, scalable, enhanced magnification platform would provide any measurable benefits to the microsurgeon. This chapter focuses on a few specific procedures that we have developed: Robotic-assisted microsurgical vasovasostomy, vasoepididymostomy, subinguinal varicocelectomy, and micro-TESE.

Preoperative Preparation

Prior to date of surgery blood thinners, aspirin or vitamin E, are appropriately held. A broad-spectrum antibiotic such as cefazolin is administered intravenously at least 30 min before skin incision. Mechanical lower extremity compression stockings are initiated for prevention of deep venous thrombosis in the preoperative area.

Operative Setup and Patient Positioning

Figure 10.1 illustrates the operative setup with the four-armed da Vinci Si system. A large high definition monitor at the foot of the patient allows the surgical assistant and the nursing team to visualize the operative field and prepare instruments and suture for each step of the procedure. The patient is placed in a supine position and prepped and draped in a standard surgical fashion. Skin incisions are made and appropriate operative tissues are exposed. The arms of the patient may be placed apart on arm boards with adequate padding to prevent any nerve compression injuries.

The robot is brought in from the right side of the patient in all our cases. Figures 10.1 and 10.2 illustrate the trocar placement and robotic arm placement. Trocars are loaded to allow the instruments to function and to stabilize their movements outside the patient's body. To optimize range of motion the instruments should be advanced 4–5 cm beyond the tip of the trocar. The fourth robotic arm may be placed lateral to the left robotic arm to minimize instrument clashes. A zero degree camera lens is used to optimize the visual field. An additional fifth arm (nitrogen powered, Karl-Storz, Inc., Tuttlingen) is utilized to hold a high definition camera (VITOM, Karl-Storz, Inc., Tuttlingen) with enhanced optical magnification

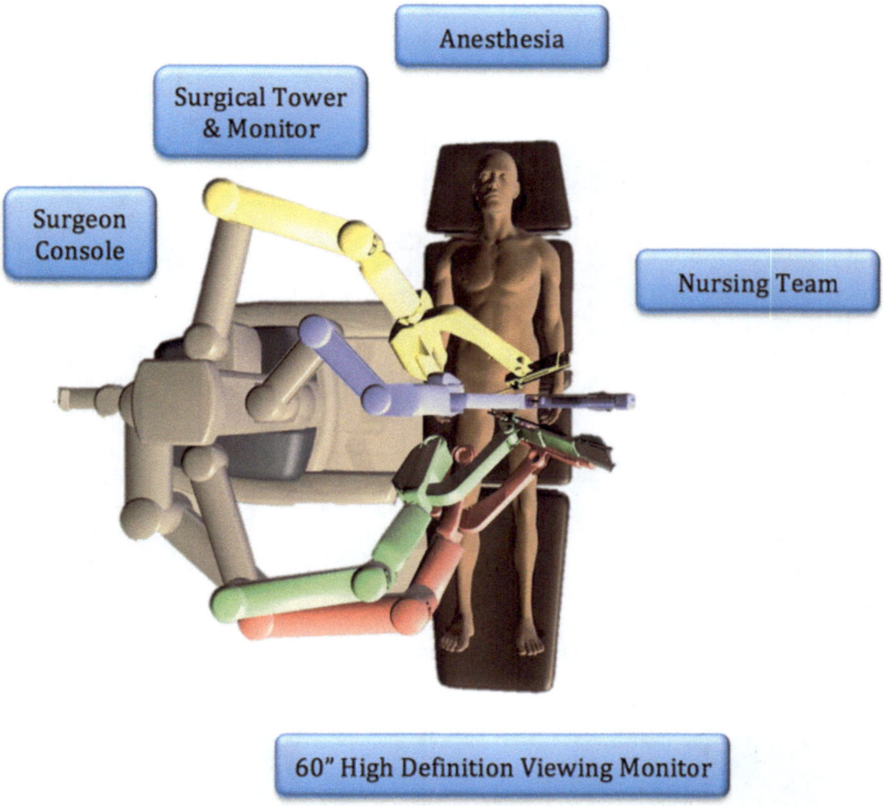

Fig. 10.1 Operative setup for robotic microsurgery cases

(16–18×) that provides the surgeon dual enhanced magnification views in the surgeon console (Fig. 10.3). This provides the surgeon with dual views of the operative field. If the case requires microscopic examination of fluid or tissues (for example examining the fluid from the proximal vas in a vasectomy reversal or examining tissue for any sperm in micro-TESE), an additional view of the microscopic field from the andrologist/embryologist's microscope can also be fed into the surgeon console so that the microsurgeon has all three views simultaneously as shown in Fig. 10.3.

Robotic-Assisted Microsurgical Vasovasostomy

Technique

The proximal and distal (beyond the previous vasectomy site) vas deferens is palpated through the scrotal skin. Through the scrotal skin the distal vas is fixed into

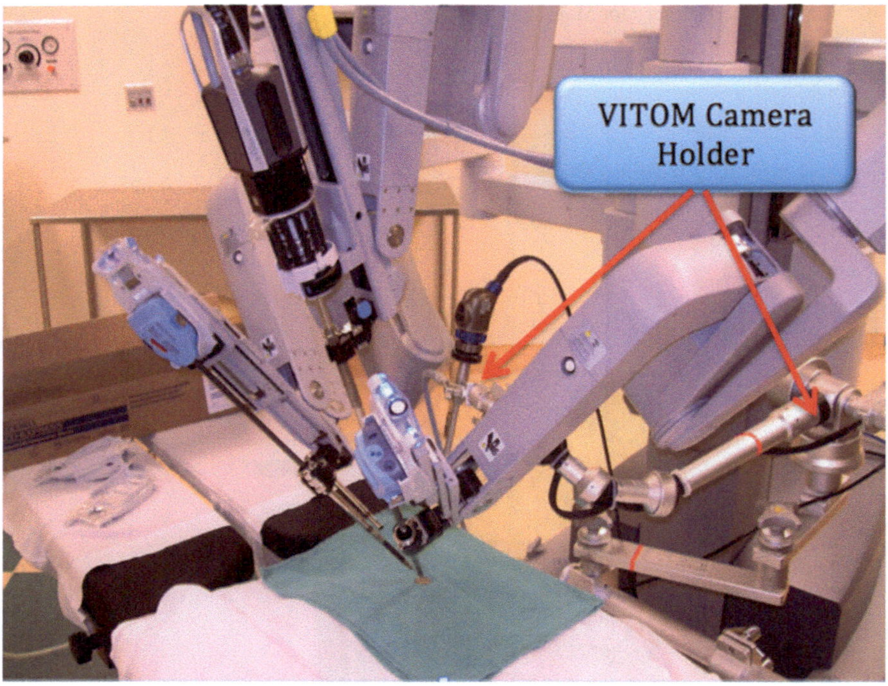

Fig. 10.2 Trocar, robotic arm, and VITOM camera placement

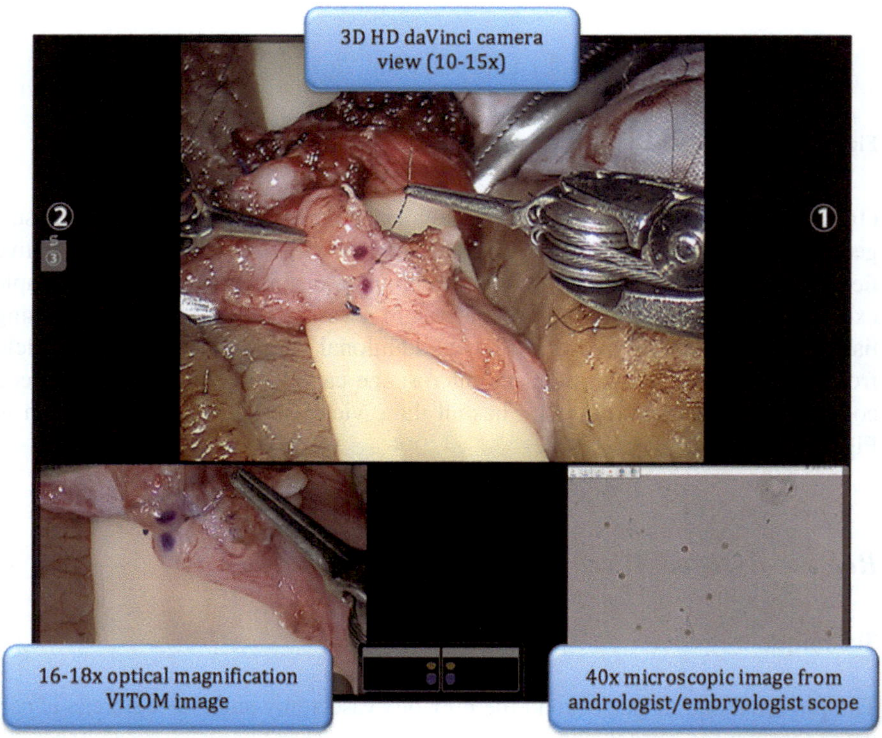

Fig. 10.3 Tri-view for the robotic microsurgeon in the surgeon console

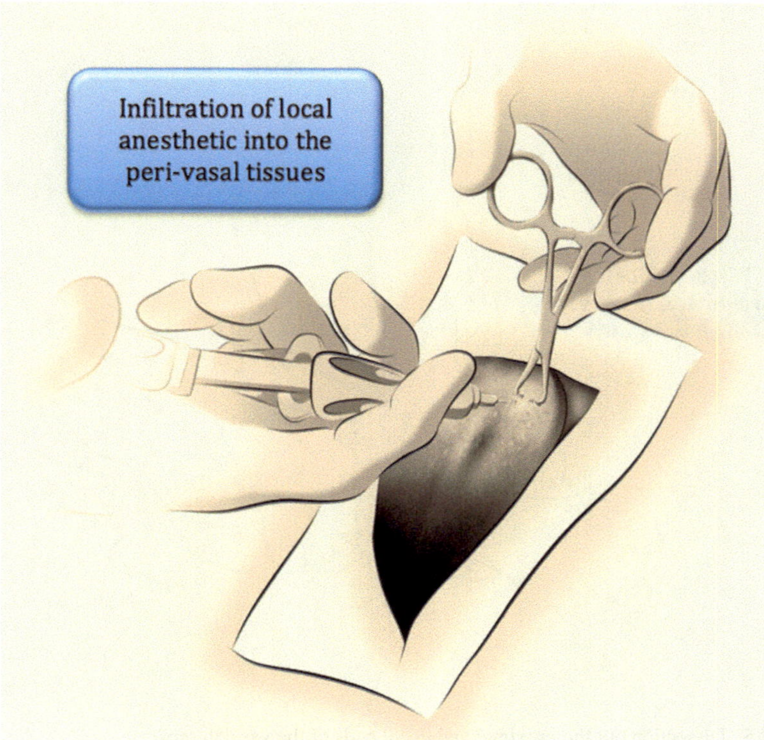

Fig. 10.4 Securing the left-sided previous vasectomy site and infiltration of local anesthesia

place with a towel clip. Local anesthesia is infiltrated into this area (Fig. 10.4). Using a #15 blade a 1–2 cm vertical incision is made over the vas starting inferiorly from the previously placed towel clip. Using fine electrocautery and sharp dissection the distal and proximal ends of the vas are dissected free (Fig. 10.5).

The proximal vas is carefully transected with an #11 blade. Efflux from the lumen is expressed and collected on a glass slide. Phase contrast microscopy is used to assess for the presence of sperm on the slides. If there is any sperm found or the efflux is copious and clear or milky, then a vasovasostomy is performed. If the efflux has no sperm and is thick and pasty, then a vasoepididymostomy is performed (described in the next section). The distal end of the vas is now transected. The two clean ends of the vas are now approximated to each other to confirm a tension-free anastomosis. The adventitia from either end of the vasa is now secured together with a 3-0 prolene suture to create a tension-free anastomosis.

The robot is now positioned to perform the microsurgical vasovasostomy. The left side vasovasostomy is generally performed first. Black diamond micro-forceps are loaded on the right and left robot arms. The zero degree camera lens is loaded onto the robot camera arm. The micro-Potts scissors are loaded onto the fourth robot arm. The two ends of the vas are placed over a 1/4″ Penrose drain. The assistant

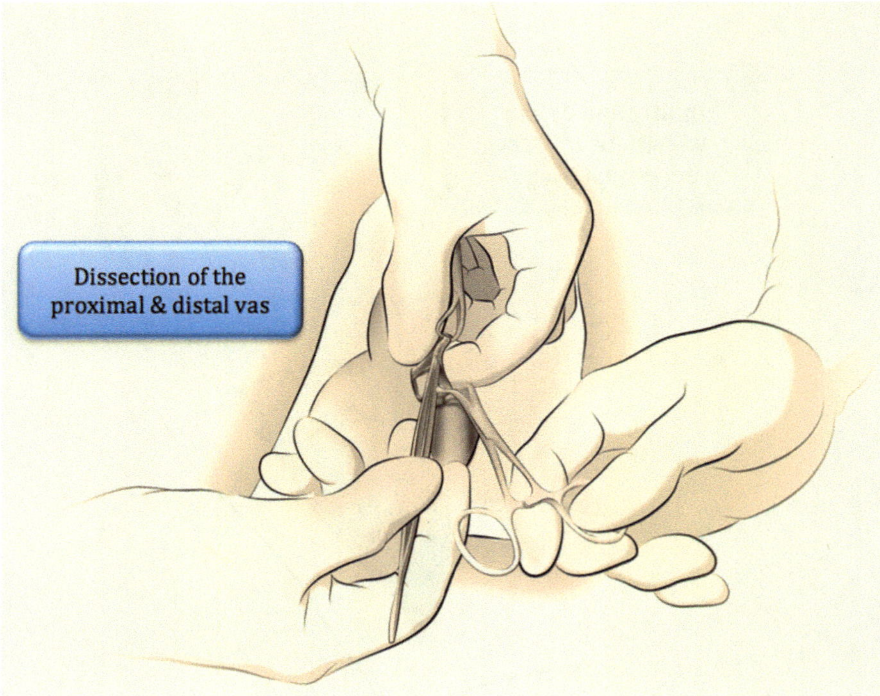

Fig. 10.5 Dissection out the proximal and distal ends of the vas deferens

irrigates the field with saline using a 10 cc syringe with an 18-gauge angiocatheter tip. Weck sponge sticks are used to dry the field.

The assistant now passes the 9-0 nylon suture that is kept in its inner packaging to the surgical field. The suture is grasped using the black diamond right hand grasper and cut to about 2 in. length using the micro-Potts scissors (left hand fourth arm). The 9-0 nylon suture is held and manipulated using the black diamond forceps in both left and right arms as needle drivers. Posterior muscularis layer of the two ends of the vas is now approximated (Fig. 10.6). Suture is cut using the micro-Potts scissors.

Two or three double-armed 10-0 nylon sutures are now placed to reanastomose the posterior mucosal lumen of the vas (Figs. 10.7 and 10.8). The sutures are placed inside out to ensure good mucosal approximation. All sutures are placed before they are tied.

Three double-armed 10-0 nylon sutures are used to close the anterior mucosal lumen of the vas. Five to six 9-0 nylon sutures are used to approximate the anterior muscularis layer of the vas. The Penrose drain is gently removed from under the repair. The vas is placed back into the scrotal cavity. The same procedure is now performed on the contralateral right side by repositioning the robot away from the patient to the right scrotum.

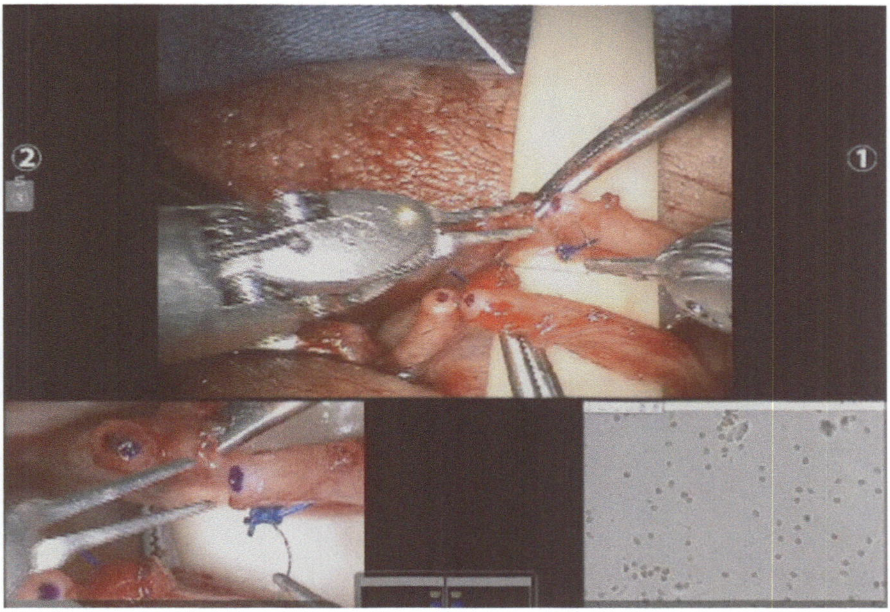

Fig. 10.6 Posterior 9-0 Nylon sutures to reapproximate the posterior muscularis layer

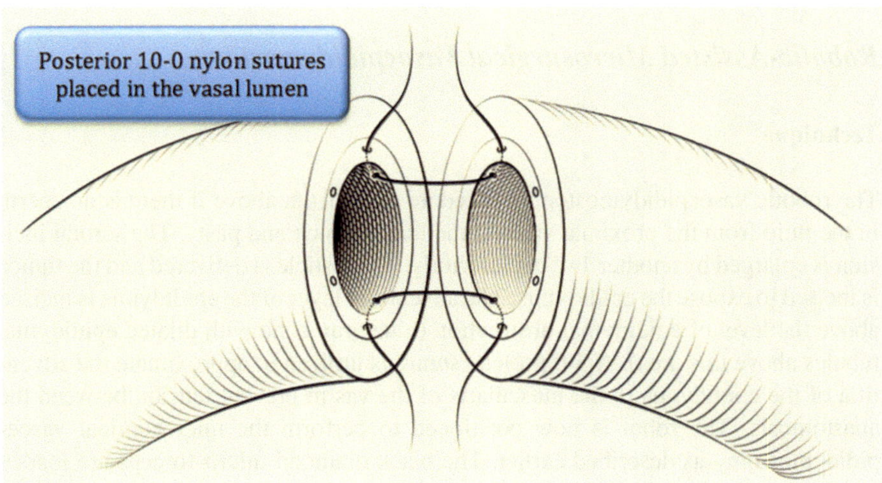

Fig. 10.7 Posterior 10-0 nylon sutures placed to reapproximate the vasal lumen (illustration)

The dartos layer is closed using a running 3-0 chromic suture. The skin is closed using a 5-0 vicryl running suture. Bacitracin ointment is applied over the incision. Fluff dressing with athletic scrotal support is applied. An ice pack is carefully applied to the scrotum in the recovery room.

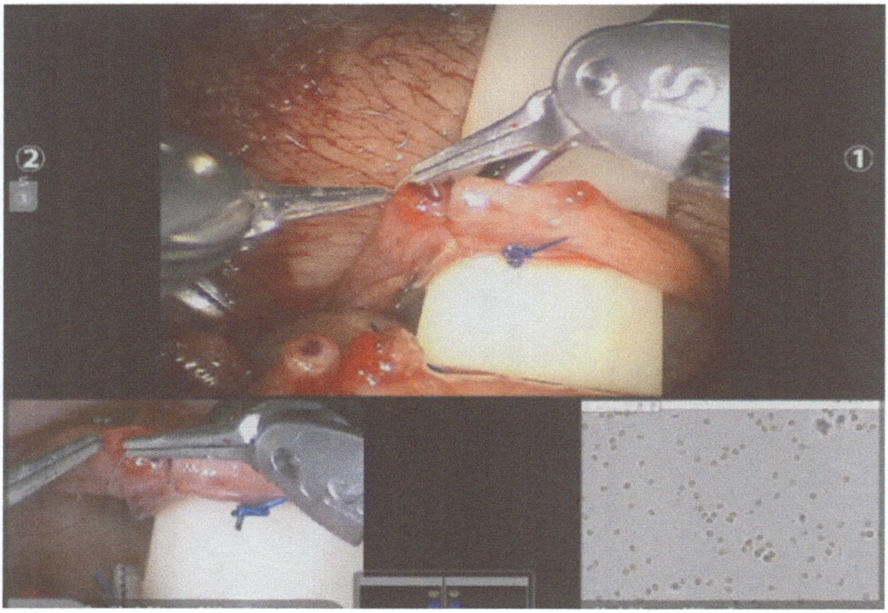

Fig. 10.8 Posterior 10-0 nylon sutures placed to reapproximate the vasal lumen (Intraoperative image)

Robotic-Assisted Microsurgical Vasoepididymostomy

Technique

The robotic vasoepididymostomy procedure starts from above if there is no sperm in the fluid from the proximal vas and the fluid is thick and pasty. The scrotal incision is enlarged by another 1–2 cm inferiorly. The testicle is delivered and the tunica is incised to expose the epididymis. The adventitial layer of the epididymis is incised above the level of epididymal obstruction (blue/gray zone with dilated epididymal tubules above this area). A 3-0 prolene suture is utilized to approximate the adventitia of the epididymis to the muscularis of the vas to prevent tension between the anastomosis. The robot is now positioned to perform the microsurgical vasoepididymostomy as described earlier. The black diamond micro-forceps are loaded on the right and left robot arms. The zero degree camera lens is loaded onto the robot camera arm. An ophthalmologic microblade is held in the fourth arm with black diamond micro-forceps or a Potts scissor may be used in the fourth arm. Two 10-0 nylon double-armed suture needles are placed longitudinally through a single epididymal tubule to expose the tubule (Fig. 10.9). This tubule is then incised longitudinally using the microblade between the two suture needles to create a lumen in the tubule. Alternatively, the tubule may be incised with a Potts scissor in the fourth robotic arm. The fluid is then aspirated (Fig. 10.10) and then examined under a separate phase contrast microscope for the presence of sperm.

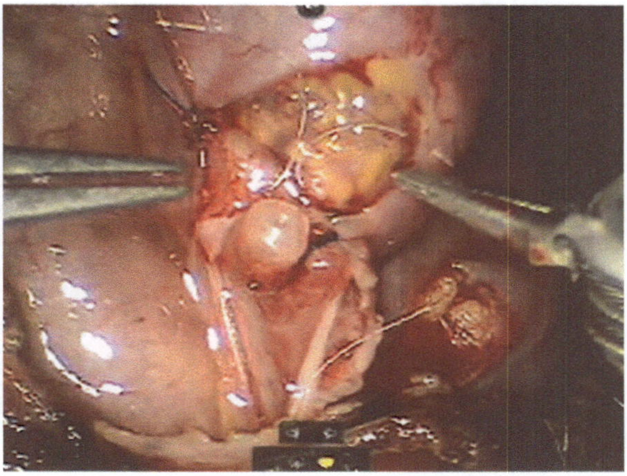

Fig. 10.9 Longitudinal intussusception vasoepididymostomy with dual armed 10-0 nylon sutures

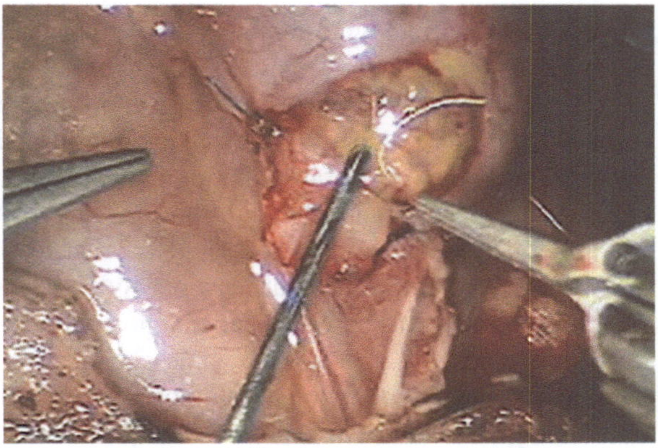

Fig. 10.10 Epididymal tubule is incised and the fluid expressed is aspirated for microscopic examination

The two double-armed 10-0 nylon needles in the epididymal tubule are advanced through and then all four of the needle ends are brought inside out on the vas mucosal lumen to involute the epididymal tubule lumen into the vas lumen. Five to six 9-0 nylon sutures are placed circumferentially to approximate the muscularis of the vas to the adventitia of the epididymal tubule (Fig. 10.11). The testicle and anastomosis are carefully delivered back into the scrotum. The dartos layer is closed using a running 3-0 chromic suture. The skin is closed using a 4-0 chromic running suture. Bacitracin ointment is applied over the incision. Fluff dressing with athletic scrotal support is applied. An ice pack is carefully applied to the scrotum in the recovery room.

Outcomes

Previous studies have shown the possible benefit in the use of robotic assistance during microsurgical procedures. Our goal was to compare robotic-assisted vasovasostomy

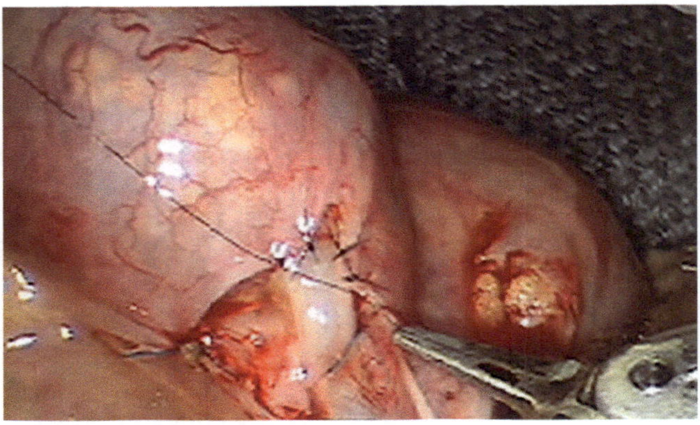

Fig. 10.11 Five to six 9-0 nylon sutures are placed circumferentially to approximate the muscularis of the vas to the adventitia of the epididymal tubule

(RAVV) and vasoepididymostomy (RAVE) to standard microsurgical vasovasostomy (MVV) and vasoepididymostomy (MVE).

A prospective control trial of 145 vasectomy reversal cases was performed from August 2007 to November 2011 by a single fellowship trained microsurgeon. The primary end point was operative duration. The secondary end point was total motile sperm count at 2, 5, 9, and 12 months postoperatively. Case breakdown was as such: 59 cases bilateral RAVV, 41 cases RAVE on at least one side, 28 cases bilateral MVV, and 17 cases MVE on at least one side. Selection of approach (robotic vs. pure microscopic) was based on patient choice. Preoperative patient characteristics were similar in both groups. The same suture materials and suturing techniques (two-layer 10-0 and 9-0 nylon anastomosis for vasovasostomy; 10-0 nylon double-armed longitudinal intussusception technique for vasoepididymostomy) were used in both approaches.

Median clinical follow-up was 16.5 months (range 1–50 months). 98% patency was achieved in the RAVV cases and 80% in MVV (>1 million sperm/high power field). Median operative duration was significantly decreased in RAVV at 90 min (40–180) compared to MVV at 120 min (60–180), $p=0.0002$. RAVE at 120 min (60–180) was significantly faster than MVE at 161 min (120–240), $p=0.0005$. Mean postoperative total motile sperm counts were not significantly higher in RAVV/RAVE versus MVV/MVE, but the rate of postoperative sperm count recovery was significantly greater in RAVV/RAVE. The improved efficiency and eliminated need for a skilled assistant in RAVV/RAVE has reduced the cost of this reversal procedure to less than the regional average cost for MVV/MVE.

The use of robotic assistance in microsurgical vasovasostomy and vasoepididymostomy may have potential benefit over MVV and MVE with regards to decreasing operative duration and improving the rate of recovery of postoperative total motile sperm counts. Further evaluation and longer follow-up is needed to assess its clinical potential and the true cost–benefit ratio.

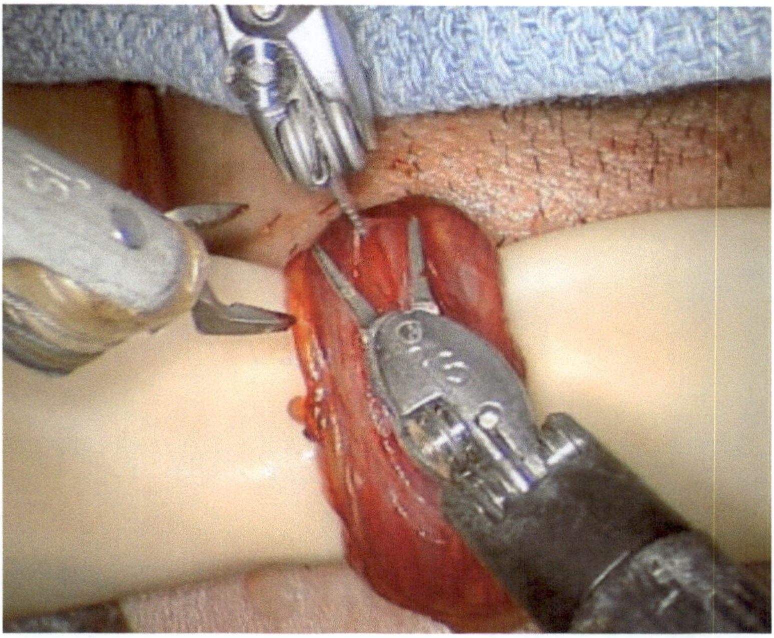

Fig. 10.12 Incision and separation of the spermatic cord sheath to reveal the varicose veins

Robotic-Assisted Microsurgical Varicocelectomy

Technique

A 2–3 cm subinguinal incision is made over the external inguinal ring. The spermatic cord is carefully dissected and then raised through the skin incision. A ½ in. Penrose drain is placed under the cord to keep it elevated. A sterile tongue blade is placed through the Penrose drain under the cord to further elevate and spread the cord. The robot is positioned from the patient's right side as described earlier. The black diamond micro-forceps are used in the right robotic arm, the micro-bipolar forceps in the left arm and the curved monopolar scissors in the fourth arm. A zero degree camera lens is utilized. The cremasteric sheath of the spermatic cord is now incised to separate the cord structures (Fig. 10.12).

Real-time intraoperative Doppler ultrasound is utilized to localize the testicular artery and ensure that no injury occurs to this vessel (Fig. 10.13). Enlarged veins are carefully dissected and then ligated using 3-0 silk suture ties (Fig. 10.14).

Doppler ultrasound verification of each vessel before it is ligated is performed to ensure that no arteries are ligated. The curved monopolar or Potts scissors in the fourth arm are used to cut the tied-off vessels. After all the veins are ligated, the

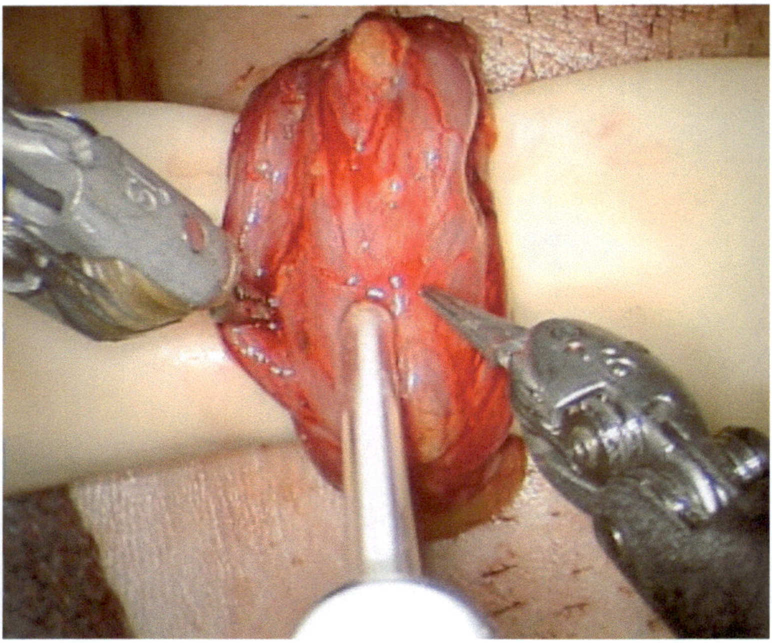

Fig. 10.13 Micro-Doppler evaluation of all the vessels to identify and preserve all arteries

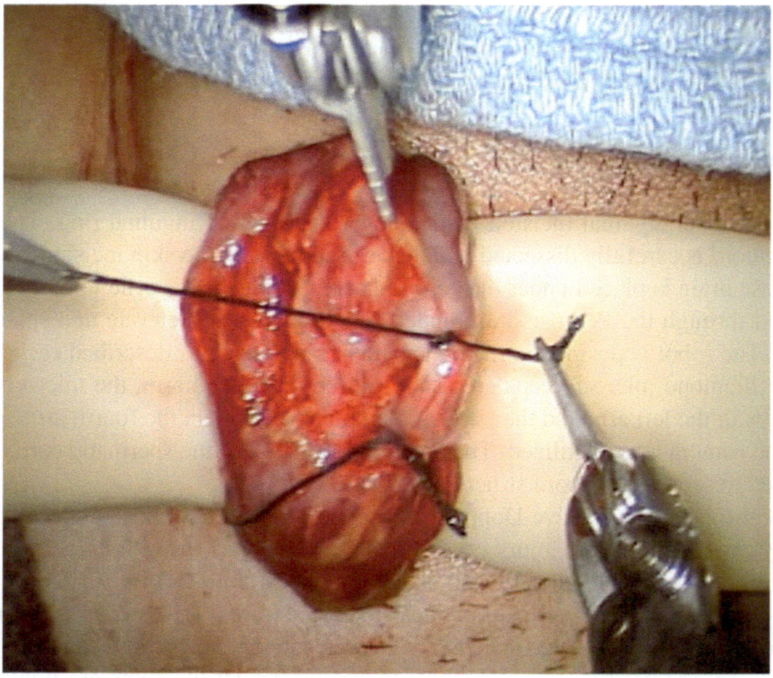

Fig. 10.14 Ligation of veins in the spermatic cord using 3-0 silk ties

spermatic cord sheath may be closed using a 6-0 prolene running suture. The tongue blade is removed from within the Penrose. The Penrose is now carefully removed and the spermatic cord is released. The testicle is gently pulled down to retract the spermatic cord completely into the incision. The skin incision is closed at the subcutaneous layer using a 3-0 monocryl suture. The skin is closed using a running subcuticular 4-0 monocryl suture and steri-strips.

Outcomes

A previous study by Shu et al. [13] has shown benefits to robotic-assisted microsurgical subinguinal varicocelectomy (RAVx) over the standard microsurgical approach (MVx). This review presents our initial clinical series. A review of a prospective clinical database of 97 RAVx cases from June 2008 to September 2010 (median follow-up 11 months: range 1–27) was performed. The median operative duration per side was 30 min (10–80). Indications for the procedure were the presence of a grade two or three varicocele and the following conditions: 10 with azoospermia, 42 with oligoospermia, and 49 with testicular pain (with or without oligoospermia, and failed all other conservative treatment options). Three-month follow-up was available for 81 patients: 75% with oligoospermia had a significant improvement in sperm count or motility, one with azoospermia was converted to oligoospermia. For testicular pain: 92% had complete resolution of pain (targeted neurolysis of the spermatic cord had been performed in addition to varicocelectomy). One recurrence or persistence of a varicocele occurred (by physical and ultrasound exam), one patient developed a small postoperative hydrocele and two patients had small postoperative scrotal hematomas (treated conservatively). The fourth robotic arm allowed the surgeon to control one additional instrument during the cases decreasing reliance on the microsurgical assistant. The fourth arm also enabled the surgeon to perform real-time intraoperative Doppler mapping of the testicular arteries while dissecting the veins with the other arms if needed.

Robotic-assisted microsurgical subinguinal varicocelectomy appears to be safe, feasible, and efficient. The preliminary human results appear promising. Further evaluation and comparative effectiveness studies are warranted.

Robotic-Assisted Microsurgical Testicular Sperm Extraction

Technique

A vertical 4–5 cm incision is made in the scrotal skin along the median raphe. The incision is carried down to the tunica vaginalis of the scrotum and then this is incised as well to deliver the testicle. The robot is now positioned from the patient's right side as described earlier. The black diamond micro-forceps are placed in the left

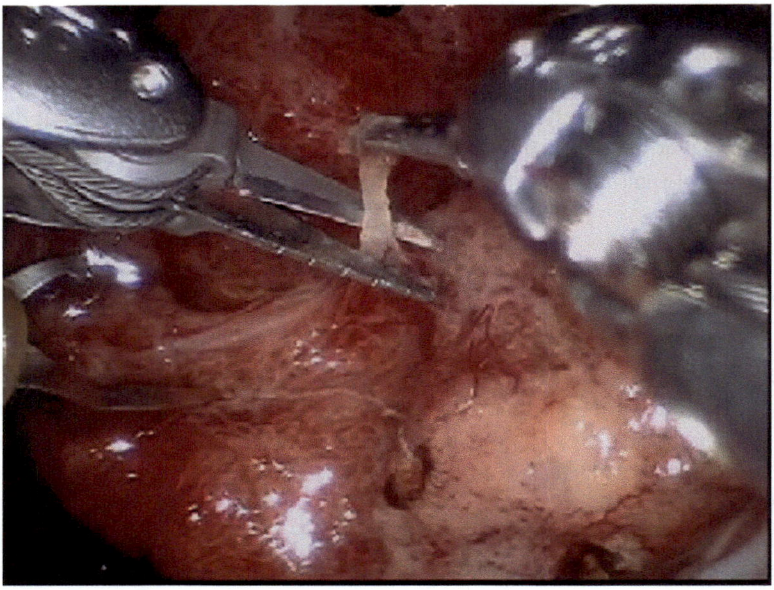

Fig. 10.15 Intraoperative image of robotic-assisted micro-TESE—sampling of the seminiferous tubules

robotic arm and fourth arm. Curved monopolar scissors are placed in the right robotic arm. Once the testicle is isolated, making a 2–3 cm transverse incision over the tunica exposes the seminiferous tubules. The tunica of the testicle is everted to fully expose all the tubules in the testicle. The testicular lobules are carefully dissected through to find areas that appear to have larger seminiferous tubules. These areas are sampled and the specimens are examined immediately with phase contrast microscopy by a trained embryologist (Fig. 10.15). Sampling is performed until sperm sufficient for multiple-assisted reproductive technique cycles are collected. These sperm are either cryopreserved or used for fresh transfer techniques.

In cases where no sperm are readily found, the testicle is thoroughly evaluated. Dissection through the deeper lobules of the testicle is performed and sampling is performed. The additional black diamond micro-forceps in the fourth robotic arm can very helpful in deep dissection to help retract the superficial lobules out of the way as the surgeon is evaluating the deeper lobules. In men who have enlarged testicles, or if the upper or lower poles of the testicle cannot be reached through the mid-transverse testicular incision, an additional 1–2 cm transverse incision is made in the upper or lower pole to assess these areas.

Once adequate sperm has been retrieved or adequate sampling has been performed, the tunical incisions in the testicle are closed with 6-0 prolene running suture. The testicle in placed back into the tunica vaginalis cavity within the scrotum and this layer is closed with running 3-0 chromic suture. The dartos muscle layer of the scrotum to closed using 3-0 chromic running suture and then the scrotal skin is closed with 4-0 chromic running suture. Bacitracin ointment is applied to the incision and fluff dressings with an athletic support are applied. An ice pack is carefully applied to the scrotum in the recovery room.

Postoperative Management

These procedures are all outpatient procedures. A scrotal support is placed prior to awaking the patient. The patient is asked to use this support for 2–3 weeks after surgery. The patient is instructed to have limited activity for about 1 week after surgery. No strenuous activity or heavy lifting is recommended for 4–6 weeks postoperatively. All patients are provided prescriptions for narcotics and antibiotics (keflex) for a few days. In the case of vasectomy reversal, patients are instructed to refrain from masturbation or ejaculation for at least 2–3 weeks postoperatively. Patients are instructed to utilize ice packs (30 min on and off) for the first week post-op to minimize the use of narcotics.

Conclusion

Robotic assisted microsurgery is still in its infancy. However, its use in microsurgery in urology and other microsurgical fields is expanding. A specialty society aimed at standardizing the training and credentialing for robotic assisted microsurgery now exists, with specialties ranging from urology, plastics, hand, reconstructive, vascular, peripheral nerve, anesthesia, ENT (ear, nose & throat) and gynecology. There are also efforts at developing more cost-effective and mobile robotic solutions that may cater to the microsurgeon. At the end of the day, the use of these technologies needs to be assessed for its true cost:benefit ratio. Hopefully, this technology will only further provide benefits for our patients.

References

1. Schultheiss D, Denil J. History of the microscope and development of microsurgery: a revolution for reproductive tract surgery. Andrologia. 2002;34(4):234–41.
2. Silber SJ. Microsurgery in clinical urology. Urology. 1975;6(2):150–3.
3. Marmar JL. Modified vasoepididymostomy with simultaneous double needle placement, tubulotomy and tubular invagination. J Urol. 2000;163(2):483–6.
4. Berger RE. Triangulation end-to-side vasoepididymostomy. J Urol. 1998;159(6):1951–3.
5. Chan PT, Li PS, Goldstein M. Microsurgical vasoepididymostomy: a prospective randomized study of 3 intussusception techniques in rats. J Urol. 2003;169(5):1924–9.
6. Fogdestam I, Fall M. Microsurgical end-to-end and end-to-side epididymovasostomy to correct occlusive azoospermia. Scand J Plast Reconstr Surg. 1983;17(2):137–40.
7. Marmar JL, Kim Y. Subinguinal microsurgical varicocelectomy: a technical critique and statistical analysis of semen and pregnancy data. J Urol. 1994;152(4):1127–32.

8. Owen ER. Microsurgical vasovasostomy: a reliable vasectomy reversal. Aust N Z J Surg. 1977;47(3):305–9.
9. Schlegel PN. Testicular sperm extraction: microdissection improves sperm yield with minimal tissue excision. Hum Reprod. 1999;14(1):131–5.
10. Silber SJ. Microscopic vasoepididymostomy: specific microanastomosis to the epididymal tubule. Fertil Steril. 1978;30(5):565–71.
11. Thomas Jr AJ. Vasoepididymostomy. Urol Clin North Am. 1987;14(3):527–38.
12. Owen ER. Microsurgical vasovasostomy: a reliable vasectomy reversal. 1977. J Urol. 2002;167(2 Pt 2):1205.
13. Shu T, Taghechian S, Wang R. Initial experience with robot-assisted varicocelectomy. Asian J Androl. 2008;10(1):146–8.

Chapter 11
The Role of Microsurgical Reconstruction in the Era of ICSI

Karen Baker and Edmund Sabanegh Jr

Abstract Even in the era of advanced assisted reproductive techniques, microsurgical reconstruction is an important and relevant treatment for obstructive azoospermia. Microsurgical reconstruction provides couples the opportunity to create a spontaneous pregnancy and thereby avoiding the expense, limitations, and risks of in vitro fertilization (IVF)/intracytoplasmic sperm injection (ICSI). The apparent ease of advanced assisted reproductive techniques should not overshadow the fact that the expense and risks of IVF/ICSI may be unjustifiable. Sperm retrieval relegates couples to IVF/ICSI and subjects fertile female partners and the offspring to potentially avoidable risk. Approximately 30% cycles in 2009 resulted in twin or higher gestation and these pregnancies are associated with higher rates of prematurity, low birth weight, and severe neonatal medical conditions [1]. Ovarian hyperstimulation syndrome is a potentially life-threatening complication of in vitro fertilization and moderate and severe ovarian hyperstimulation syndrome are estimated to occur in 3–6% and 0.1–2% of IVF cycles, respectively [2]. Every surgeon will encounter couples for whom the best option for pregnancy is sperm retrieval paired IVF/ICSI. For couples with amenable conditions, however the safety of a natural conception remains a compelling justification for microsurgical reconstruction.

Keywords Vasovasostomy • Microsurgery • Male infertility • Sterilization reversal • Cost effectiveness • Vasoepididymostomy • Obstructive interval • Sperm granuloma • Intravasal azoospermia • Female age • Male age • Previous pregnancy • Length of proximal vas remnant

K. Baker, M.D. (✉) • E. Sabanegh Jr, M.D.
Center for Male Fertility, Glickman Urological and Kidney Institute, Cleveland Clinic, 9500 Euclid Ave, Cleveland, OH 44195, USA
e-mail: bakerk8@ccf.org

J.I. Sandlow (ed.), *Microsurgery for Fertility Specialists: A Practical Text*,
DOI 10.1007/978-1-4614-4196-0_11, © Springer Science+Business Media New York 2013

Introduction

Even in the era of advanced assisted reproductive techniques, microsurgical reconstruction is an important and relevant treatment for obstructive azoospermia. Microsurgical reconstruction provides couples the opportunity to create a spontaneous pregnancy and thereby avoiding the expense, limitations, and risks of in vitro fertilization (IVF)/intracytoplasmic sperm injection (ICSI). The apparent ease of advanced assisted reproductive techniques should not overshadow the fact that the expense and risks of IVF/ICSI may be unjustifiable. Sperm retrieval relegates couples to IVF/ICSI and subjects fertile female partners and the offspring to potentially avoidable risk. Approximately 30% cycles in 2009 resulted in twin or higher gestation and these pregnancies are associated with higher rates of prematurity, low birth weight, and severe neonatal medical conditions [1]. Ovarian hyperstimulation syndrome is a potentially life-threatening complication of in vitro fertilization and moderate and severe ovarian hyperstimulation syndrome are estimated to occur in 3–6% and 0.1–2% of IVF cycles, respectively [2]. Every surgeon will encounter couples for whom the best option for pregnancy is sperm retrieval paired IVF/ICSI. For couples with amenable conditions, however the safety of a natural conception remains a compelling justification for microsurgical reconstruction.

The success of vasal reconstruction has improved with refinements in techniques and favorable patency rates are reported after a decade or more of obstruction and for a variety of etiologies to include iatrogenic injury, inflammatory, and congenital conditions. Reconstruction is cost competitive as compared to sperm retrieval and cryopreservation, and the cost per newborn is significantly less for vasal reconstruction and natural pregnancy as compared to sperm retrieval and ICSI [3–7]. Vasal reconstruction should not be dismissed in couples with known female factor infertility as postoperative semen parameters are typically adequate for intrauterine insemination. In couples for whom female factor indicate a low chance of natural pregnancy, men who undergo reconstruction are able to provide fresh ejaculated specimens, thus avoiding the expense of sperm cryopreservation and sperm retrieval. Postoperative complications are acceptably infrequent and minor and the recovery is short. Microsurgical reconstruction, therefore, remains an important option for couples overcoming obstructive azoospermia.

In this chapter, we compare the cost of vasectomy reversal to IVF/ICSI and review the preoperative factors that influence the outcomes of vasal reconstruction. Our goal is to arm the surgeon with the information necessary to guide couples through their decision of electing vasal reconstruction versus sperm retrieval paired with IVF/ICSI. Later chapters will discuss the operative techniques.

Cost Comparison

There are no controlled trial comparing efficacy and cost between vasal reconstruction and sperm retrieval paired with IVF/ICSI, nor is it realistic to expect such a study to be conducted. The available analytical models and retrospective reviews conclude that reconstruction is less expensive than, and at least as effective as, sperm retrieval paired with IVF/ICSI for the majority of couples. Of interest, none of these analyses account for the preference of many couples to have multiple pregnancies over time—a preference which would compound the cost benefit of vasectomy reversal over ART. Further discussion is warranted to familiarize the reader with the additional limitations, assumptions, and outcomes contained within the published literature.

Pavlovich and Schlegel performed an extensive analysis of cost effectiveness of vasectomy reversal compared to sperm retrieval via microsurgical epididymal sperm aspiration (MESA) paired with IVF/ICSI based on 1994 costs [8]. The model included direct cost and indirect costs such as male and female pretreatment costs, anesthetic/ambulatory surgery fees, complications, and lost work costs. Expenses were based on fees charged at four established fertility centers in the USA. Outcomes (such as live delivery rates and complications) were based on published literature and/or telephonic contact with established fertility centers and were limited to female age of 39 or less. The authors chose to evaluate the cost per live delivery however the model accounted for costs resulting from multiple gestations. The analysis determined that sperm retrieval paired with IVF/ICSI was 2.8 times more expensive than vasectomy reversal with an average cost of $72,521 versus $25,475 per live delivery. Subset analysis revealed bilateral vasovasostomy and bilateral vasoepididymostomy were more cost effective than either percutaneous and testicular sperm retrieval or MESA paired with IVF/ICSI. The cost advantage of vasectomy reversal persisted despite increasing obstructive interval and across the range of reported pregnancy rates with IVF/ICSI.

Heidenreich et al. compared the expense and outcomes of 112 couples who underwent vasectomy reversal to 69 couples who underwent MESA or testicular sperm extraction paired with IVF/ICSI at a single institution [3]. The analysis considered the costs associated with multiple gestations. Reported patency and pregnancy rates after vasectomy reversal were 77% and 53%, respectively. Pregnancy rates for sperm retrieval paired with IVF/ICSI were 24.5% and the rates of miscarriage and multiple gestations were higher in the IVF/ICSI versus the vasectomy reversal cohort (miscarriage 15.8% versus 2.4% and multiple gestations 15.8% versus 1.2%, respectively). The cost per live delivery using sperm retrieval paired with IVF/ICSI was five times the cost calculated for vasectomy reversal (14,547€ versus 2,793€, respectively). The authors concluded that pregnancy rates, cost per delivery, and rates of multiple births and female complications strongly favor vasectomy reversal and recommended that only couples not amenable to vasal reconstruction be considered candidates for sperm retrieval paired with IVF/ICSI.

The cost advantage of vasectomy reversal over sperm retrieval paired with IVF/ICSI extends to repeat vasal reconstructions and vasoepididymostomy. Donovan et al. retrospectively compared a single institution series of 18 men undergoing repeat vasal reconstruction after failed vasectomy reversal to nine couples undergoing MESA paired with IVF/ICSI. The indications for MESA included congenital etiologies and men with obstruction not amenable to surgical reconstruction. The authors did not consider repeat vasal reconstruction in patients with a history of bilateral vasoepididymostomies. The repeat reconstruction required bilateral vasovasostomy in four patients, vasovasostomy and contralateral vasoepididymostomy in five patients, bilateral vasoepididymostomy in four patients, solitary vasovasostomy in four patients, and solitary vasoepididymostomy in one patient. Patency and pregnancy rates after repeat vasal reconstruction were 78% and 44%, respectively. There were 12 pregnancies in the repeat vasal reconstruction cohort; however two of the pregnancies were achieved through IVF/ICSI. Notably the authors' cost comparison included the expense of these IVF/ICSI cycles in the analysis of repeat vasal reconstructions. The authors demonstrated a clear cost advantage for repeat vasal reconstruction versus MESA paired with IVF/ICSI. The average cost per delivered baby or ongoing pregnancy was 2.3 times more expensive for MESA paired with IVF/ICSI as compared to repeat vasal reconstruction ($14,892 versus $35,570, respectively). The authors conclude that repeat vasal reconstruction was the rationale choice for couple with previous failed vasectomy reversal.

Kolettis and Thomas reviewed the outcome of 55 patients who underwent bilateral or unilateral, solitary vasoepididymostomy [4]. Forty-five patients in the cohort (82%) were repeat surgery after failed vasal reconstruction consisting of vasovasostomy in 41 patients and vasoepididymostomy in four patients. The authors reported an overall patency, pregnancy, and delivery rate of 85%, 44%, and 36%, respectively. The reconstruction cohort was compared to a model for outcomes and expense of MESA paired with IVF/ICSI based the average institutional expense for the procedure and published rates for live delivery and complications for MESA and IVF/ICSI. The cost analysis included calculations for time off work, delivery costs, and estimated complications. The authors reported a cost advantage for vasoepididymostomy as compared to MESA paired with IVF. MESA paired with IVF was 1.6 times more expensive than vasectomy reversal requiring vasoepididymostomy. The authors concluded that vasoepididymostomy was less expensive and equally efficacious as MESA paired with IVF/ICSI.

Meng et al. performed a cost analysis comparing vasal reconstruction to sperm retrieval paired with IVF/ICSI across a range of female fecundity rates and postoperative patency rates after vasal reconstruction [9]. The model presumed a baseline postoperative patency of 80% and pregnancy of 30% after vasectomy reversal, and presumed that 50% of couples who failed to achieve a pregnancy after primary therapy would continue to ART. The authors concluded that vasectomy reversal was more cost effective than sperm retrieval paired with IVF/ICSI independent of female fecundity when postoperative patency was 78% or greater. The model further predicted that sperm retrieval and IVF/ICSI was cost advantageous when postoperative patency was anticipated to be less than 60%, such as may been seen after vasoepididymostomy.

Hsieh et al. performed Markov modeling based on published outcomes of sperm retrieval paired with IVF/ICSI and vasal reconstruction. The intent of the Markov model is to account for change in outcomes over time. The model examined the cost effectiveness and impact of out of pocket expense for each option for a couple initiating treatment after a 14-year obstructive interval and female age of 34. The model assumed a base cost of $12,400 per IVF/ICSI cycle and $8,500 per vasectomy reversal and used published and conservative rates for outcomes following surgery and ART. The authors concluded that ART yielded a slightly higher cumulative pregnancy rate than vasectomy reversal (99.4% versus 95.3%, respectively), albeit at a higher cost. Effectiveness of treatment was negatively influence by increasing female age and, to a lesser degree, by obstructive interval. Perhaps the most sobering conclusion of this study is the potential out of pocket expense facing couples attempting to achieve a pregnancy. For couples willing to pay up to $65,000 for a pregnancy, vasectomy reversal was more cost effective than ART for all female ages. For couples willing to pay up to $100,000 for a pregnancy, however, immediate assisted reproductive techniques were more cost effective than vasectomy reversal for women age 33.1–38 years in this model. These potential expenses would be daunting for the average family considering treatment for postvasectomy obstruction and should remind fertility specialists of the economic realities facing these couples.

Obstructive Interval

Obstructive interval was once seen as a major determinant for the technical success of vasal reconstruction. Recent publications report minimal decline in patency with increasing obstructive interval, however, pregnancy rates do decline as the obstructive interval increases. The landmark article of the Vasovasostomy Study Group reviewed the outcomes of 1,247 men undergoing initial vasovasostomy and reported overall patency and pregnancy rates of 86% and 52%, respectively [10]. Patency and pregnancy rates decreased in a stepwise fashion when outcomes were grouped by obstructive interval but pregnancy rates declined more rapidly. Patency was 97% and pregnancy achieved in 76% of couples with obstructive intervals of less than 3 years. By comparison, patency and pregnancy rates were 88% and 53%, respectively, for intervals of 3–8 years, 79 and 44% for intervals of 9–14 years and 71 and 30% for intervals of 15 years or more. [10] In 2004, Boorjian et al. published a review of 213 patients randomly selected from a single surgeon's 17 year operative experience of bilateral vasal reconstructions. The authors reported patency rates of 91%, 88%, 91%, and 89% after obstructive intervals of less than 5, 5–10, 10–15, and greater than 15 years, respectively [11]. The overall pregnancy rate was 81% for the entire cohort, but pregnancy rates dropped precipitously to 44% for the cohort with an obstructive interval greater 15 years. Magheli et al. published the results of retrospective review of a single surgeon's series of 334 vasectomy reversals. Overall patency was 97% in the 251 patients in whom the results of semen analysis were available and the pregnancy rate was 62% for the entire cohort [12]. Patency and pregnancy rates were not influenced by obstructive interval. Multivariate analysis revealed longer obstructive intervals were associated with an increased need to perform vasoepididymostomy and increased female age was significantly associated with a decrease in pregnancy rate. Kolettis et al. examined outcomes 74 vasectomy reversal performed by three surgeons after obstructive interval of 10 years or longer. The mean obstructive interval was 14.5 years (range from 10 to 24 years) and overall patency and pregnancy rates were 77% and 37%, respectively. When grouped by obstructive interval, patency and pregnancy rates were 74 and 40% after 10–15 years of obstruction, 87 and 36% after 16–19 years, and 75 and 27% after 20 or more years of obstruction [13]. Notably, the pregnancy rates for up to 15 years of obstruction are on par with per cycle pregnancy rates with IVF/ICSI [3].

Age

The age of the female partner clearly impacts pregnancy rates after reconstruction with the most precipitous decrease occurring at age 40. Gerrard et al. compared patency and pregnancy rates based on age of the female partner in 249 vasal reconstructions and confirmed that pregnancy rates decreased dramatically after age 40. The patency rates were 90%, 89%, 90%, 86%, and 83% while the pregnancy rates were 67%, 52%, 57%, 54%, and 14% for patients with female partners aged 20–24, 25–29, 30–34, 35–39, and 40+ years, respectively [14]. Deck and Berger reviewed outcomes for vasectomy reversals for male partners with an ovulating female partner aged 38 or older. The median male age was 46 and the median female age was 40. Overall patency was 69% and the pregnancy rate and live birth rate for couples with at least 1 year of follow-up were 22% and 17%, respectively [7]. Kolettis et al. examined the outcomes of vasectomy reversal for couples in whom the female was 35 years or older. Pregnancy was achieved by 35% of couples with sufficient follow-up with 46% of females age 35–39 achieving pregnancy but only 14% of females 40 or older [15]. Of the preoperative factors that can predict postoperative pregnancy, older female age is consistently associated with lower pregnancy rates even when the impact of female age is not the primary research question [12–16].

Age of the male by itself does not appear to be a significant predictor of postoperative patency or pregnancy. Magheli et al. found that older age of the male at the time of reversal was associated with a longer obstructive interval and the need for a vasoepididymostomy (VE) [12]. Parekatti et al. found male age at the time of reversal to be a significant predictor for the need to perform VE during univariate analysis but multivariate logistical regression found only obstructive interval to be predictive of the need to perform VE [17].

Previous Paternity and Pregnancy

In the absence of previous paternity, a focused history and physical exam should be performed and men with findings concerning for impaired spermatogenesis, such as small testicles, should be evaluated further. Men with previous paternity and normal genitourinary examination require no additional infertility evaluation prior to reversal. There are conflicting results regarding the impact of previous pregnancies between the partners on the pregnancy rates after vasectomy reversal. Chan et al. reviewed 1,048 vasectomy reversals and identified 27 couples with a history of previous pregnancies together. Patency and spontaneous pregnancy rates among these couples were 100% and 86%, respectively [18]. In a retrospective review of 747 vasectomy reversal, Bolduc et al. found previous pregnancy as a couple was associated with higher pregnancy rates [19]. Kolettis et al. examined the outcomes of 34 men who underwent vasectomy reversal and had the same partner. Twenty-nine of the couples had a previous pregnancy together. Mean obstructive interval was 5 years and the mean female age was 31.9 years. Overall patency was 93% and pregnancy occurred in 60% of the couples with sufficient follow-up [20]. Hernandez and Sabanegh reported higher pregnancy rates in couples with previous history of pregnancies together in a series of 41 couples undergoing repeat reconstruction after failed attempt at vasectomy reversal. Pregnancy rates were 80% in couples with previous pregnancies together ($n=5$) versus 17% in remarried couples ($n=26$) [21]. Kim et al. reviewed their series of 44 couples electing vasectomy reversal and determined that age of the female partner, not a history of pregnancy together, was a significant predictor of pregnancy [22].

Sperm Granuloma

The presence of a sperm granuloma at the vasectomy site has been suggested by some to portend better patency rates after vasectomy reversal. The rationale being the granuloma is evidence of sperm leaking from the testicular vas and the leakage decreases the back pressure and, therefore, the damage to the epididymis. While there are conflicting results in the literature, the weight of the evidence suggests that sperm granuloma does not improve pregnancy rates and is unlikely to improve patency rates. The Vasovasostomy Study Group reported no statistically significant difference between patency and pregnancy rates in patients with and without a histologically proven sperm granuloma [10]. The presence of a granuloma at the vasectomy site positively correlated with patency in a review performed by Bolduc et al. of 747 vasectomy reversals performed over a 16-year period [19]. In 2009, Hinz et al. reported the presence of a sperm granuloma was associated with better patency rates but not improved pregnancy rates in a series of 351 vasectomy reversals performed by a single surgeon [23]. Boorjian reported the presence of a sperm granuloma on a least one side had no impact on patency or pregnancy rates in 213 vasectomy reversals performed by a single surgeon [11]. Magheli et al. reviewed the outcomes of 334 vasectomy reversal and found no correlation between presence of sperm granuloma and patency or pregnancy rates [12].

Length of Proximal Vas Remnant

Witt et al. examined the length of the postvasectomy testicular vas remnant of 26 men undergoing vasectomy reversal. The vas length was measured from the cauda of the epididymis to the vas defect for each operative side ($n=52$ vas remnants) and the length correlated with the presence of whole sperm in the intravasal fluid. Whole sperm were present in the intravasal fluid in 30 of 32 (94%) vas remnants 2.7 cm or greater in length but only 3 of 20 (15%) vas remnants less than 2.7 cm in length [24]. Conceptually the notion that a longer vas remnant may afford the epididymis protection against back pressure is in keeping with current thinking. Some have argued that preoperative assessment of the remnant length is imprecise, however, the information gleaned from this study may prove useful when counseling couples in whom the length of the testicular vas is concerningly short during physical exam.

Previous Reconstruction

Previous attempt at reconstruction does not preclude success on repeat surgery. In 2007, Hollingsworth published the results of 49 repeat vasectomy reversal performed by four surgeons. The average obstructive interval before the first reversal was 10.5 years and the average obstructive interval between the first and second reversal was 2.7 years. Thirty-four percent of the patients underwent at least a unilateral VE and the percentage of patients undergoing VE was not statistically different between patients with obstructive intervals of less than 10 years and those with obstructive intervals of 10 years or longer. Overall patency and pregnancy rates were 85% and 44%, respectively and there was no statistically significant difference in these rates between patients with obstructive intervals of less than 10 years and patients with obstructive intervals of 10 years or longer [25]. Paick et al. published the outcomes of 62 patient undergoing unilateral VV ($n=2$), bilateral VV ($n=58$), or combination of VV and VE ($n=2$) after a failed previous attempt at vasal reconstruction [16]. Unless technically not feasible, a repeat vasovasostomy was performed regardless of the quality of the intravasal fluid or the presence of sperm. Overall patency was 92% and natural birth rate was 52% [16]. The authors examined potential predictors of patency and pregnancy and found that increased age of the female negatively influenced pregnancy rates. Univariate analysis of the presence or absence of sperm in the intravasal fluid, the presence or absence of motile sperm, obstructive interval, the type of reconstruction (bilateral VV versus all others), and anastomotic level (straight versus convoluted vas) did not confer a statistically significant difference in patency or pregnancy. Hernandez and Sabanegh reviewed the outcomes of 41 couples undergoing repeat reconstruction after one or more attempts at vasectomy reversal. Reconstruction consisted of bilateral VV in 7, unilateral VV in 4, bilateral VE in 16, unilateral VE in 4, and a combination of unilateral VE and unilateral VV in 10 patients. Overall patency rates were 79% and pregnancy rates were 31% in the 33 and 31 couples in whom follow-up was available [21]. Pasqualotto reviewed the outcomes of repeat vasal reconstruction in 18 patients who underwent 10 unilateral and 8 bilateral microsurgical VE. The patency was confirmed in 66.7 and 25% of couples reported spontaneous pregnancy [26]. Patients with a congenital etiology for their obstruction demonstrated a high patency rate (85.7%) as compared to patients with a history of vasectomy or inflammation (patency rates of 75% and 43%, respectively) as the etiology of their obstruction, but this difference did not reach statistical significance. Fox reported on 28 patients who underwent VE after failed vasectomy reversal and reported patency and pregnancy rates of 57% and 32%, respectively [27]. The published literature support the decision to offer repeat vasal reconstruction to couples with azoospermia after failed reconstruction as reasonably high patency and pregnancy rates are expected.

Vasovasostomy Versus Vasoepididymostomy

The small and delicate epididymal tubule is a challenging surgical target and the surgical techniques for performing vasoepididymostomy are described in later chapters. Patency rates reported in most modern series are encouragingly high. In 1998 Berger described a triangulated intussusception technique for VE and reported 11 of 12 patients (92%) had motile sperm in the postoperative ejaculate [28]. Pregnancy data was not reported. Marmar subsequently reported the outcomes of 19 men who underwent a two suture intussusception VE. Patency and pregnancy rates were 78 and 22% in 9 men who underwent bilateral VE and 83 and 28% in the 7 men with unilateral VE paired with contralateral VV during a follow-up period of less than 12 months (mean follow-up not reported) [29]. In 2005, Schiff et al. retrospectively compared the outcomes of two needle longitudinal intussusception VE (LIVE), triangulation intussusception VE (TIVE), conventional end to side (ES) and end to end (EE) VE in 153 VE performed by a single surgeon. The series was not limited to postvasectomy obstructive azoospermia and included patients with primary epididymal obstruction. Motile sperm were detected in 67% of LIVE, 68% of TIVE, 37% of ES, and 49% of EE patients. Pregnancy rates were 24% for LIVE, 16% for TIVE, 11% for ES, and 6% for EE but the difference in rates was not statistically significant [30]. This experience was extended by Chan et al. who identified and prospectively followed 68 patients who underwent either LIVE or TIVE by the same surgeon. Mean patient age was 39.8, mean obstructive interval was 18.8 years (range 3–28) and, again, the series was not limited to postvasectomy obstructive azoospermia. Overall patency (defined as ≥ 10,000 sperm/ml) was 84%. Natural pregnancy was achieved in 40% of couples with >1 year of follow-up and the median time to pregnancy of 14.2 months [31]. These modern series report encouragingly high patency rates with evolution of microsurgical techniques, however overall pregnancy rates after VE are lower than after VV. It is important to note that not all published series report patency rates this high which likely speaks to the technical difficulty of the VE [32, 33].

Surgical Approaches

Silber and Owen are credited with independently describing the microscopic vasovasostomy in 1977 and thereby revolutionizing the surgical approach to obstructive azoospermia [34, 35]. Overall surgical outcomes are superior with the use of the microscope but a few authors report competitive patency and pregnancy rates with Loupe magnification and unmagnified vasovasostomy in the modern era. Gopi and Townell retrospectively reviewed 70 consecutive vasovasostomies performed by a single surgeon over a 12-year period. The median obstructive interval was 8.5 years. The surgeon performed a spatulated end to end vasovasostomy with 6-0 prolene and without the aid of magnification. Overall patency and pregnancy rates were 90% and 54%, respectively, with high rates in patients whose obstructive intervals were 10 years or less. [36] Hsieh et al. retrospectively compared the outcomes of 42 bilateral microsurgical vasovasostomies (group 1) with 32 bilateral vasovasostomies performed with Loupe magnification (group 2). All surgeries were performed by one surgeon and both techniques used interrupted 9-0 nylon sutures in a one layer vasovasostomy. Patency and pregnancy rates were 91 and 43% for group 1 and 89 and 39% for group 2 and the difference in rates was not statistically significant between the two groups [37]. Urquhart-Hay reported patency (defined as sperm concentrations >20mil/ml) in 86% and pregnancy rate of 51% in 125 men undergoing vasectomy reversal with ×3.5 Loupe magnification [38].

The microsurgical approach is considered the gold standard for vasal reconstruction. Operative times are shorter with Loupe magnification or no magnification as compared to microsurgery, but the precise mucosal to mucosal approximation afforded by microsurgery is generally believed to result in superior patency. Jee and Hong retrospectively reviewed 25 men undergoing microsurgical vasovasostomy to 25 men who underwent vasectomy reversal with the aid of ×4 Loupe magnification by a single surgeon over a 22-month period. A one layer vasovasostomy technique utilizing interrupted 9-0 nylon was used. Patency was statistically significantly increased in the microsurgery group (91%) versus the loupe-assisted group (72%, $p=0.021$). Pregnancy rates were higher for the microsurgical group versus the loupe-assisted group (40% versus 28%) but this difference was not statistically significant. Mean age of the patient, mean age of the wife, obstructive interval, postoperative sperm concentration, and percent motility were comparable between the two groups [39]. Dewire and Lawson reviewed 32 men who underwent vasal reconstruction utilizing loupe magnification and found a patency rate comparable to microsurgery at 89%, but a pregnancy rate of only 41% [40]. Lee and McLoughlin compared 41 patients who underwent a single layer unmagnified vasovasostomy utilizing 4-0 to 6-0 absorbable suture to 26 patient who underwent microsurgical two layer vasovasostomy utilizing 8-0 to 10-0 synthetic suture. Outcomes favored the microscopic approach with slightly higher patency and pregnancy rates (96% and 54%, respectively) for microsurgery patient as compared to the unmagnified repairs (patency 90% and pregnancy 46%) [41].

There is little published data regarding the use and outcomes of robotic-assisted microsurgery reconstruction. Several institutions published findings supporting the feasibility of robotic-assisted vasal reconstruction in animal and ex vivo fresh human vas models [42–44]. Fleming reported the personal experience of two surgeons who performed robot-assisted microsurgical vasovasostomy, but outcomes data was not included [45]. Parekattil et al. recent published preliminary outcomes for a prospective study comparing microsurgical vasovasostomy to robot-assisted microsurgical vasovasostomy performed by a single fellowship trained surgeon over a 37-month period. Mean operative time was significant lower for robot-assisted cases (90 min versus 120 min for microsurgical approach). Patency (defined as >1 million sperm per milliliter) was 94% in the robot group and 79% in the microsurgical group. Pregnancy rates were not included in this publication [46]. In light of the increased cost and reduced optical magnification of robotic-assisted surgery as compared to standard microsurgical techniques, the advantages to robotic-assisted reconstruction remain to be established.

Complex Vasal Reconstruction

Obstruction of the vas deferens within the inguinal canal from previous surgery is a reality that will be faced by many microsurgeons. Matsuda reviewed the outcomes of 22 men with azoospermia or oligospermia (sperm density <5 mil/ml) who underwent vasal reconstruction for obstruction due to inguinal hernia repair. The distal end of the vas was found at or above the internal inguinal ring in 57% of the repairs and 3 cm or more of vas was reported missing by the authors in 37% of the repairs. Eighteen patients underwent inguinal microsurgical VV and four underwent crossed vasovasostomy wherein the distal vas, once freed, was passed directly through the abdominal wall at the level of the external inguinal ring. Patency was reported as 89% however this included patients who remained azoospermic after surgery but had a patent anastomosis by vasography [47]. Pasqualotto reviewed the outcomes of 13 men with azoospermia or severe impairment of semen parameters underwent vasal reconstruction for post-herniorrhaphy obstruction. Overall patency was 65% and pregnancy rates for patients with greater than 12 months follow-up was 40% [48]. Of note six men required a second procedure due to failure of the first reconstruction. Shaeer and Shaeer reviewed their experience with vasal reconstruction in 25 men with a history of inguinal herniorrhaphy in whom vasography confirmed unilateral ($n=15$) or bilateral ($n=10$) obstruction of the vas deferens at the level of the inguinal canal. After dividing the vas at the internal ring, the authors mobilize the pelvic portion of the vas deferens laparoscopically and route the mobilized vas to the scrotum through a tunnel created through the conjoint tendon and/or abdominus rectus. The authors then performed either a single layer vasovasostomy using 8-0 nylon or a formal two layer vasovasostomy using 10-0 and 9-0 nylon. Overall patency was 68% with 60% patency for unilateral repairs and 80% patency for bilateral repairs [49]. Sabanegh and Thomas reported a series of 12 microsurgical crossed transseptal vasoepididymostomies performed for irreparable ipsilateral ductal obstruction with a normal testis and poorly functioning or absent contralateral testis. Patency was confirmed in eight of nine (88%) patients with 6 months or greater follow-up and two couple achieved spontaneous pregnancies [50]. Mean postoperative sperm concentration and motility were 98 M/ml and 13%, respectively. Two patients required reoperation. The authors noted that as compared to other etiologies for vasal obstruction, agenesis of the vas was associated with lower postoperative sperm concentrations.

Conclusion

Microsurgical reconstruction of the vas deferens will continue to play a vital role in fertility restoration in the era of IVF/ICSI. Reconstruction provides couples more options for reproduction and in many situations will be cost advantageous for couples. The minimal postoperative side effects and low risk of complication are on par with sperm retrieval and postoperative recovery is acceptably brief. Previous attempts at vasectomy reversal and the need for complex repair do not preclude success. While many factors may influence the outcomes after vasal reconstruction, couples should be counseled that female age remains the most significant predictor of postoperative pregnancy.

References

1. Anon. Clinic Summary Report. Available at: https://www.sartcorsonline.com/rptCSR_PublicMultYear.aspx?ClinicPKID=0. Accessed 15 Sept 2011.
2. Delvigne A. Symposium: update on prediction and management of OHSS. Epidemiology of OHSS. Reprod Biomed Online. 2009;19(1):8–13.
3. Heidenreich A, Altmann P, Engelmann UH. Microsurgical vasovasostomy versus microsurgical epididymal sperm aspiration/testicular extraction of sperm combined with intracytoplasmic sperm injection. A cost-benefit analysis. Eur Urol. 2000;37(5):609–14.
4. Kolettis PN, Thomas Jr AJ. Vasoepididymostomy for vasectomy reversal: a critical assessment in the era of intracytoplasmic sperm injection. J Urol. 1997;158(2):467–70.
5. Lee R, Li PS, Goldstein M, et al. A decision analysis of treatments for obstructive azoospermia. Hum Reprod. 2008;23(9):2043–9.
6. Donovan Jr JF, DiBaise M, Sparks AE, Kessler J, Sandlow JI. Comparison of microscopic epididymal sperm aspiration and intracytoplasmic sperm injection/in-vitro fertilization with repeat microscopic reconstruction following vasectomy: is second attempt vas reversal worth the effort? Hum Reprod. 1998;13(2):387–93.
7. Deck AJ, Berger RE. Should vasectomy reversal be performed in men with older female partners? J Urol. 2000;163(1):105–6.
8. Pavlovich CP, Schlegel PN. Fertility options after vasectomy: a cost-effectiveness analysis. Fertil Steril. 1997;67(1):133–41.
9. Meng MV, Greene KL, Turek PJ. Surgery or assisted reproduction? A decision analysis of treatment costs in male infertility. J Urol. 2005;174(5):1926–31. discussion 1931.
10. Belker AM, Thomas AJ, Fuchs EF, Konnak JW, Sharlip ID. Results of 1,469 microsurgical vasectomy reversals by the Vasovasostomy Study Group. J Urol. 1991;145(3):505–11.
11. Boorjian S, Lipkin M, Goldstein M. The impact of obstructive interval and sperm granuloma on outcome of vasectomy reversal. J Urol. 2004;171(1):304–6.
12. Magheli A, Rais-Bahrami S, Kempkensteffen C, et al. Impact of obstructive interval and sperm granuloma on patency and pregnancy after vasectomy reversal. Int J Androl. 2010;33(5):730–5.
13. Kolettis PN, Sabanegh ES, D'amico AM, et al. Outcomes for vasectomy reversal performed after obstructive intervals of at least 10 years. Urology. 2002;60(5):885–8.
14. Gerrard ER, Sandlow JI, Oster RA, et al. Effect of female partner age on pregnancy rates after vasectomy reversal. Fertil Steril. 2007;87(6):1340–4.
15. Kolettis PN, Sabanegh ES, Nalesnik JG, et al. Pregnancy outcomes after vasectomy reversal for female partners 35 years old or older. J Urol. 2003;169(6):2250–2.

16. Paick J-S, Park JY, Park DW, et al. Microsurgical vasovasostomy after failed vasovasostomy. J Urol. 2003;169(3):1052–5.
17. Parekattil SJ, Kuang W, Agarwal A, Thomas AJ. Model to predict if a vasoepididymostomy will be required for vasectomy reversal. J Urol. 2005;173(5):1681–4.
18. Chan PTK, Goldstein M. Superior outcomes of microsurgical vasectomy reversal in men with the same female partners. Fertil Steril. 2004;81(5):1371–4.
19. Bolduc S, Fischer MA, Deceuninck G, Thabet M. Factors predicting overall success: a review of 747 microsurgical vasovasostomies. Can Urol Assoc J. 2007;1(4):388–94.
20. Kolettis PN, Woo L, Sandlow JI. Outcomes of vasectomy reversal performed for men with the same female partners. Urology. 2003;61(6):1221–3.
21. Hernandez J, Sabanegh ES. Repeat vasectomy reversal after initial failure: overall results and predictors for success. J Urol. 1999;161(4):1153–6.
22. Kim SW, Ku JH, Park K, Son H, Paick J-S. A different female partner does not affect the success of second vasectomy reversal. J Androl. 2005;26(1):48–52.
23. Hinz S, Rais-Bahrami S, Weiske WH, et al. Prognostic value of intraoperative parameters observed during vasectomy reversal for predicting postoperative vas patency and fertility. World J Urol. 2009;27(6):781–5. Available at: http://www.ncbi.nlm.nih.gov/pubmed/19255761. Accessed 6 Mar 2011.
24. Witt MA, Heron S, Lipshultz LI. The post-vasectomy length of the testicular vasal remnant: a predictor of surgical outcome in microscopic vasectomy reversal. J Urol. 1994;151(4):892–4.
25. Hollingsworth MR, Sandlow JI, Schrepferman CG, Brannigan RE, Kolettis PN. Repeat vasectomy reversal yields high success rates. Fertil Steril. 2007;88(1):217–9.
26. Pasqualotto FF, Agarwal A, Srivastava M, Nelson DR, Thomas AJ. Fertility outcome after repeat vasoepididymostomy. J Urol. 1999;162(5):1626–8.
27. Fox M. Failed vasectomy reversal: is a further attempt using microsurgery worthwhile? BJU Int. 2000;86(4):474–8.
28. Berger RE. Triangulation end-to-side vasoepididymostomy. J Urol. 1998;159(6):1951–3.
29. Marmar JL. Modified vasoepididymostomy with simultaneous double needle placement, tubulotomy and tubular invagination. J Urol. 2000;163(2):483–6.
30. Schiff J, Chan P, Li PS, Finkelberg S, Goldstein M. Outcome and late failures compared in 4 techniques of microsurgical vasoepididymostomy in 153 consecutive men. J Urol. 2005;174(2):651–5. quiz 801.
31. Chan PTK, Brandell RA, Goldstein M. Prospective analysis of outcomes after microsurgical intussusception vasoepididymostomy. BJU Int. 2005;96(4):598–601.
32. Ho KL, Wong MH, Tam PC. Microsurgical vasoepididymostomy for obstructive azoospermia. Hong Kong Med J. 2009;15(6):452–7.
33. Kumar R, Mukherjee S, Gupta NP. Intussusception vasoepididymostomy with longitudinal suture placement for idiopathic obstructive azoospermia. J Urol. 2010;183(4):1489–92.
34. Silber SJ. Microscopic technique for reversal of vasectomy. Surg Gynecol Obstet. 1976;143(4):631.
35. Owen ER. Microsurgical vasovasostomy: a reliable vasectomy reversal. Aust N Z J Surg. 1977;47(3):305–9.
36. Gopi SS, Townell NH. Vasectomy reversal: is the microscope really essential? Scott Med J. 2007;52(2):18–20.
37. Hsieh M-L, Huang HC, Chen Y, Huang ST, Chang PL. Loupe-assisted vs microsurgical technique for modified one-layer vasovasostomy: is the microsurgery really better? BJU Int. 2005;96(6):864–6.
38. Urquhart-Hay D. A low-power magnification technique for the re-anastomosis of the vas–further results in a personal series of 125 patients. Aust N Z J Surg. 1984;54(1):73–4.
39. Jee SH, Hong YK. One-layer vasovasostomy: microsurgical versus loupe-assisted. Fertil Steril. 2010;94(6):2308–11.
40. Dewire DM, Lawson RK. Experience with macroscopic vasectomy reversal at the Medical College of Wisconsin. Wis Med J. 1994;93(3):107–9.

41. Lee L, McLoughlin MG. Vasovasostomy: a comparison of macroscopic and microscopic techniques at one institution. Fertil Steril. 1980;33(1):54–5.
42. Kuang W, Shin PR, Oder M, Thomas Jr AJ. Robotic-assisted vasovasostomy: a two-layer technique in an animal model. Urology. 2005;65(4):811–4.
43. Schiff J, Li PS, Goldstein M. Robotic microsurgical vasovasostomy and vasoepididymostomy in rats. Int J Med Robot. 2005;1(2):122–6.
44. Kuang W, Shin PR, Matin S, Thomas Jr AJ. Initial evaluation of robotic technology for microsurgical vasovasostomy. J Urol. 2004;171(1):300–3.
45. Fleming C. Robot-assisted vasovasostomy. Urol Clin North Am. 2004;31(4):769–72.
46. Parekattil SJ, Cohen MS. Robotic microsurgery 2011: male infertility, chronic testicular pain, postvasectomy pain, sports hernia pain and phantom pain. Curr Opin Urol. 2011;21(2): 121–6.
47. Matsuda T, Muguruma K, Hiura Y, et al. Seminal tract obstruction caused by childhood inguinal herniorrhaphy: results of microsurgical reanastomosis. J Urol. 1998;159(3):837–40.
48. Pasqualotto FF, Pasqualotto EB, Agarwal A, Thomas Jr AJ. Results of microsurgical anastomosis in men with seminal tract obstruction due to inguinal herniorrhaphy. Rev Hosp Clin Fac Med Sao Paulo. 2003;58(6):305–9.
49. Shaeer OKZ, Shaeer KZ. Pelviscrotal vasovasostomy: refining and troubleshooting. J Urol. 2005;174(5):1935–7.
50. Sabanegh Jr E, Thomas Jr AJ. Effectiveness of crossover transseptal vasoepididymostomy in treating complex obstructive azoospermia. Fertil Steril. 1995;63(2):392–5.

Chapter 12
Tubal Microsurgery

Jeffrey M. Goldberg and Tommaso Falcone

Abstract Tubal anastomosis is a minimally invasive outpatient procedure that can be performed by minilaparotomy or laparoscopy, with or without robotic assistance. Success rates are high even in older women. Although the cost to achieve a pregnancy is generally less with tubal anastomosis than with IVF, the advantages and disadvantages of each needs to be discussed with the patient.

Keywords Fallopian tubes • Tubal anastomosis • Tubal ligation reversal • Female sterilization reversal • Microsurgery • Robotic surgery

Tubal Anastomosis Versus IVF

The only indication for microsurgery in gynecology is reversal of tubal ligation. Among women who underwent tubal sterilization, 0.9–26% regret their decision [1]. For women who desire future fertility, several factors must be weighed in deciding between tubal anastomosis and IVF. These include the age of the patient, ovarian reserve, number of children desired, presence of other infertility factors, experience

J.M. Goldberg, MD (✉)
Department of Obstetrics and Gynecology, Cleveland Clinic,
9500 Euclid Avenue, Cleveland, OH 44195, USA
e-mail: goldbej@ccf.org

T. Falcone, MD
Ob/Gyn and Women's Health Institute, Cleveland Clinic,
9500 Euclid Avenue A81, Cleveland, OH 44195, USA
e-mail: falcont@ccf.org

J.I. Sandlow (ed.), *Microsurgery for Fertility Specialists: A Practical Text*,
DOI 10.1007/978-1-4614-4196-0_12,

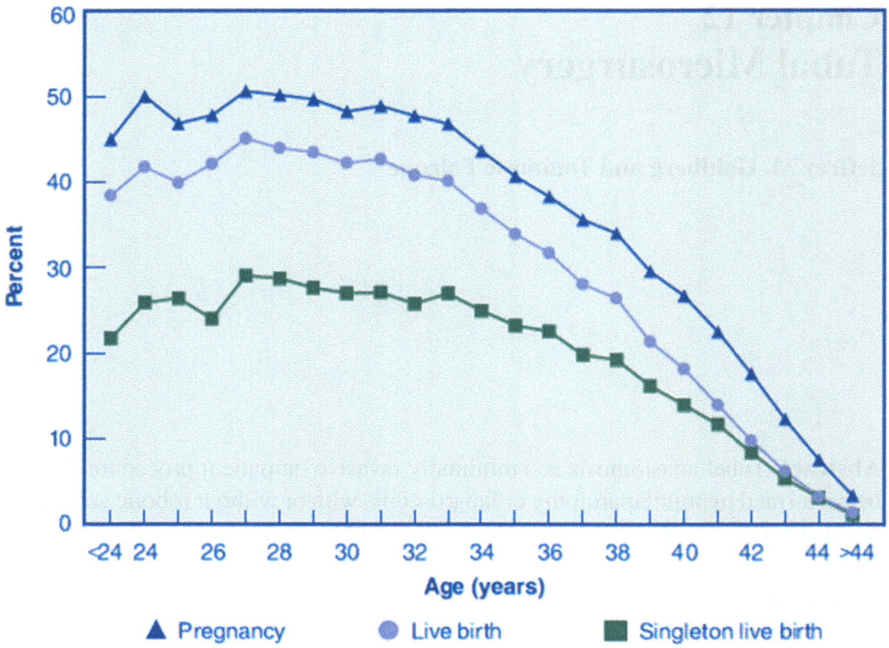

Fig. 12.1 Pregnancy, live birth, and singleton live birth rates based on IVF cycles initiated in 2008 (2404 Centers for Disease Control 2008)

of the surgeon, and success rate of the IVF program. The patient's preferences, religious beliefs, cost, and insurance coverage must also be considered.

The age of the woman is the strongest predictor of success with tubal anastomosis [2–5]. The 2-year cumulative intrauterine pregnancy rate is from 70% to more than 90% after microsurgical reversal of tubal sterilization in women under age 40 [3, 6, 7]. Even women 40–45 years old have excellent cumulative intrauterine pregnancy rates of 41.7–70.6% [3, 4, 6–11].

The women's age is also the factor most predictive of IVF success (Fig. 12.1). The current national IVF registry data from 2008 reported a 30.0% live birth rate per cycle initiated [12]. Therefore, multiple IVF cycles must be attempted to attain the same cumulative pregnancy rate achieved with tubal anastomosis. There are no randomized controlled trials comparing tubal anastomosis with IVF [13]. Retrospective studies noted that tubal anastomosis had a significantly higher cumulative pregnancy rate for women less than 37 years of age but no difference in women ≥37 [14]. The average cost per live birth with IVF was 2–10 times higher than for tubal anastomosis [11, 14].

IVF would be the preferred treatment if less than 4 cm of tubal length is available for repair and there are significant tubo-ovarian adhesions, stage 3–4 endometriosis, or more than a mild male factor. Otherwise, the advantages and disadvantages of both treatment options must be reviewed in order for the patient to make an informed decision. The advantages of tubal anastomosis are that it is a one-time (usually minimally invasive outpatient) procedure, and patients may attempt conception every month without further intervention and they may conceive more than once. It is more cost-effective than IVF and the risks associated with IVF are avoided.

The disadvantages are the risks for surgical complications such as bleeding, infection, organ damage, and reaction to anesthesia. There is also postoperative discomfort during the short recovery phase. The rate of ectopic pregnancy following tubal anastomosis ranges from 2 to 10% versus 1–2% for IVF [3, 4, 6–8, 10, 12].

The primary advantage of IVF is that it is nonsurgical. IVF can also decrease the time to pregnancy assuming that the patient is willing to try multiple cycles in succession. Its disadvantages are greater cost (especially if more than one cycle is required) and the need for frequent injections and monitoring over several weeks. IVF is associated with a high rate of multiple pregnancy. In 2008, the twin and triplet or more rates in the USA were 29 and 3.5%, respectively [12].

Multiple pregnancies greatly increase the risks of perinatal mortality, cerebral palsy, and other severe disabilities due to premature delivery. The medical costs for delivery and ongoing care can place a huge financial burden on the patient and the health care system as a whole. Several studies have identified a higher incidence of adverse perinatal outcomes such as perinatal mortality, preterm delivery, low and very low birth weights, intrauterine growth retardation, and congenital malformations even among singleton infants conceived with IVF [15–19]. In addition, IVF places the patient at risk for ovarian hyperstimulation syndrome which can be potentially life threatening in severe cases.

Preoperative Evaluation

An attempt should always be made to acquire the operative and pathology reports from the tubal ligation. If the procedure was performed in a way that would not provide sufficient tubal length for repair, or significant pelvic disease was noted, the patient should be counseled to go directly to IVF. If the operative report indicates that the pelvis was normal and the tubal ligation was performed with Fallope rings or Filshie clips, or a postpartum ligation was performed with only short segments of excised tubes measured on the pathology report, tubal anastomosis can be performed without a prior diagnostic laparoscopy. In all other cases, diagnostic laparoscopy should be performed just prior to the anastomosis as 3.8–27% of patients who desired tubal anastomosis did not have repairable tubes [20–22].

Although a preoperative HSG is useful for revealing intrauterine pathology, a diagnostic hysteroscopy can be performed just prior to the tubal anastomosis without putting the patient through a painful HSG procedure. A semen analysis is always advised prior to scheduling tubal anastomosis as IVF is the procedure of choice if a significant male factor is present. For women 35 years of age and older, day 3 FSH and estradiol levels, a Clomid challenge test, anti-mullerian hormone level, or antral follicle count can be performed to rule out diminished ovarian reserve which may indicate a poorer prognosis for success with both tubal anastomosis and IVF.

Technique

Our standard approach to microsurgical tubal anastomosis is by minilaparotomy as an outpatient procedure, though it may not be feasible in obese patients. The patient is placed in modified lithotomy position. After diagnostic hysteroscopy is performed, a uterine manipulator is placed to help elevate the fundus to the incision as well as to perform chromotubation. Diagnostic laparoscopy is then performed if indicated.

A 5 cm transverse incision is made about 2 fingerbreadths above the symphysis through the skin and subcutaneous fat to the level of the fascia. The fascia and peritoneum are incised vertically in the midline. A Mobius abdominal retractor (CooperSurgical, Trumbull, CT) is then placed through this cruciate incision. This single-use device provides excellent exposure and protects the wound edges without the risk of nerve compression injuries associated with metal retractors. Packs and sponges are not used and frequent irrigation is performed with Lactated Ringer's with 5,000 units of heparin per liter to reduce postoperative adhesion formation. Hemostasis may be achieved with micro-bipolar forceps or ophthalmic cautery.

The uterine fundus is delivered to the incision and the tubal segments are identified. Dilute vasopressin (20 units/100 ml of injectable saline) is infiltrated in the mesosalpinx beneath the occluded ends. The operating microscope is draped and brought into the operative field. The tubes are then mobilized using the unipolar microneedle. The occluded ends are opened with iris scissors. Transcervical chromotubation is performed by injecting indigo carmine through the uterine manipulator to demonstrate patency of the proximal tubal segments. Successive thin slices may be made with the iris scissors until free flow of dye is noted. A Beaver blade may be used instead in cases of cornual occlusion. Patency of the distal segments is documented by retrograde injection of dye using a 14 gauge angiocath (with needle removed) through the fimbria.

A single interrupted 6-0 Vicryl suture is placed through the mesosalpinx to align the tubal ends and take tension off the actual anastomosis. The anastomosis is performed with interrupted 8-0 Vicryl sutures placed such that the knots are tied extraluminally. There are no data to indicate that it makes a difference whether or not the tubal lumen is included. The first stitch is placed by the mesosalpinx (6:00 position). Additional stitches are then placed at 3, 9, and 12:00. It may be preferred to tie the knots after the stitches have been placed if visibility of the lumens is limited. Transcervical chromotubation is again performed to assess tubal patency. It is not necessary for the anastomosis to be watertight as long as spill of dye is seen through the fimbriated ends. Additional stitches may be required if there is an anastomotic leak but no distal spill. Finally, interrupted 8-0 Vicryl sutures are used to reapproximate the tubal serosa. Most patients are discharged within two hours.

Laparoscopic and Robotic Tubal Anastomosis

The quest for an even less invasive approach led to the first published reports of tubal ligation reversal by laparoscopy in the 1990s. However, the results were poor until proper instrumentation was available. Recent publications with conventional laparoscopy show excellent outcomes using a standard two-layer anastomosis. This approach was not widely adopted because of the great technical difficulties in learning laparoscopic microsurgery. Modifications of the technique were introduced such as the use of a one- or two-stitch repair with good results. A robotic approach was initially reported in 1999 with the ZEUS (Computer Motion Inc) robot, which is no longer available [23]. Robotic tubal reversals are now solely performed with the daVinci robot (Intuitive Surgical Inc, Sunnyvale, CA).

If a minimally invasive approach is chosen, we prefer to use robotic-assisted laparoscopy rather than conventional laparoscopy because the robotic system eliminates the fulcrum effect and the motion scaling reduces tremor. This is critical when working with fine sutures. Furthermore, the physician is comfortably seated with elbows placed on the resting area with robotic surgery. The only motion is at the wrist, which is the standard microsurgery approach. Robotic microsurgery's main limitation is the lack of haptic feedback that leads to needle bending and suture breaking. Visual cues are typically used to gauge the appropriate movements. This procedure requires experience to minimize these limitations.

Surgical Technique for Robotically Assisted Tubal Ligation Reversal

The components of the daVinci surgical robot include the surgeon's console, a video cart, and a surgical cart or tower. The surgical tower has four robotic arms that attach to specifically designed robotic trocars. The trocars that are used for tubal ligation reversal are 8 mm for the surgical instruments and 12 mm for the laparoscopic port. The console, placed anywhere in the operating room, provides the surgeon a three-dimensional vision of the operative field, as well as the ability to move the camera and manipulate surgical instruments (Fig. 12.2). The console settings should be adjusted to provide fine movements and extra magnification. Magnification can be easily adjusted and scaling is usually set at very fine (1:3). The surgeon's arms are placed comfortably on the arm rest so that only the wrists and fingers are moving (Fig. 12.3). The main advantage of the robot over conventional laparoscopy is the seven degrees of freedom of wrist movement.

The patient is placed in dorsal lithotomy position in Allen stirrups and a RUMI uterine manipulator is placed transcervically. The robot tower is "side docked" to allow access to the vagina and cervix for possible adjustments of the uterine manipulator or for performing a hysteroscopy (Fig. 12.4). Furthermore, it provides more space for an assistant to sit and manipulate the uterus comfortably. After establishing

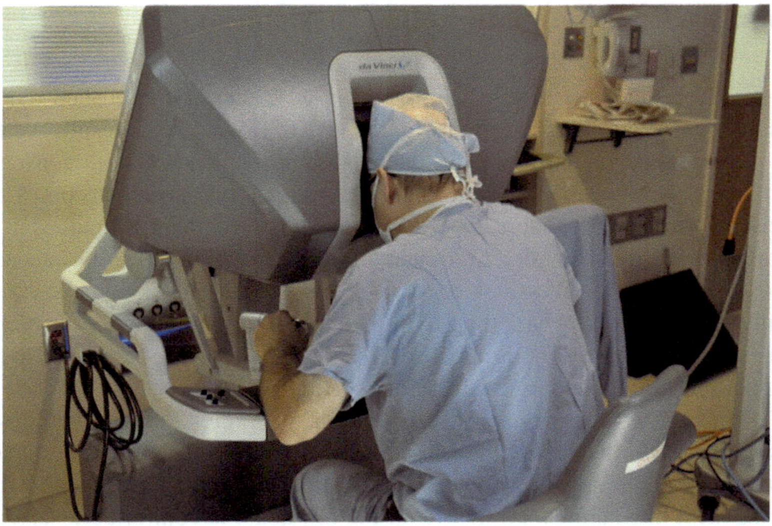

Fig. 12.2 daVinci surgical console

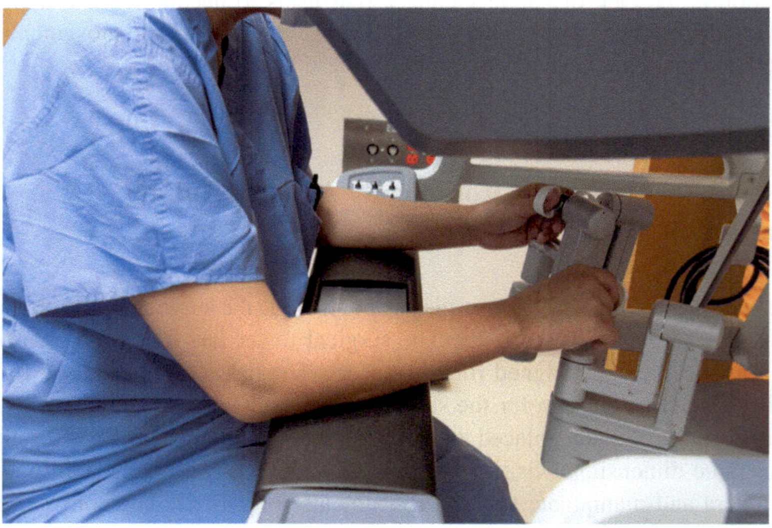

Fig. 12.3 Surgeon's arms are supported while the fingers control the "joysticks"

a pneumoperitoneum, a 12 mm port is placed in the umbilicus. The proper placement of accessory trocars for robotic surgery is critical so as to avoid collision. We typically use three accessory robotic ports and one accessory conventional port for the introduction of needles, suction–irrigation, and other conventional laparoscopic instruments. The robotic ports need to be placed 8–10 cm away from each other. The conventional accessory laparoscopic port is placed in the lower quadrant, usually on the right side. A 12 mm port is typically used as the small needles can get stuck in

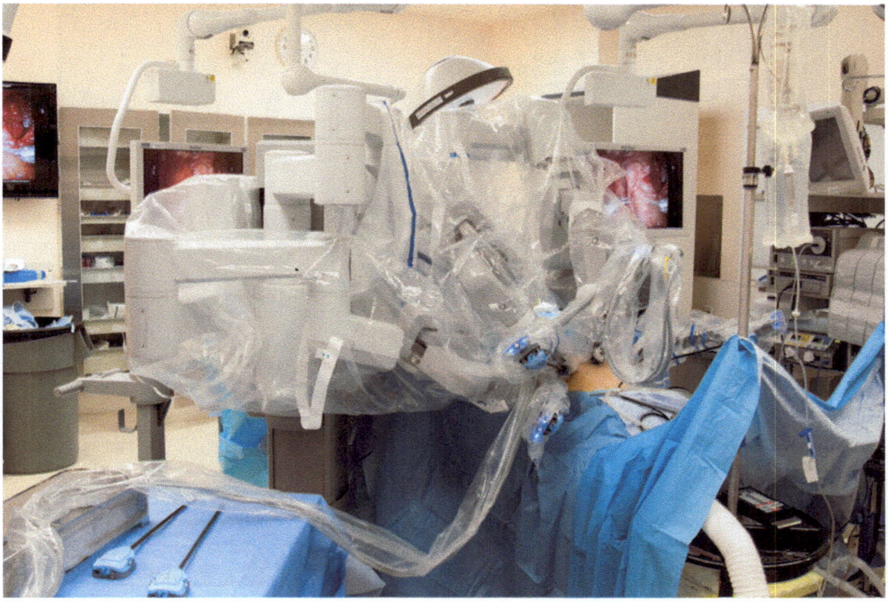

Fig. 12.4 The instrument tower is docked to the side of the operating table

smaller ports. It is important that needles are visualized as they enter and leave the trocar since it is easy to lose one of these fine needles.

Our standard robotic instruments are the Prograsp forceps, Potts scissors, micro-bipolar cautery, and the black diamond microforceps. We also use conventional robotic monopolar scissors for macro-dissection of the surgical site and the Potts scissors for the micro-dissection of the anastomosis site. Figure 12.5 shows the typical setup with the Prograsp in arm 3, the micro-bipolar in arm 2, and the Potts or robotic monopolar scissors in arm 1. Power settings should be at 15 W. The serosa is usually dissected 5 mm from the tip so that the muscularis is seen.

We use a laparoscopically placed stent through the proximal and distal lumen to facilitate the suturing. This stent can be either the inner catheter of the Novy cornual cannulation set (Cook Medical Inc, Bloomington, IN) or a graduated ERCP cannula. The surgery starts with the preparation of the proximal and distal anastomosis site. Dilute vasopressin (20 units in 200 ml) is injected into the mesosalpinx. The area is trimmed and the proximal and distal anastomosis site prepared. Suturing is accomplished with the use of the black diamond forceps. An 8 cm length of 6-0 Vicryl is introduced to suture the mesosalpinx layer. This stitch should be no closer than 5 mm from the tube so as to keep a gap between the proximal and distal sites (Fig. 12.6). A 6 cm length of 7-0 or 8-0 polypropylene on a BV 175-6 or BV 130-needle is then introduced to suture the first layer. The first stitch is placed at 6 o'clock and tied (Fig. 12.7). Additional sutures are placed at 3 and 9 o'clock but not tied until the 12 o'clock stitch is placed and then they are all tied. Dilute indigo carmine is then injected transcervically to confirm patency. The fascial layer of

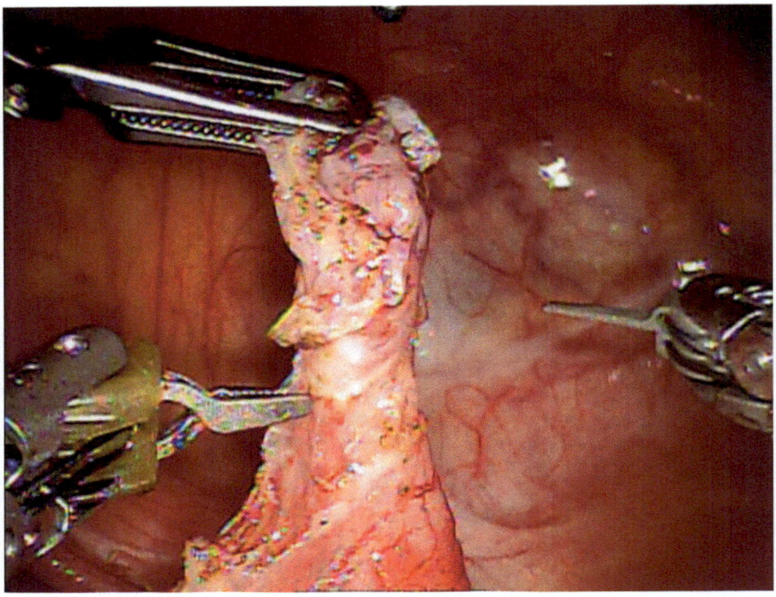

Fig. 12.5 daVinici instrument tips; Prograsp top, micro-bipolar lower left, scissors on right

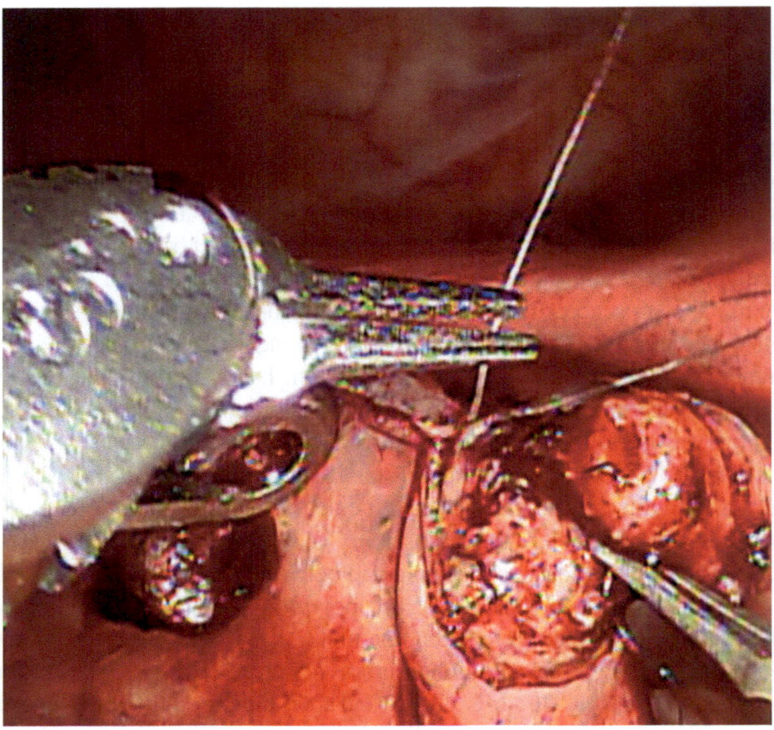

Fig. 12.6 Suture placed through the mesosalpinx of the proximal tubal segment

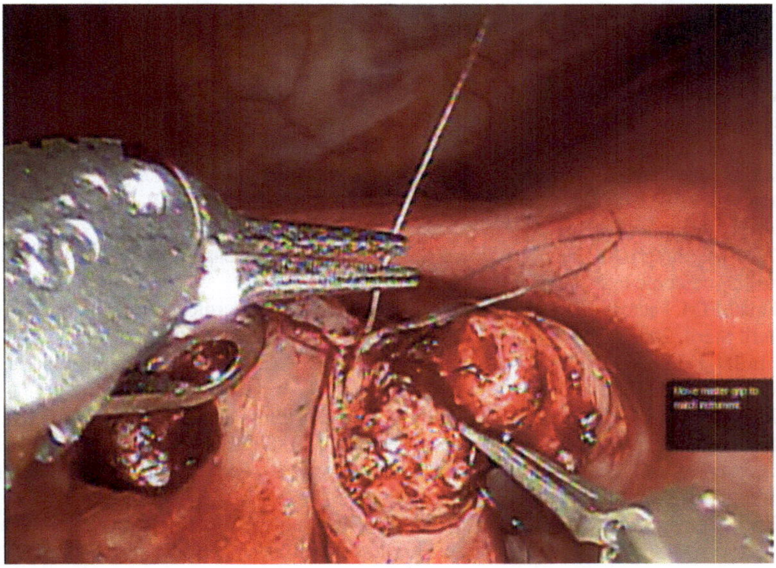

Fig. 12.7 The 6:00 suture are placed through the tubal lumen of the proximal segment

the 12 mm ports are closed while only the skin is closed at the 8 mm trocar sites. The patient is discharged the same day.

Perioperative and Reproductive Outcomes

The original case series of eight patients who underwent tubal anastomosis with the daVinci robot was published in 2000 [24]. Since then, there have been 4 case series with over 140 patients with pregnancy rates between 61 and 80% [25–28]. In comparison with laparotomy, surgical times are longer and costs are higher. In our institution, we conducted a retrospective comparison of tubal anastomosis by minilaparotomy and robotic-assisted laparoscopy, both performed as an outpatient. This revealed average surgical and anesthesia times of 181 and 205 min for the minilaparotomy group versus 229 and 283 min for the robotic group. The robotic group returned to work in 0.8 weeks compared with 2.8 weeks in the laparotomy group. It is unclear if the increased costs of robotic surgery ($1,446 additional mean cost per robotic case) are offset by the faster return to work.

In the retrospective study by Dharia-Patel, outpatients treated robotically were compared with patients that had a laparotomy with a 6–8 cm incision and were admitted overnight. The length of hospital stay in this group was of course longer [27]. Time to recovery was 11 days in the robotic group and 28 days in the laparotomy group. It seems that the robot may not have an advantage over minilaparotomy outpatient microsurgery but may be superior to traditional laparotomy. The robot may be especially advantageous in patients with previous pelvic surgery and adhesions and obese patients where a minilaparotomy may be more challenging.

References

1. ACOG Committee on Practice Bulletins-Gynecology. ACOG practice bulletin. Benefits and risks of sterilization. Obstet Gynecol. 2003;102:647–58.
2. Putman JM, Holden AE, Olive DL. Pregnancy rates following tubal anastomosis: Pomeroy partial salpingectomy versus electrocautery. J Gynecol Surg. 1990;6:173–8.
3. Dubuisson JB, Chapron C, Nos C, Morice P, Aubriot FX, Garnier P. Sterilization reversal: fertility results. Hum Reprod. 1995;10:1145–51.
4. Yoon TK, Sung HR, Kang HG, Cha SH, Lee CN, Cha KY. Laparoscopic tubal anastomosis: fertility outcome in 202 cases. Fertil Steril. 1999;72:1121–6.
5. Hanafi MM. Factors affecting the pregnancy rate after microsurgical reversal of tubal ligation. Fertil Steril. 2003;80:434–40.
6. Kim JD, Kim KS, Doo JK, Rhyeu CH. A report on 387 cases of microsurgical tubal reversals. Fertil Steril. 1997;68:875–80.
7. Gordts S, Campo R, Puttemans P, Gordts S. Clinical factors determining pregnancy outcome after microsurgical tubal reanastomosis. Fertil Steril. 2009;92:1198–202.
8. Trimbos-Kemper TC. Reversal of sterilization in women over 40 years of age: a multicenter survey in The Netherlands. Fertil Steril. 1990;53:575–7.
9. Glock JL, Kim AH, Hulka JF, Hunt RB, Trad FS, Brumsted JR. Reproductive outcome after tubal reversal in women 40 years of age or older. Fertil Steril. 1996;65:863–5.
10. Cha SH, Lee MH, Kim JH, Lee CN, Yoon TK, Cha KY. Fertility outcome after tubal anastomosis by laparoscopy and laparotomy. J Am Assoc Gynecol Laparosc. 2001;8:348–52.
11. Petrucco OM, Silber SJ, Chamberlain SL, Warnes GM, Davies M. Live birth following day surgery reversal of female sterilisation in women older than 40 years: a realistic option in Australia? Med J Aust. 2007;187:271–3.
12. Centers for Disease Control. Assisted reproductive technology (ART) report: section 2—ART cycles using fresh, nondonor eggs or embryos. Atlanta: Centers for Disease Control; 2008.
13. Yossry M, Aboulghar M, D'Angelo A, Gillett W. In vitro fertilisation versus tubal reanastomosis (sterilisation reversal) for subfertility after tubal sterilisation. Cochrane Database Syst Rev. 2006;3:CD004144.
14. Boeckxstaens A, Devroey P, Collins J, Tournaye H. Getting pregnant after tubal sterilization: surgical reversal or IVF? Hum Reprod. 2007;22:2660–4.
15. Hansen M, Bower C, Milne E, de Klerk N, Kurinczuk JJ. Assisted reproductive technologies and the risk of birth defects—a systematic review. Hum Reprod. 2005;20:328–38.
16. McDonald SD, Murphy K, Beyene J, Ohlsson A. Perinatel outcomes of singleton pregnancies achieved by in vitro fertilization: a systematic review and meta-analysis. J Obstet Gynaecol Can. 2005;27:449–59.
17. Jackson RA, Gibson KA, Wu YW, Croughan MS. Perinatal outcomes in singletons following in vitro fertilization: a meta-analysis. Obstet Gynecol. 2004;103:551–63.
18. Kallen B, Finnstrom O, Lindam A, Nilsson E, Nygren KG, Otterblad PO. Congenital malformations in infants born after in vitro fertilization in Sweden. Birth Defects Res A Clin Mol Teratol. 2010;88:137–43.
19. El-Chaar D, Yang Q, Gao J, et al. Risk of birth defects increased in pregnancies conceived by assisted human reproduction. Fertil Steril. 2009;92:1557–61.
20. Opsahl MS, Klein TA. The role of laparoscopy in the evaluation of candidates for sterilization reversal. Fertil Steril. 1987;48:546–9.
21. Seiler JC. Factors influencing the outcome of microsurgical tubal ligation reversals. Am J Obstet Gynecol. 1983;146:292–8.
22. Taylor PJ, Leader A. Reversal of female sterilization: how reliable is the previous operative report? J Reprod Med. 1982;27:246–8.
23. Falcone T, Goldberg J, Garcia-Ruiz A, Margossian H, Stevens L. Full robotic assistance for laparoscopic tubal anastomosis: a case report. J Laparoendosc Adv Surg Tech A. 1999;9: 107–13.

24. Degueldre M, Vandromme J, Huong PT, Cadiere GB. Robotically assisted laparoscopic microsurgical tubal reanastomosis: a feasibility study. Fertil Steril. 2000;74:1020–3.
25. Rodgers AK, Goldberg JM, Hammel JP, Falcone T. Tubal anastomosis by robotic compared with outpatient minilaparotomy. Obstet Gynecol. 2007;109:1375–80.
26. Vlahos NF, Bankowski BJ, King JA, Shiller DA. Laparoscopic tubal reanastomosis using robotics: experience from a teaching institution. J Laparoendosc Adv Surg Tech A. 2007;17: 180–5.
27. Dharia Patel SP, Steinkampf MP, Whitten SJ, Malizia BA. Robotic tubal anastomosis: surgical technique and cost effectiveness. Fertil Steril. 2008;90:1175–9.
28. Caillet M, Vandromme J, Rozenberg S, Paesmans M, Germay O, Degueldre M. Robotically assisted laparoscopic microsurgical tubal reanastomosis: a retrospective study. Fertil Steril. 2010;94:1844–7.

Chapter 13
Microsurgical Penile Revascularization, Replantation, and Reconstruction

Jeffrey Lee Rosenblum and Arthur L. Burnett

Abstract Microsurgery, in a general sense, can be defined as surgery with optical enhancement. Certainly, nuances with regard to various specialties and their respective domain's microsurgical procedures exist. In the field of urology, urologists initially were exposed to microsurgery as it related to male-factor fertility (Silber, Urology 6:150–3, 1975), such as vasovasostomy, vasoepididymostomy, and microsurgical scrotal and groin explorations. However, just as the field of andrology encompasses fertility issues as well as erectile dysfunction, so too does microsurgery have applications in the latter. Microsurgical techniques have formed an essential component of penile revascularization and venous surgery for erectile dysfunction in a select group of patients (Crespo et al., Urology 20:271–5, 1982; Goldlust et al., J Urol 128:821–2, 1982; Goldstein et al., J Sex Med 5:2018–21, 2008; Munarriz, ScientificWorldJournal 10:1–9, 2010; Munarriz et al., J Urol 182:643–8, 2009; Montague et al., The management of erectile dysfunction: an update. Baltimore, MD: American Urological Association Education and Research, 2005; Munarriz et al., Glenn's urologic surgery. Philadelphia, PA: Lippincott Williams & Wilkins, 2004; Lewis and Munarriz, Campbell-Walsh urology, Philadelphia, PA: Saunders Elsevier, 2007; Sharaby et al., Urol Clin North Am 22(4):821–32, 1995). Extrapolating this further, penile microvascular surgery is relevant in the armamentarium of techniques for penile replantation and reconstruction. In this chapter, we elucidate microsurgical techniques as applied to the continuum of genital disorders requiring penile revascularization, replantation, and reconstruction.

J.L. Rosenblum, M.D. (✉)
The Rosenblum Center for Urologic Care, Medical Arts Building,
80 West Welsh Pool Road, Suite 100, Exton, PA 19341, USA
e-mail: urology@comcast.net

A.L. Burnett, M.D.
Department of Urology, The Johns Hopkins Hospital,
600 North Wolfe St., Marburg 407, Baltimore, MD 21287, USA

J.I. Sandlow (ed.), *Microsurgery for Fertility Specialists: A Practical Text*,
DOI 10.1007/978-1-4614-4196-0_13,

Keywords Amputated penis • Erectile dysfunction • Flap • Forearm flap • Hypogastric-cavernosal system • Microarterial bypass • Microsurgery • Penile reconstruction • Penile replantation • Penile revascularization • Penile venous surgery

Anatomy of the Penis and Male Perineum

In order to fully comprehend penile microvascular surgery, the infrastructure of the male genitalia and its anatomic and functional interrelationships must be understood.

Penis

The penile shaft consists of three erectile structures (Fig. 13.1): bilateral corpora cavernosa dorsally and the corpus spongiosum encasing the urethra ventrally [1]. Each corpus cavernosum contains erectile tissue within a dense, elastic connective tissue sheath—the tunica albuginea (Fig. 13.2). The tunica albuginea is composed of an inner circular and outer longitudinal layer of elastic fibers. Communication between the two corpora cavernosa occurs through an incompetent midline septum. The fibers of the septal strands interweave with those of the inner circular layer of the tunica albuginea dorsally and ventrally. The corpora cavernosa split apart proximally and become independent chambers to form the crura resembling an inverted "Y" (Fig. 13.1). Each crus attaches to its ipsilateral inferior pubic ramus and ischium. The erectile tissue of each corpus consists of trabeculae (from the tunica albuginea), arteries, veins, nerves, muscle, and flat endothelial-lined venous sinusoids [2]. A layer of areolar connective tissue lies between this erectile tissue and the inner wall of the tunica albuginea. Each corpus cavernosum has a cavernosal artery running through its center.

The corpus spongiosum contains the urethra throughout the penile shaft [3]. It is positioned in a ventral groove between the corpora cavernosa. Similar to the corpora cavernosa, the corpus spongiosum has a tunica albuginea covering. The erectile tissue within the corpus spongiosum is less robust than that of the corpora cavernosa. The corpus spongiosum expands at its distal end to form the glans penis covering the tips of the corpora cavernosa (Fig. 13.1). The urethral meatus is positioned ventrally at the glans tip. Beyond where the corpora cavernosa split and become the crura, the corpus spongiosum widens to form the bulbospongiosus (bulb of the penis) within the perineum [4] (Fig. 13.3).

The Urethra

The urethra is divided into six segments [4] (Fig. 13.4):

1. The *fossa navicularis* is within the glans penis. It is lined with stratified squamous epithelium.

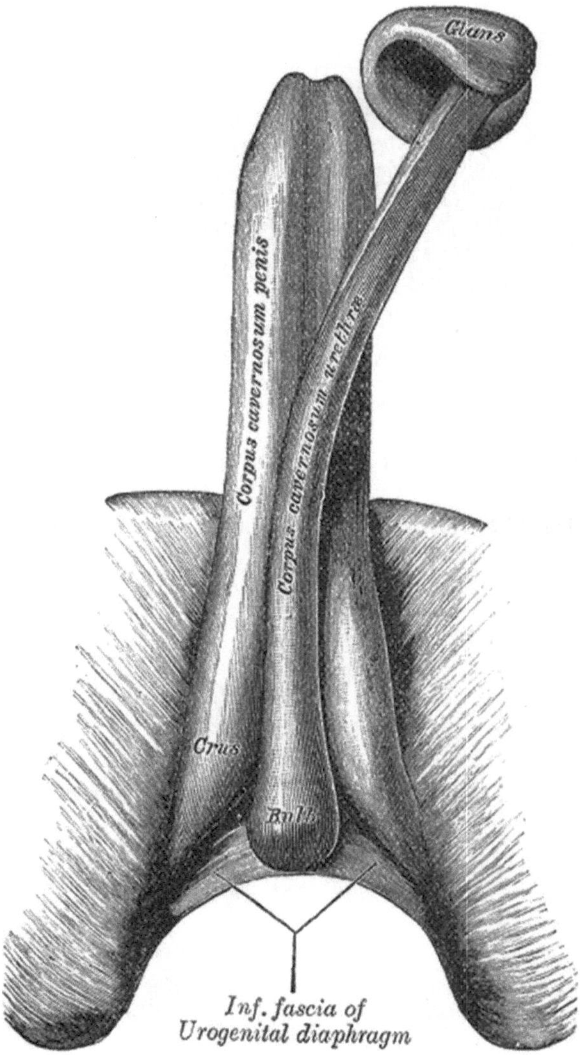

Fig. 13.1 The three corpora of the penis. The glans penis is an expansion of the distal corpus spongiosum (Gray's Anatomy, 1918)

2. The *penile or pendulous urethra* extends from where the fossa navicularis begins to where the bulbospongiosus ends. Simple squamous epithelium makes up the lining of this area.
3. The *bulbous urethra* is that portion proximal to the penile urethra and is covered by the bulbospongiosus muscle. Its proximal extent is where the bulbospongiosus attaches to the perineal body. It is lined distally with squamous epithelium that gradually changes to transitional epithelium as it slopes up to the membranous urethra.

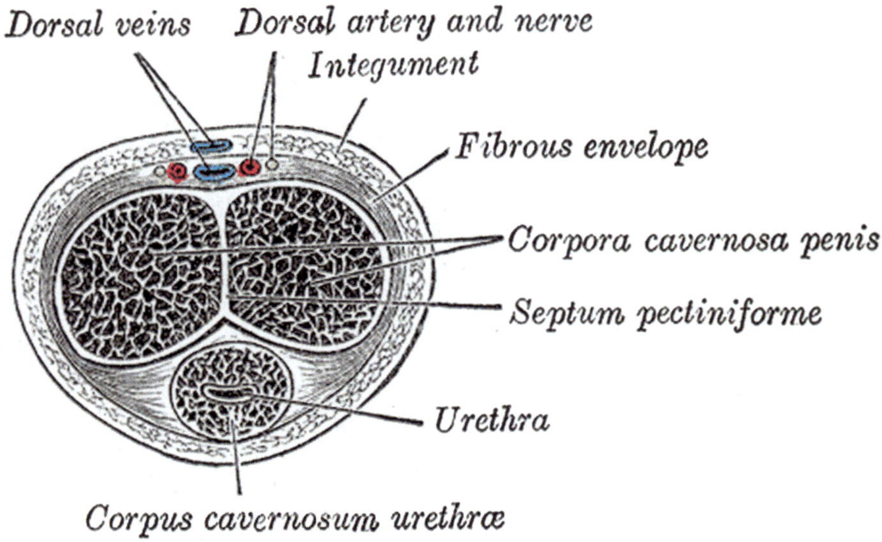

Fig. 13.2 Cross section of penis. Each corpora is surrounded by a tunica albuginea (Gray's Anatomy, 1918)

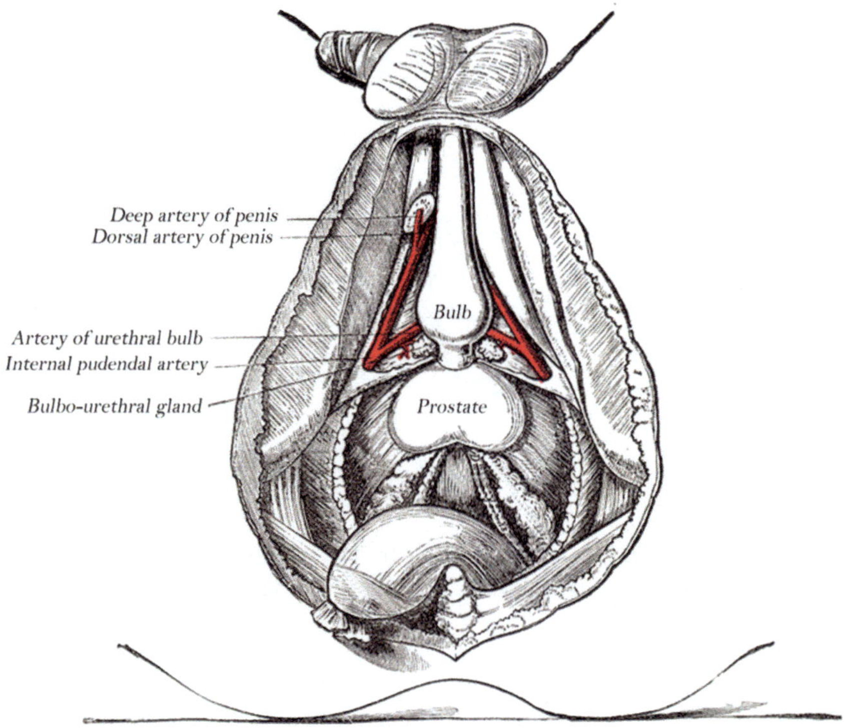

Fig. 13.3 The male perineum demonstrating the urethral bulb and surrounding structures (Gray's Anatomy, 1918)

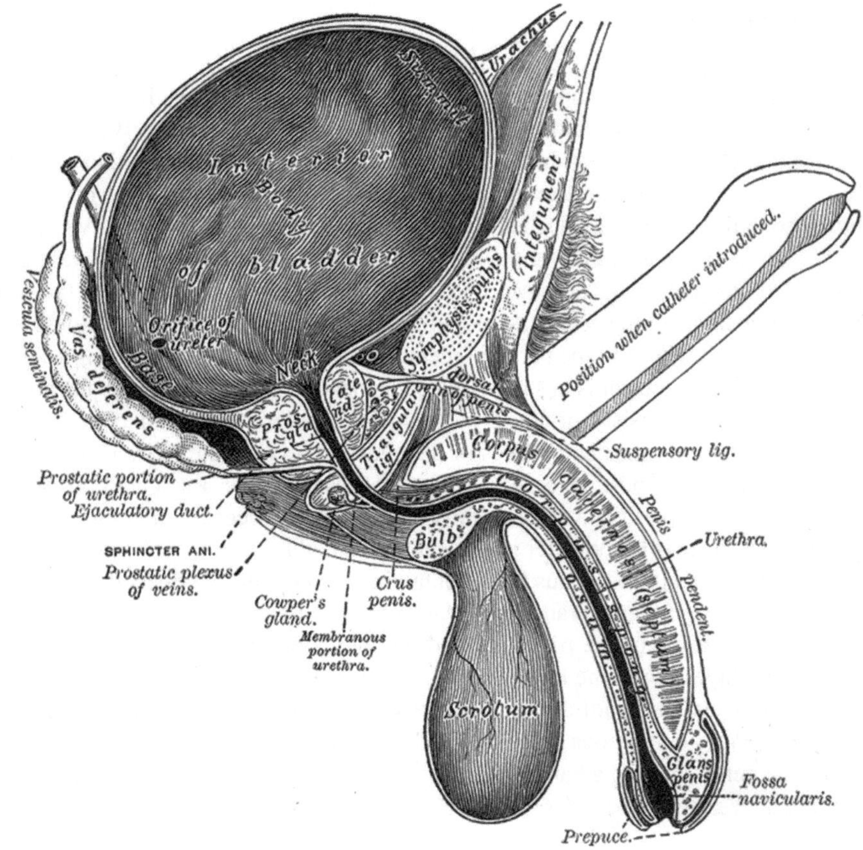

Fig. 13.4 Sagittal view of the male perineum and penis. The urethral segments are shown (Gray's Anatomy, 1918)

4. The *membranous urethra* is surrounded by the external urethral sphincter complex and is lined with transitional epithelium.
5. The *prostatic urethra* is proximal to the membranous urethra and surrounded by prostate tissue. Transitional epithelium lines the prostatic urethra and extends into the bladder.
6. The *bladder neck* is the area circumferentially distal to the trigone adjacent and variably including the prostate.

Five sphincter-type areas are found surrounding the male posterior urethra [4–6]. These are (1) the *bladder neck*, (2) the *prostate* itself with its muscular stroma, (3) the *external smooth muscle sphincter* at the level of the membranous urethra, (4) the *external rhabdosphincter*, and (5) *muscles of recruitment* in the area of the membranous urethra. These sphincters have continence correlations with regard to various types of injuries and subsequent penile and urethral reconstructive procedures.

Fascial Layers

Two main fascial coverings surround the three erectile bodies [4, 5]. Buck's fascia is the deep penile fascia. The dartos fascia is the superficial penile fascia. Buck's fascia is a resilient elastic layer that immediately surrounds all three corpora. Dorsally on the corpora cavernosa, the deep dorsal vein, dorsal arteries, and dorsal nerves lie above the tunica albuginea attached to the inner surface of Buck's fascia. Ventrally, Buck's fascia splits surrounding the corpus spongiosum. Distally, Buck's fascia is attached to the glans penis at the corona. Proximally, it covers each crus of the corpora cavernosa attaching to the ischiopubic rami. Buck's fascia also encloses the bulb and is fixed with it to the perineal membrane or urogenital diaphragm [4, 7].

Dartos fascia of the penis lies immediately beneath the penile skin and just above Buck's fascia. It consists of loosely arranged alveolar tissue and contains the superficial arteries, veins, and nerves of the penis. Unique to the penis is that there is no subcuticular adipose layer. The superficial fascia of the perineum consists of two layers: the superficial, areolar, fatty layer and the deeper, more substantial membranous layer [6]. The latter is also known as *Colles' fascia*. The tunica dartos of the scrotum is a subcutaneous layer containing smooth muscle fibers that give the scrotal skin its rugose appearance. The dartos fascia of the penis is continuous with the superficial fascia of the perineum and the tunica dartos of the scrotum. These three fascial layers combine at the base of the penis to form the suspensory structures of the penis: the fundiform and suspensory ligaments [4, 7]. The outer fundiform ligament is continuous with the caudal portion of the linea alba and travels around the penis creating a hammock underneath it. The inner suspensory ligament is triangularly shaped and secures the dartos fascia of the penis to the anterior aspect of the pubic bone.

Arterial Supply

The arterial blood supply of the penile skin is from the left and right inferior external pudendal vessels arising from the first portion of the femoral artery [4, 7]. These inferior external vessels traverse the upper medial portion of the femoral triangle and divide into two main branches. They traverse the penile shaft within the dartos fascia running dorsolaterally and ventrolaterally with extensive collaterals across the midline. These fine branches form an extensive subdermal vascular plexus. Venous tributaries accompany the arteries. This rich vascular supply concomitant with the penile skin's mobility imparts the ideal characteristics for its use in urethral substitution [3, 4]. The scrotal wall and ventral penile skin derive their blood supply from posterior scrotal artery which is a superficial branch from the internal pudendal artery. Tributaries for this system travel within the tunica dartos.

The blood supply to the deep penile structures emanates from the common penile artery, the continuation of the internal pudendal artery after it gives off its perineal

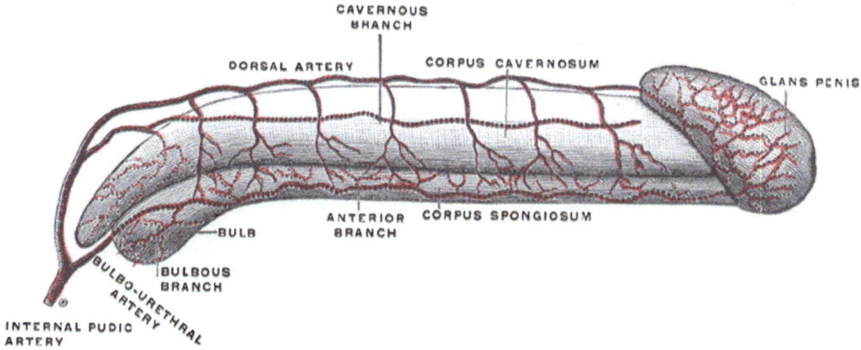

Fig. 13.5 The three terminal branches of the common penile artery: the bulbourethral, dorsal, and cavernosal arteries (Gray's Anatomy, 1918)

branch [7]. After traversing the perineal membrane, the common penile artery abuts the inferior pubic ramus medially and then divides into its terminal branches near the urethral bulb. However, there can be variations in this blood supply. These terminal penile branches can originate from an accessory pudendal artery arising from the obturator artery or the internal pudendal artery prior to its entrance into the greater sciatic foramen. The accessory pudendal artery makes its way to the root of the penis by traveling along the lower detrusor area anterolateral to the prostate.

The three terminal branches of the common penile artery are (Fig. 13.5):

1. The *bulbourethral artery*—a short artery or arteries which pierce the perineal membrane and Buck's fascia entering the bulb of the penis. A variation is when it arises as a branch of the dorsal or cavernosal artery. The urethral artery, stemming from the bulbourethral artery or as a separate branch of the common penile artery, travels in the corpus spongiosum ventrolateral to the urethra. It terminates in the glans anastomosing with the terminal branches of the dorsal arteries.
2. The *dorsal artery*—the terminal branch of the internal pudendal or accessory pudendal artery. The dorsal artery travels along the dorsum of the penis between the deep dorsal vein medially and the dorsal nerve laterally. It has a coiled configuration which straightens out as the penis elongates with erection [4, 6]. Along its course, it gives off three to ten circumflex cavernosal arteries that accompany circumflex veins around the lateral surface of the corpora cavernosa. These circumflex arterial branches supply the corpus spongiosum. The dorsal artery's terminal branches arborize in the glans. This dual blood supply to the corpus spongiosum is of paramount importance in reconstructive surgical procedures, permitting the urethra to be divided with its distal vascularity coming retrograde from the glans unless disease, trauma, or previous surgery has altered or obstructed these vessels [3]. Sometimes, dorsal artery branches perforate the tunica albuginea and connect to the cavernosal arteries, though the functional significance of these anastomoses varies with regard to erectile function [8, 9].

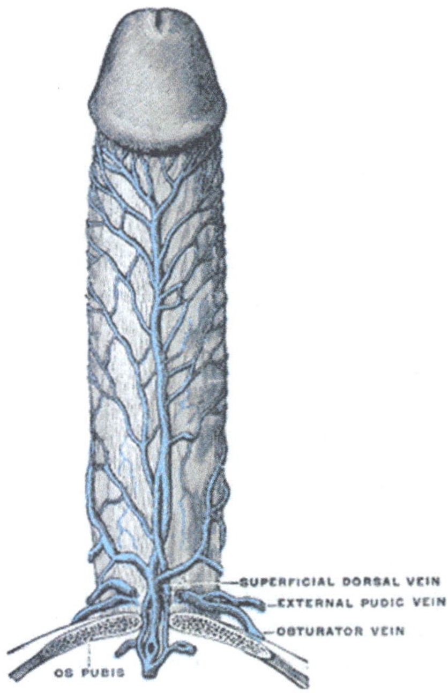

Fig. 13.6 Venous drainage of the penis (*penile view*) (Gray's Anatomy, 1918)

3. The *cavernosal artery*—usually a single artery on each side that arises as the terminal branch of the common penile artery. It enters the corpus cavernosum at the hilum running the length of the penile shaft. The cavernosal artery gives off the many helicine arteries that comprise the arterial component of the corporal erectile process. The helicine arteries empty directly into the cavernous sinusoidal spaces. Numerous types of variations have been seen on diagnostic evaluations assessing erectile function [8, 9]. These have included variations in the origin and number of cavernosal arteries. Cavernosal arteries have been seen to arise from an accessory pudendal artery and frequently the cavernosal arteries branch before entering the corpora. A branch can enter the contralateral corpus cavernosum or a single cavernosal artery can branch within the ipsilateral corpus to supply both corpora. Hypoplasia of cavernosal arteries has been seen on diagnostic studies as well [8].

Venous Drainage

Three venous systems drain the penis (Figs. 13.6 and 13.7) [4, 5, 7]:

1. *Superficial*. The superficial veins are contained in the dartos fascia, run dorsolaterally, and unite at the base of the penis to form a single superficial dorsal vein. The superficial dorsal vein usually drains into the left saphenous vein. Rarely, it can drain into the right saphenous vein or form two trunks that can drain into both saphenous veins. Some superficial veins may drain into the superficial

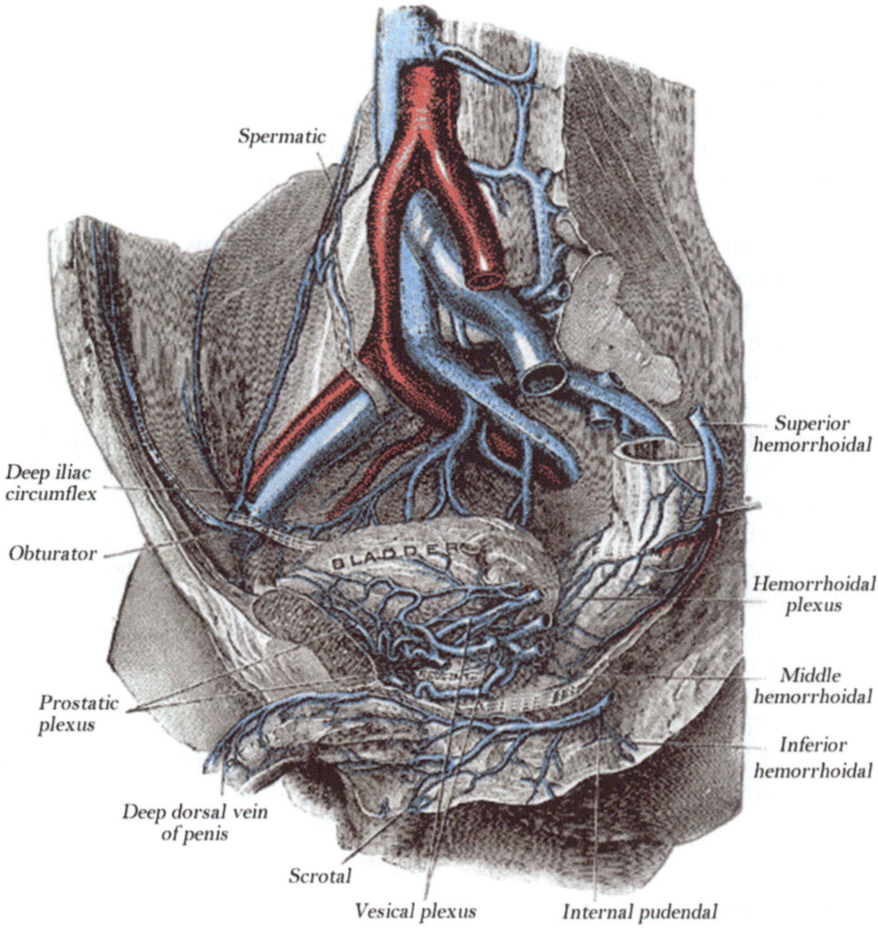

Fig. 13.7 Venous drainage of the penis (*pelvic view*) (Gray's Anatomy, 1918)

external pudendal veins. Still further, connections between the superficial veins and the deep dorsal vein of the penis can occur.

2. *Intermediate*. The intermediate venous system consists of the deep dorsal vein and circumflex veins lying within and beneath Buck's fascia and the venae comitantes that travel with the dorsal arteries. Blood from the sinusoids of the erectile spaces is drained via venules into a subtunical venous network. Emissary veins from this subtunical network pierce the tunica albuginea emerging on the dorsolateral surface of the corpora cavernosa to drain into the circumflex veins or directly into the deep dorsal vein. The circumflex veins, more prominent in the distal two thirds of the penis, arise from the corpus spongiosum. The emissary veins drain into the circumflex veins as the circumflex veins pass around the lateral aspect of the corpora cavernosa beneath the dorsal arteries and nerves to empty into the deep dorsal vein. The circumflex veins communicate with each

other ispilaterally and contralaterally to form between 3 and 12 common venous channels that are usually accompanied by branches of the dorsal nerve and artery. The circumflex veins can also communicate ventrally forming bilateral periurethral veins. These latter veins must be identified as they can be important in the surgical treatment of veno-occlusive dysfunction-related impotence. Five to eight small veins from the glans penis form a retrocoronal plexus. This plexus drains into the deep dorsal vein which sits in a midline groove between the corporal bodies. As noted earlier, connections can exist between the deep and superficial dorsal veins. The deep dorsal vein may consist of a number of anastomosing tributaries along the penile shaft. The deep dorsal vein receives blood from the emissary and circumflex veins and passes beneath the pubis at the level of the suspensory ligament. It leaves the shaft of the penis to drain into the periprostatic plexus known as *Santorini's plexus*.

3. *Deep*. The deep venous system consists of the cavernosal and crural veins. In the proximal third of the corpora cavernosa, emissary veins join together to form multiple thin-walled trunks on the dorsomedial surface of each crus adjacent to the ischial tuberosities. They merge into one or two cavernosal veins bilaterally in the penile hilum medial to the cavernosal arteries and nerves. The cavernosal veins drain into Santorini's plexus or may diverge laterally between the bulbospongiosus and the penile crus to drain into the internal pudendal veins. Small veins from the penile bulb also empty into the cavernosal veins. Small crural veins from the dorsolateral surface of the crura drain into the internal pudendal veins. The internal pudendal veins along with the internal pudendal artery and pudendal nerve enter Alcock's canal. The internal pudendal veins then drain into the internal iliac vein [1, 4, 7].

Lymphatic Drainage (Fig. 13.8)

The lymphatic drainage of the prepuce and penile shaft skin converges dorsally and then divides at the base of the penis to drain into the right and left superficial inguinal nodes [4, 7]. The glans' lymph tributaries collect at the frenulum, then encircle the corona dorsally. These lymph vessels then traverse the penis below Buck's fascia to drain into the femoral triangle's deep inguinal lymph nodes. Some of these lymph vessels drain into the presymphyseal lymph nodes and via this route drain into the superficial inguinal lymph nodes and the lateral external iliac lymph nodes [10].

Nerve Supply (Fig. 13.9)

The afferent and efferent nerve supply of the penis is derived from the pudendal and cavernosal nerves [4, 7, 11]. The pudendal nerves supply somatic motor and sensory innervation. The cavernosal nerves are the autonomic nerve supply controlling erectile

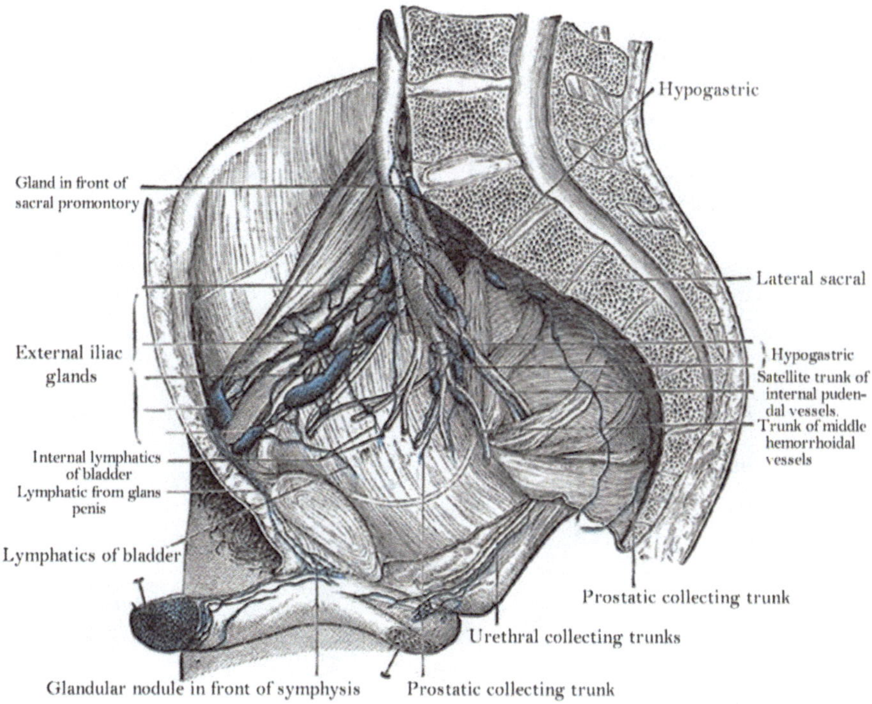

Fig. 13.8 Lymphatic drainage of the penis (Gray's Anatomy, 1918)

function [12]. The autonomic nerves consist of the parasympathetic and sympathetic efferent and visceral afferent nerve fibers. Along with the internal pudendal vessels noted earlier, the pudendal nerves enter the perineum through the lesser sciatic notch at the posterior border of the ischiorectal fossa and enter the fibrofascial sheath of Alcock's canal to the posterior perineal membrane [4, 7].

The dorsal nerve of the penis is the first branch of the pudendal nerve in Alcock's canal [4, 7]. It courses ventral to the main trunk of the pudendal nerve traveling above the obturator internus muscle and below the levator ani. The dorsal nerve continues dorsally on the penile shaft lateral to the dorsal artery on the inner surface of Buck's fascia. Multiple nerve branches from the dorsal nerve supply proprioceptive and sensory nerve terminals on the surface of the tunica albuginea and sensory terminals in the skin and glans.

The autonomic innervation of the penis arises from the pelvic plexus. This plexus consists of preganglionic parasympathetic efferent fibers from the sacral center (S2–S4), pre- and postganglionic sympathetic efferent fibers from the thoracolumbar center (T11–L2), and visceral afferents to both centers. The cavernous nerves arise from the pelvic plexus, run lateral to the tips of the seminal vesicles, posterolateral to the prostate and through the wall of the membranous urethra just lateral to the striated sphincter. They pierce the perineal membrane innervating Cowper's

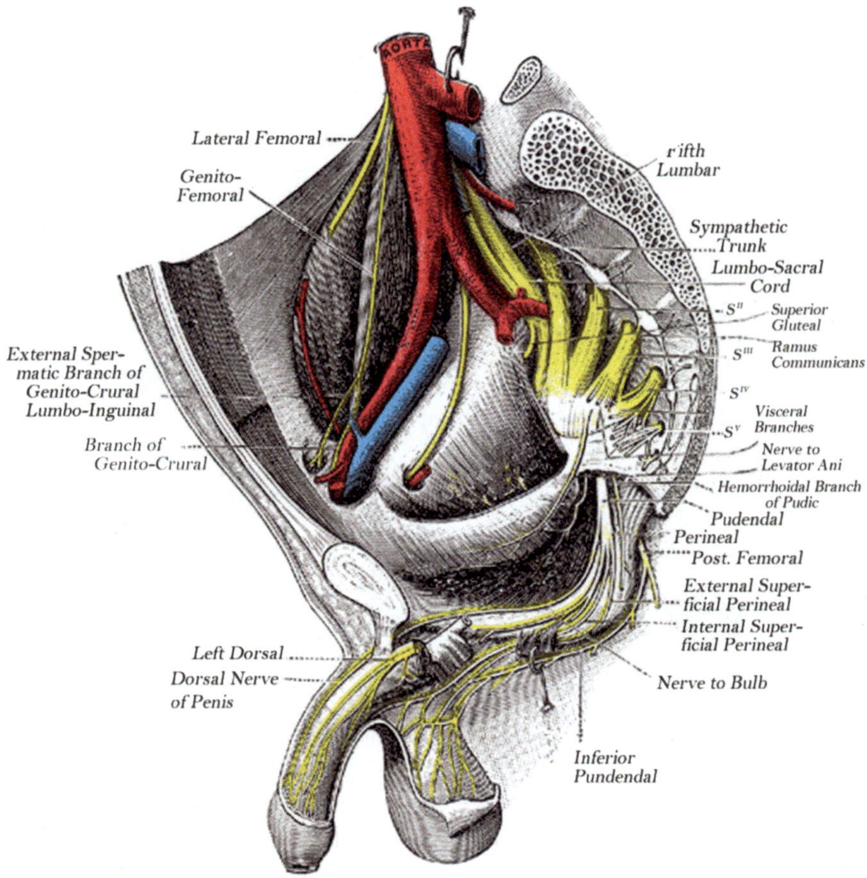

Fig. 13.9 Nerve supply of the penis (Gray's Anatomy, 1918)

glands, then enter the corpora cavernosa. The cavernosal nerve is dorsomedial to the cavernosal artery within each corpus [1, 3–5, 7].

Microvascular Erectile Dysfunction Surgery

Surgical restoration of blood flow to the corpora has been utilized for vascular erectile dysfunction in a select minority of patients [13–19]. Conversely, venous leak surgery has been performed for corporal veno-occlusive dysfunction. However, venous surgery has fallen out of favor as will be discussed below. In both of these scenarios, appropriate candidate selection and diagnostic testing are imperative. Even with strict adherence to these criteria, variable rates of success have been achieved with these procedures [19]. The American Urological Association Clinical Guidelines

Panel on Erectile Dysfunction [16] has recommended that the only standard of care surgical alternative for patients with acquired organic erectile dysfunction is implantation of a penile prosthesis. Penile vascular surgery is still considered experimental. However, the members of the Panel listed the following optional treatment: "Arterial reconstructive surgery is a treatment option only in healthy individuals with recently acquired erectile dysfunction secondary to a focal arterial occlusion and in the absence of any evidence of generalized vascular disease" [16].

Microvascular Arterial Bypass Surgery

The main objective of penile microvascular revascularization is to bypass obstructive lesions in the hypogastric-cavernosal system, thereby increasing cavernosal arterial perfusion pressure [13–15, 17, 18]. As will be discussed below, this is best achieved in younger patients who have sustained a traumatic blunt pelvic/perineal injury, resulting in damage to vessels leading to the corpora cavernosa.

The initial experience with penile revascularization surgery is credited to Michal et al. [20] in the 1970s. They initially used the inferior epigastric artery as the donor vessel anastomosed directly to the corpus cavernosum (Michal I procedure). This resulted in flow rates of more than 100 mL/min and intraoperative erections. Unfortunately, nearly all of the cases had anastomotic stenosis and poor success rates [14]. Subsequently, they anastomosed the inferior epigastric artery to the dorsal artery of the penis in an end-to-side manner (Michal II procedure). Here, a 56% success rate was achieved [14, 20]. Virag et al. [21] modified this procedure in the early 1980s by arterializing an isolated segment of dorsal vein. Here, the donor inferior epigastric artery was anastomosed to the deep dorsal vein increasing penile perfusion in a retrograde fashion. They reported a 49% success rate and an additional 20% improvement rate [14, 21]. Furlow and Fisher [22] also reported dorsal vein arterialization with ligation of its circumflex branches to prevent glanular hyperemia. Their success rate was 62% [22]. Sharaby et al. [19] created a side-to-side fistula between the dorsal artery and deep dorsal vein. They then used a spatulated inferior epigastric artery as the input source to this arteriovenous combination realizing an 80% success rate [14]. A variety of modifications were utilized (Table 13.1). A lack of patient eligibility criteria and standardized protocols and techniques likely contributed to the variable results and subsequent low popularity of these procedures. Current microarterial bypass surgical techniques involve anastomosing the inferior epigastric artery to either the dorsal vein or artery [13–15]. Although the artery-to-vein anastomosis is technically easier than that of artery-to-artery, the former is more likely to fail. The dorsal vein has valves that can retard penile reperfusion. These valves may also cause anastomotic thrombosis. A valvulotome or Fogarty balloon catheter can be used to remove the valves but may also cause endothelial injury, resulting in activation of the clotting system's intrinsic pathway leading to thrombosis and failures. Artery-to-artery microarterial bypass surgery obviates the penile hyperemia seen with dorsal vein arterializations noted earlier [13–15, 17, 18].

Table 13.1 Modifications of microvascular penile revascularization procedures

Michal I	Inferior epigastric artery to corpus cavernosum
Michal II	Inferior epigastric artery to dorsal artery
Crespo	Femoral artery to central artery of the corpus cavernosum or dorsal artery with autologous venous graft interposed between the two
Virag I	Inferior epigastric artery to deep dorsal vein
Virag II	Inferior epigastric artery to deep dorsal vein (proximal vein ligated)
Virag III	Inferior epigastric artery to deep dorsal vein via saphenous vein bypass (proximal vein ligated)
Virag IV	Virag I plus a shunt between the deep dorsal vein and cavernous body
Virag V	Virag II plus a shunt between the deep dorsal vein and cavernous body
Virag VI	Virag III plus a shunt between the deep dorsal vein and cavernous body
Hauri	Inferior epigastric artery with one anastomosis to deep dorsal vein and one dorsal artery
Furlow–Fisher	Modification of Virag II with ligation of both proximal and distal ends of deep dorsal vein

Adapted from Sharaby JS, Benet AE, Melman A. Penile revascularization. Urol Clin North Am. 1995;22(4):821–32

Venous Leak Surgery

Surgical correction of veno-occlusive erectile dysfunction has included penile venous ligation, crural banding, and spongiolysis in a small subset of patients [18, 23, 24].

Microvascular penile venous surgery is utilized to correct venous leak [18, 23, 24]. As the corpora expand during erection, the subtunical venules are compressed creating venous outflow resistance. This is the corporal veno-occlusive mechanism. Venous leak impotence equates with the inability to maintain an erection secondary to abnormal venous outflow from the corpora cavernosa. Penile trauma, Peyronie's disease, urethral stricture incision/excision, congenital corpora cavernosal venous drainage abnormalities, and priapism surgery can all result in focal defects in the corporal veno-occlusive mechanism.

Penile venous reconstructive surgery to limit the venous outflow of the penis is not recommended according to the American Urological Association Clinical Guidelines Panel on Erectile Dysfunction [16]. The Panel cites the difficulty in distinguishing functional smooth muscle dysfunction from anatomical tunical abnormalities. They also describe the difficulty in determining the proportion of erectile dysfunction secondary to a veno-occlusive etiology independent of general arterial hypofunction and how to diagnose and treat this subset of patients.

Presently, venous leak surgery has been nearly abandoned since the predominant pathology is smooth muscle dysfunction and ligating the draining veins does not remedy the veno-occlusive dysfunction [25].

In appropriately selected erectile dysfunction patients with both poor arterial inflow and veno-occlusive dysfunction, a combination of surgical revascularization and venous ligation procedure can be performed. However, despite a patent anastomosis and adequate veno-occlusion, significant failure rates may be seen secondary to end-organ corporal disease and poor distal arterial runoff beyond the anastomosis [18, 25, 26].

Other Treatment Options

Evaluation of the patient with erectile dysfunction should proceed along a patient-centered evaluation using a goal-directed approach as described by Lue [27] in 2007. Alternative nonsurgical and surgical treatment modalities should be discussed with the patient. Patients with mild to moderate vascular disease may benefit from oral PDE-5 inhibitors or intracavernosal vasoactive injection therapy. Similarly, vacuum devices and penile prostheses are alternative therapies for patients with arterial and/or veno-occlusive dysfunction etiologies.

Patient Selection for Microvascular Penile Revascularization

Medical History

The optimal patient for penile revascularization is a younger patient, less than 55 years of age, with focal arterial lesions limiting flow to the corpora cavernosa [13–18]. A comprehensive history and physical examination is performed. He should be psychologically stable and understand alternative treatment choices as mentioned earlier. First-line, less-invasive treatments are usually tried first. Blunt perineal trauma or pelvic fracture should be the likely culprit of the arterial lesions. Using a narrow bicycle seat with a protruding nose extension during bicycle riding causes compression of the ischiopubic rami, perineum, and the contents of Alcock's canal [13, 28–30]. Resultant suprasystolic perineal compression pressures occlude penile perfusion and potentially induce endothelial injury, resulting in arterial vasculogenic erectile dysfunction. A wide bicycle seat without a nose extension results in pressure applied to the ischial tuberosities, thus sparing compression of the perineum allowing penile arterial inflow [30]. Vascular risk factors such as atherosclerosis, diabetes, hypertension, and coronary artery disease should be absent as these portend more diffuse disease with a worse prognosis after revascularization. Tobacco use needs to be eliminated at least 6 months prior to surgery. A normal libido, reduction in erectile rigidity during sexual activity, improved rigidity and sustaining ability in the morning, and poor spontaneous erections requiring increased stimulation to achieve these are characteristics of the ideal patient's history.

Physical Examination

Physical examination should reveal appropriate penile geometry with normal penile extensibility during stretching maneuvers [17, 18]. No Peyronie's plaques or intracavernosal lesions should be present. A neurologic examination without evidence of a sensory neuropathy is mandatory [13–15, 17, 18].

Laboratory Examination

Routine endocrinologic evaluation is undertaken to confirm that the hormonal milieu, including serum testosterone, is within normal limits [13–15, 17, 18].

Specialized Testing

Nocturnal penile tumescence testing is performed to rule out a psychogenic cause [13–15, 17, 18]. Tumescence, rigidity, and number of erectile episodes are recorded. Duplex Doppler ultrasonography with intracavernous vasodilator injection reveals functional and anatomic information [8, 9, 31]. Redosing of the vasodilating agent may be necessary. If the cavernosal artery peak systolic velocity is less than 25 cm/s, a vascular etiology is highly likely and corresponds with abnormal pudendal angiography [8, 9, 13–15, 17, 18, 27, 31]. Peak systolic velocities between 25 and 30 cm/s are borderline for arterial insufficiency but values are age dependent [8, 9, 13–15, 17, 18, 27, 31]. End diastolic velocities less than 5 cm/s are consistent with normal corporo-occlusive function [8, 9, 13–15, 17, 18, 27, 31]. Anatomically, the presence of communicating branches between the dorsal artery and cavernosal artery distal to the occlusive lesions is evaluated. This is necessary so that when new blood flow is restored to the dorsal artery, it will result in increased intracorporal pressure. Dorsal artery diameters and flow direction through septal communicators are also assessed. Hence, the best recipient dorsal artery can be chosen. Subsequently, dynamic infusion cavernosometry/cavernosography (DICC) is performed to demonstrate arterial pressure gradients between the cavernosal and brachial arteries [8, 9, 13–15, 17, 18, 27]. A gradient of more than 30 mmHg between the penile occlusion pressure and mean brachial pressure demonstrates functional arterial disease. DICC is also used to rule out veno-occlusive dysfunction. Flows to maintain less than 5 cc/min and pressure decays less than 45 mmHg over 30 s essentially rule out venous leak [8, 9, 13–15, 17, 18, 27, 31].

A common iliac arteriogram and a selective internal pudendal arteriogram are mandatory to identify the location of the obstructive arterial lesion as well as the best-suited donor vessel usually the inferior epigastric artery [8, 9, 13–15, 17, 18]. The inferior epigastric artery should be of sufficient length to allow a tension-free anastomosis to the dorsal artery. Common trunks between the inferior epigastric artery and the obturator arteries should be absent to avoid diminution of inferior epigastric artery perfusion pressures via the steal syndrome. The distal occlusive lesion in one or both hypogastric-cavernous arterial beds is usually located within the common penile or cavernosal artery and should be less than 2 mm in diameter [13]. Blockages in the internal pudendal arteries that are between 2 and 4 mm can be treated with endovascular stents. However, occlusive lesions in the internal pudendal arteries have a significant association with systemic atherosclerotic disease which portends a worse prognosis with regard to patency and success [25].

Surgical Technique of Microvascular Penile Revascularization

Technically, the operation consists of three stages [13–15, 17, 18] (1) dorsal artery or recipient vessel dissection, (2) inferior epigastric artery or donor vessel harvesting, and (3) microsurgical anastomosis.

Preoperative prophylactic antibiotics are administered, usually a third-generation cephalosporin or vancomycin if a penicillin allergy exists. The patient is positioned supine with both upper extremities padded and secured next to his body to minimize pressure-induced and nerve-related injuries. The lower extremities and all dependent areas are likewise protected. Sequential compression devices are placed around each lower extremity. General endotracheal anesthesia with muscle relaxation is utilized as this facilitates harvesting the donor inferior epigastric vessel artery off of the rectus muscle. The genitalia and abdomen are shaved, prepped, and draped. A 16 French Foley catheter is placed in the usual sterile fashion.

Recipient Vessel (Dorsal Artery) Dissection

A curvilinear inguinoscrotal incision is made on the side opposite to the planned abdominal incision for the donor inferior epigastric artery harvesting (Fig. 13.10). This incision provides optimal proximal and distal exposure of the dorsal neurovascular bundle, and penile shortening is prevented by preserving the fundiform ligament. Additionally, better cosmesis is achieved by obviating postoperative scars on the penile shaft or base. The incision is made approximately two finger breadths from the base of the penis, from a point opposite the ventral root, to the scrotal median raphe. A Scott ring retractor with elastic hooks maximizes exposure. Blunt dissection deepens the incision through the dartos layer. The ipsilateral tunica albuginea is identified at the midshaft. The penis is then stretched and blunt finger dissection along the tunica albuginea is performed distally deep and inferior to the spermatic cord along the lateral aspect of the penile shaft. Injury to the fundiform ligament is avoided. The penis, including the glans, is inverted completely through the incision. A plane is created between Buck's and Colles' fascia around the distal penile shaft using blunt finger dissection. A Penrose drain is placed in this area. The neurovascular bundle is exposed. As noted in "Anatomy of the Penis and Male Perineum" section, the dorsal arteries of the penis are lateral to the deep dorsal vein and medial to the respective dorsal nerves. Dissection of the dorsal artery is limited at this point in the procedure to minimize ischemic, mechanical, and thermal trauma to these vessels. Topical papaverine hydrochloride irrigation is applied liberally to the vessels to prevent vasospasm-induced vasoconstriction and resultant endothelial and smooth muscle cell injury. In the past, both dorsal arteries were dissected and anastomosed to the bifurcation of the inferior epigastric artery. However, a significant improvement in erectile function was not made manifest in patients who underwent a bilateral anastomosis compared to those who had a unilateral anastomosis. Hence, the current consensus is that performing a single anastomosis minimizes surgical

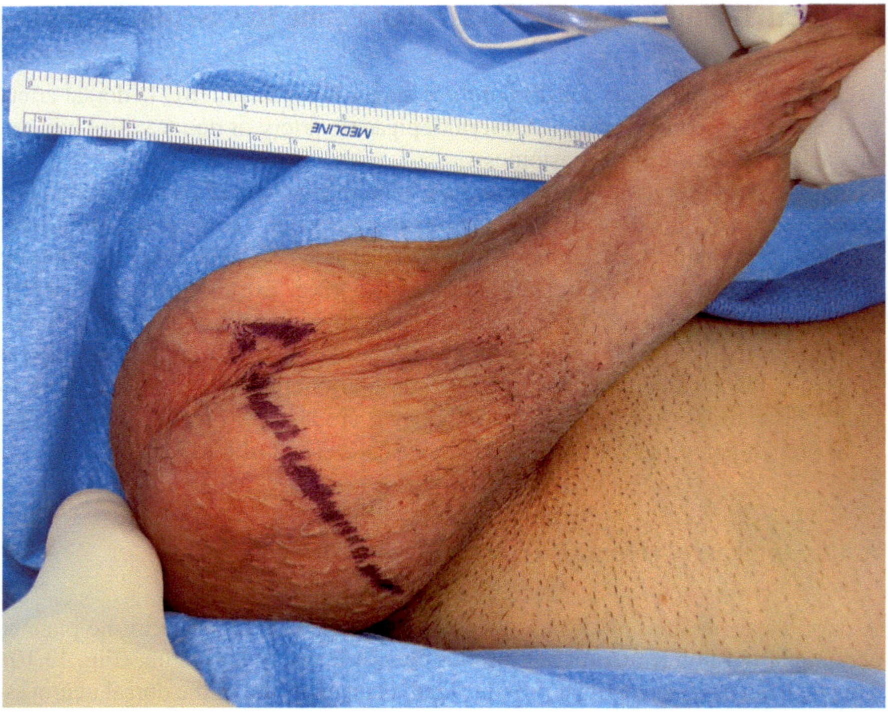

Fig. 13.10 A curvilinear inguinoscrotal incision is marked in preparation for recipient vessel dissection. This provides optimal exposure of the dorsal neurovascular bundle and better cosmesis by obviating penile scars (photo courtesy of Irwin Goldstein, M.D., Director of Sexual Medicine at Alvarado Hospital, San Diego, CA; Clinical Professor of Surgery at University of California at San Diego; and Director of San Diego Sexual Medicine)

time and preserves the contralateral dorsal artery in case a second penile revascularization is required. The preselected right or left dorsal artery is identified and its course is bluntly followed proximally underneath the fundiform ligament. The fundiform ligament is left intact during this dissection allowing the penis to maintain elasticity during postoperative erection. Blunt dissection is performed between the proximal fundiform ligament and the pubic bone toward the external ring on the side of the preselected inferior epigastric artery. This dissection creates a transfer route allowing the inferior epigastric artery access to the dorsal artery of the penis while preserving the fundiform ligament. The penis is reverted back to its normal anatomic position and the inguinoscrotal incision is closed temporarily with skin staples.

Donor Vessel (Inferior Epigastric Artery) Harvesting

A transverse semilunar abdominal skin incision along Langer's lines provides excellent inferior epigastric artery exposure and heals with better cosmesis than a para-

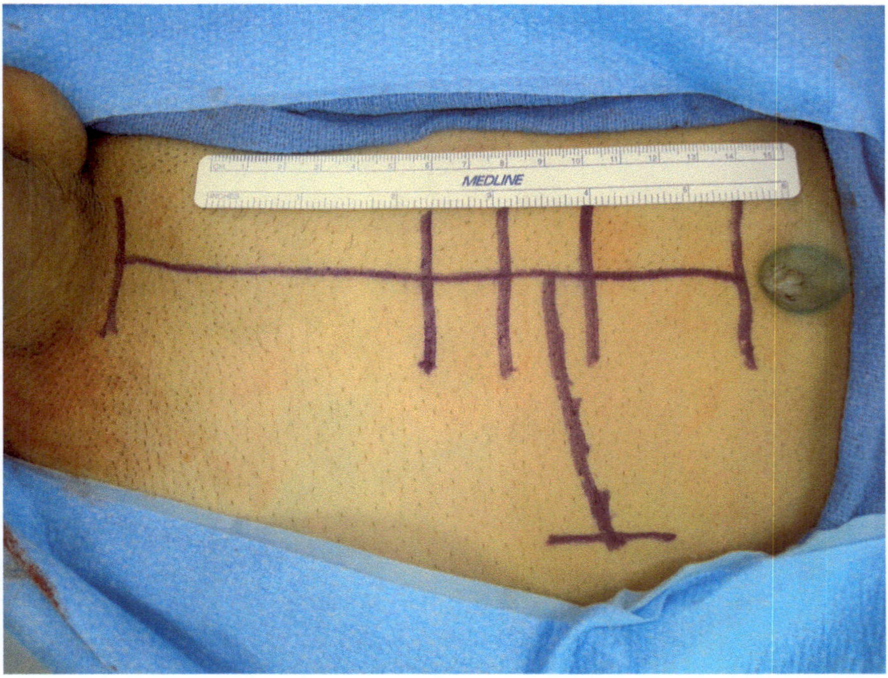

Fig. 13.11 A transverse semilunar incision is marked three fourths of the distance up from the pubic bone to the umbilicus. It extends laterally for approximately 5 cm to the side of the preselected inferior epigastric artery (photo courtesy of Irwin Goldstein, MD, Director of Sexual Medicine at Alvarado Hospital, San Diego, CA; Clinical Professor of Surgery at University of California at San Diego; and Director of San Diego Sexual Medicine)

median incision. This transverse incision is started in the midline approximately three fourths of the total distance up from the pubic bone to the umbilicus. It extends laterally for approximately 5 cm to the side of the preselected inferior epigastric artery (Fig. 13.11). The incision is carried down to the rectus fascia which is incised vertically. The junction between the rectus muscle and underlying preperitoneal fat is identified and the preperitoneal plane is entered. The rectus muscle is reflected medially using retractors and the ring retractor. The inferior epigastric artery and its two accompanying veins are identified beneath the rectus muscle in this preperitoneal plane. Sufficient length of inferior epigastric artery must be harvested to create a tension-free anastomosis. Similar to the dorsal artery dissection, topical papaverine is utilized on the vessel to prevent injurious vasospasm and endothelial damage. Low-current bipolar cautery is used sparingly to avoid thermal damage and ischemia. The vasa vasorae are preserved by performing an en bloc dissection of the inferior epigastric artery with its surrounding veins and fat. The inferior epigastric artery is dissected from its origin from the external iliac artery to the level of the umbilicus. It is not transected at this time (Fig. 13.12).

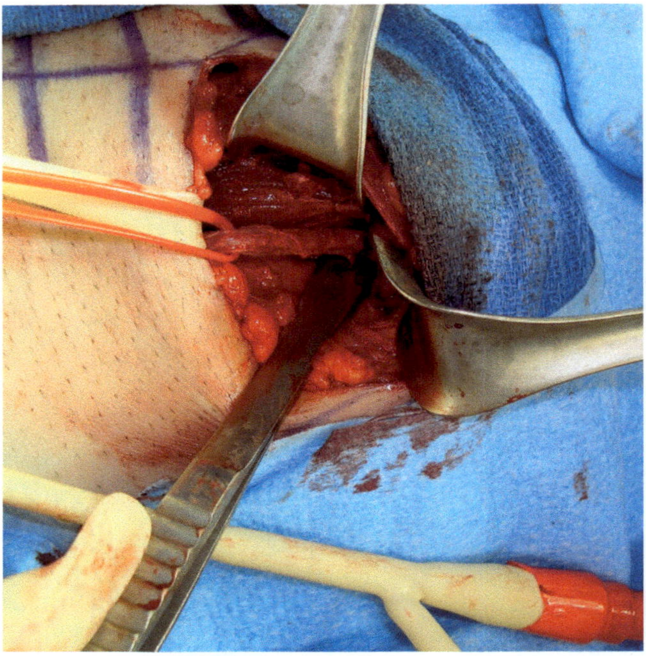

Fig. 13.12 The inferior epigastric artery and surrounding vascular structures are dissected off the rectus muscle from the external iliac artery to the umbilicus. It is not transected at this time (photo courtesy of Irwin Goldstein, M.D., Director of Sexual Medicine at Alvarado Hospital, San Diego, CA; Clinical Professor of Surgery at University of California at San Diego; and Director of San Diego Sexual Medicine)

The temporary inguinoscrotal staples are removed and the penis is reinverted. The transfer route is now created. Blunt finger dissection is utilized through the ipsilateral inguinal canal. A long fine vascular clamp is passed through the fenestration in the fundiform ligament, the external ring, and the internal ring lateral to the origin of the inferior epigastric artery. A Penrose drain is then placed through this transfer route for identification purposes.

The donor inferior epigastric artery vascular bundle is transected at the level of the umbilicus between two ligaclips (Fig. 13.13). The area is inspected for any bleeding points and hemostasis is achieved according to the principles above. Donor artery pulsations should be observed. Retroperitoneal attachments are removed prior to donor vessel transfer to avoid tension, kinking, and vascular compromise. The long fine vascular clamp is again passed up the inguinal canal through the transfer route delineated by the Penrose drain. The end of the transected inferior epigastric artery vascular bundle is grasped and transferred down to the base of the penis. There should be sufficient length without any kinking. Donor artery pulsations should be brisk. After adequate hemostasis is achieved, the abdominal incision is closed in two layers. The rectus fascia is closed with a running 0 polyglycolic acid suture. ON-Q Silversoaker catheters (I-Flow Corporation, Lake Forest, CA) are placed below and

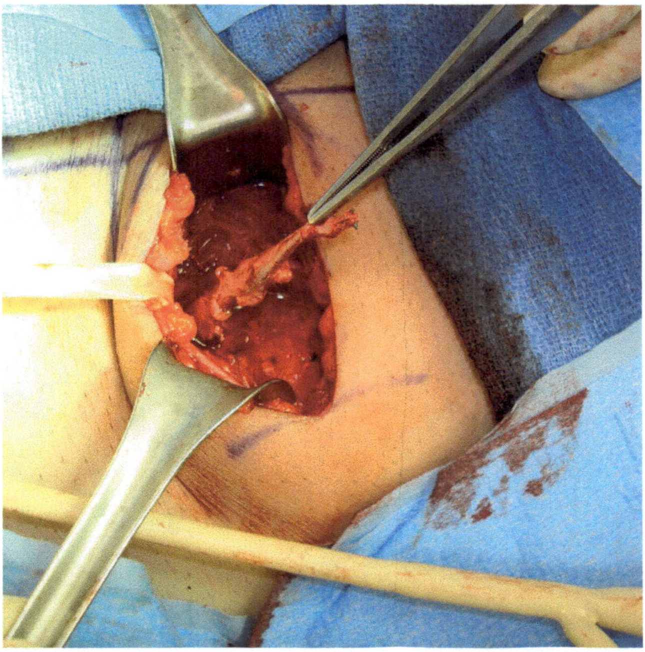

Fig. 13.13 The donor inferior epigastric artery is clipped and transected distally in preparation for its transfer down the inguinal canal to the dorsal penile vessels (photo courtesy of Irwin Goldstein, M.D., Director of Sexual Medicine at Alvarado Hospital, San Diego, CA; Clinical Professor of Surgery at University of California at San Diego; and Director of San Diego Sexual Medicine)

above the rectus fascia. 0.5% Marcaine analgesia is delivered at 2 mL/h through each catheter for 48–72 h postoperatively. The skin is closed in layers using 4–0 Monocryl with Dermabond applied over the incision or with skin staples.

Microsurgical Anastomosis

Attention is once again directed to the inguinoscrotal incision. The ring retractor and elastic hooks are again placed to retract the skin and the fenestration of the fundiform ligament to expose the proximal dorsal neurovascular bundle. The inferior epigastric artery is placed adjacent to the dorsal arteries. The location for anastomosis is based on the preoperative arteriographic and duplex Doppler ultrasound findings. An end-to-end anastomosis transfers perfusion pressure more effectively and with less turbulence than an end-to-side anastomosis. Intraluminal arterial irrigation with a dilute solution of papaverine, heparin, and electrolytes inhibits myointimal proliferative lesions during surgical preparation. The preselected dorsal penile artery segment is dissected and freed from the tunica albuginea without injuring its communicating branches to the cavernosal artery. Hemostasis of this segment can be achieved with gold-plated (low-pressure) aneurysm vascular clamps or vessel loops

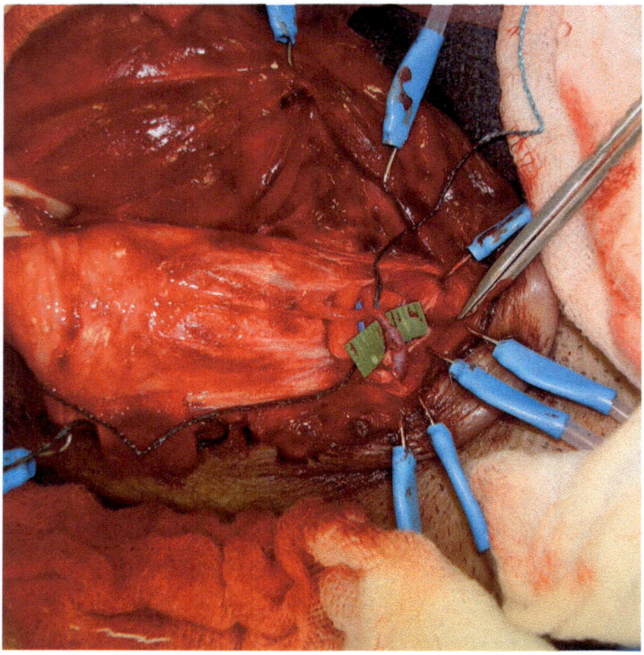

Fig. 13.14 The microsurgical anastomosis between the inferior epigastric artery and the dorsal penile artery is completed (photo courtesy of Irwin Goldstein, M.D., Director of Sexual Medicine at Alvarado Hospital, San Diego, CA; Clinical Professor of Surgery at University of California at San Diego; and Director of San Diego Sexual Medicine)

with a minimum of tension for the shortest time possible. The adventitia of the vessels is only removed focally at the site where the anastomosis is to be performed to avoid subsequent thrombosis. Portions of adventitia entering the anastomosis can activate clotting factors from the extrinsic clotting system, resulting in thrombosis. Preservation of the remaining adventitia is important for an intact vasa vasorum and vessel innervation.

A plastic colored background is placed behind the vessels to be anastomosed for better visualization with the surgical microscope. An end-to-end anastomosis between the inferior epigastric artery and the dorsal artery is performed using interrupted 10–0 nylon sutures (single-armed, 100 μm, 149° curved needle) under 10× magnification. Sutures are passed out-to-in on the inferior epigastric artery and then from in-to-out on the dorsal artery. All suture bites are taken 1 mm from the cut edge. The anastomotic sutures are placed in a circumferential fashion equidistant from each other to create an even anastomosis. Usually, 15 or more sutures are required to create a watertight closure. The temporary occluding vascular clamp or vessel loop is removed from the dorsal penile artery. Arterial pulsations should now be seen across the anastomosis, implying patency. Next, the vascular clamp is removed from the inferior epigastric artery and the intensity of the arterial pulsations increases (Fig. 13.14).

The application of a small amount of hemostatic material may occasionally be required to aid in hemostasis from vessel wall suture needle holes.

Modifications of the anastomosis exist. A common alternative is the end-to-side inferior epigastric artery to the dorsal penile artery anastomosis. Again, as noted earlier, the adventitia is removed only focally from the vessels where the anastomosis will be performed. A 10–0 suture is placed along the longitudinal axis of the dorsal penile artery to secure a 1-mm segment in the region of the intended anastomosis. Tension is placed on this suture to elevate a section of the artery wall. An oval section of the artery wall is excised from this raised area with curved microscissors, resulting in a 1.2- to 1.5-mm horizontal arteriotomy. A temporary 2 French silastic stent is placed within the arteriotomy for improved visualization of the vessel lumen and back wall. 10–0 nylon sutures are initially placed at each apex of the anastomosis. Subsequent interrupted sutures (usually three to five) are placed into each side wall in an equidistant manner to avoid an uneven anastomosis. One side of the anastomosis is completed before commencing the other side. The temporary vascular stent is removed following suture placement.

The inguinoscrotal incision is closed by approximating the dartos layer using a running 3–0 polyglycolic acid suture. Similar to the abdominal skin closure, the inguinoscrotal skin is closed using 4–0 Monocryl with Dermabond applied over the incision or with skin staples. Patency of the anastomosis can be confirmed by Doppler ultrasound. The ON-Q catheters are secured to the skin with Tegaderm. A compressive scrotal dressing is placed. The Foley catheter remains to closed-system gravity drainage overnight.

The patient refrains from vigorous movements initially, then gradually increases his activity level. He abstains from sexual activity involving the erect penis for a minimum of 6 weeks postoperatively.

Minimally Invasive Harvesting of the Donor Vessel

Minimally invasive techniques have been utilized to harvest the donor vessel for microvascular penile revascularization. Laparoscopic and daVinci (Intuitive Surgical, Sunnyvale, CA) robotic harvesting of the inferior epigastric artery have been reported [32–34]. Enhanced magnification facilitates this process. Once the donor vessel is mobilized and transected, its free end is transposed down for the anastomosis which takes place through a small incision. In the robotic cases, the daVinci system with its wristed instruments can be utilized for the anastomosis as well. Successful outcomes have been achieved but the patient numbers were small. These approaches negate the necessity of open abdominal incisions and their inherent morbidity. Recovery time can be shortened as less pain and tissue trauma is experienced by the patient. Further studies with increased patient accrual and longer follow-up are required to fully evaluate this minimally invasive technology as it relates to penile revascularization.

Table 13.2 Penile arterial surgery: criteria for article selection

Patient age	55 years or less
Exclusion criteria	Diabetes mellitus and cigarette smoking
Length of follow-up	12-month minimum
Inclusion criteria	Normal serum testosterone
	Failed pharmacologic erection test or documentation of organicity by either abnormal nocturnal penile tumescence or abnormal blood flow studies (duplex Doppler ultrasonography or dynamic infusion cavernosometry)
	Abnormal penile arteriogram
	Artery-to-artery or artery-to-dorsal vein anastomosis used in surgical technique
	Objective follow-up data reported by either duplex Doppler ultrasonography, penile arteriogram, or validated outcome questionnaire

Montague DK, Jarow J, Broderick GA, Dmochowski RR, Heaton JPW, Lue TF, et al. The management of erectile dysfunction: an update. American Urological Association Education and Research; 2005. http://www.auanet.org/content/guidelines-and-quality-care/clinical-guidelines.cfm?sub=ed

Results

Success rates for microvascular penile revascularization have been variable [13–15, 17–19]. Lack of standardization with regard to appropriate candidate selection, diagnostic testing, and surgical technique has contributed to this. Limited long-term follow-up and the lack of validated outcome data have made the comparison of patient results and surgical procedures difficult.

The American Urological Association Clinical Guidelines Panel on Erectile Dysfunction established criteria for the Arterial Occlusive Disease Index Patient [16] (Table 13.2). The Panel reviewed the English-language literature from 1966 to 2003 for reports pertaining to penile vasculature surgery. Articles reporting penile arterial surgery on the Arterial Occlusive Disease Index Patient were analyzed. Thirty-one manuscripts describing penile arterial surgery contained hundreds of patients. However, only four articles met the Panel's criteria for acceptance. These four articles represented a total of 50 patients (Table 13.3). Of these 50 patients, 42 had anastomosis of the inferior epigastric artery to the dorsal penile artery; the remaining 8 had anastomosis of the inferior epigastric artery to the dorsal penile vein. The Panel concluded that the total of 50 patients with reported outcomes was too small to determine if penile arterial revascularization is effective.

Reported successful outcomes spanned a wide range of between 36 and 91% [16].

Recently, as of this chapter's writing, the largest long-term outcome microvascular penile revascularization study using validated instruments was published in 2009 by Munarriz et al. [15]. It was a single-institution, retrospective, institutional review board-approved study from the Center for Sexual Medicine, Department of Urology, Boston University School of Medicine. This is a center of excellence—the only center doing these types of surgeries on a continuous basis for more than two

Table 13.3 Penile arterial reconstructive surgery: summary of studies published subsequent to the 1996 *report* literature analysis

References	Type of surgery	Number of patients	Months of follow-up overall: range (mean)	Success rate, % (*N*)	Success criteria
Ang and Lim (1997)	Doral vein	6	8–37 (20)	66 (4)	NPT, Doppler
DePalma et al. (1995)	Dorsal artery	11	12–48	60 (7)	Doppler
Grasseo et al. (1992)	Dorsal artery	22	1 year for all	68 (15)	NPT
				36 (8)	Doppler
Jarow and DeFranzo (1996)	Mixed	11	12–84 (50)	91 (10)	Doppler, DUS

DUS duplex ultrasonography, *NPT* nocturnal penile tumescence
Montague DK, Jarow J, Broderick GA, Dmochowski RR, Heaton JPW, Lue TF, et al. The management of erectile dysfunction: an update. American Urological Association Education and Research; 2005. http://www.auanet.org/content/guidelines-and-quality-care/clinical-guidelines.cfm?sub=ed

decades. The study consisted of 71 men (mean age 30.5 ± 9.2 years) who underwent microvascular arterial bypass surgery between 1996 and 2007 (mean follow-up 34.5 ± 18 months). Mean preoperative penile rigidity assessed by an analog scale with and without phosphodiesterase type 5 inhibitors was 41% and 77%, respectively; and 71% and 90.8% postoperatively. Mean total International Index of Erectile Function Score, Erectile Function Domain, and question 3 and 4 scores preoperatively were 35.5 ± 14.8, 13.7 ± 6.7, 2.2 ± 1.4, and 2.1 ± 1.3, respectively; and 56.2 ± 16.6, 23.8 ± 6.6, 4.1 ± 1.4, and 3.9 ± 1.5 postoperatively. Center for Epidemiologic Studies Depression Scale scores were 42.0 ± 10.0 preoperatively and 33.7 ± 6.1 postoperatively. Treatment satisfaction assessed by the Erectile Dysfunction Inventory of Treatment Satisfaction was high. 87.7% of patients would recommend or undergo surgery again. 88.7% of patients reported significant improvement in their erectile function. All differences were statistically significant.

Complications

Complications of microvascular penile revascularization [13–15, 17, 18, 32] can be divided into immediate, short-term (<6 months), and delayed (>6 months).

Intraoperative hemorrhage can occur from donor or recipient vessel branches that are missed during ligation. Strict adherence to good vascular surgical technique is mandatory. The integrity of all vascular clamps and vessel loops should be assessed prior to placement on any vessel. Microsurgical expertise is a necessity for microsurgical penile revascularization procedures.

Penile edema is a common occurrence immediately postoperatively. A nonstrangulating elastic circumferential penile dressing for 24 h postoperatively reduces the edema. Any residual edema usually resolves within the ensuing weeks.

Genital ecchymoses and hematomas are not uncommon and usually resolve spontaneously. Occasionally, a drain may be placed to avoid serious wound hematomas and then removed within 2 days postoperatively.

In the largest long-term outcome penile microarterial bypass surgery study by Munarriz et al. [15], short-term complications included: infection (2 of 71), fevers (1 of 71), nausea/emesis (2 of 71), urinary problems (5 of 71), and penile pain (6 of 71). Penile pain occurred more commonly with nocturnal tumescence and resolved within 6 weeks postoperatively.

Mechanical disruption of the microvascular anastomosis with subsequent hemorrhage can occur within the first few weeks postoperatively [35]. This may occur from blunt trauma related to coitus, masturbation, or accidents. Therefore, resumption of sexual activity should not begin until after 6 weeks postoperatively.

Long-term complications of microvascular penile revascularization include penile shortening and penile numbness (hypoesthesia). Loss of penile length can occur from scar entrapment and loss of compliance with fibrosis of the fundiform and suspensory ligaments. Preservation of the fundiform ligament, as discussed in "Surgical Technique of Microvascular Penile Revascularization" section, has theoretically minimized penile shortening. Penile shortening was documented in 20 of 71 (28%) patients in the study by Munarriz et al. [15]. Average loss of penile length was 0.91 in. However, about 90% of the patients would recommend or undergo surgery again, suggesting that the loss of penile length was not critical in their satisfaction with the procedure. Vascular factors such as anastomotic tension were thought not to be a factor in the penile shortening. Munarriz et al. [15] extensively mobilize the inferior epigastric artery and dorsal artery to minimize penile shortening, bleeding, and early occlusion. Redundant inferior epigastric artery is routinely used to minimize potential penile shortening. Preoperative and postoperative penile length is being documented to assess this common complication. Occasionally, penile shortening from scar entrapment may require surgical scar release and relaxing Z-plasty incisions or scrotal flap coverage.

Penile hypoesthesia occurs secondary to dorsal nerve denervation during dissection [13–15, 17, 18, 35]. Penile sensation usually returns within 18 months postoperatively if no major penile sensory nerve has been severed. Approximately, 25% (17 of 71) of the patients in the Munarriz series reported loss of penile sensation. However, their orgasmic function was improved according to postoperative Orgasmic Function domain scores. This was explained by a significant improvement in overall sexual function while concomitantly ruling out significant dorsal neuropathy. Despite using 10× magnification and meticulous technique, small neurotomies were hypothesized as the potential cause of penile hypoesthesia. An ongoing prospective study with preoperative and postoperative biothesiometric evaluation was suggested to glean a better understanding of this complication [15].

Glans hyperemia, seen with deep dorsal vein arterialization, occurs when a communicating vein from the deep dorsal vein to the glans is missed and left unligated [13–15, 17, 18]. Surgical re-exploration with ligation of the arterialized communicator resolves the problem. However, the artery-to-vein type of anastomosis is not commonly performed anymore, so this complication is no longer seen [13–15, 17, 18, 36].

Hernias can occur postoperatively [15]. A surgeon familiar with microarterial bypass surgery and the postoperative anatomy should be the one performing the hernia repair if it is required. If the inferior epigastric artery is not readily identified, intraoperative Doppler ultrasound should be used to prevent vascular compromise [15].

Conclusion

Microvascular arterial bypass surgery for penile revascularization is best utilized for focal lesions in the hypogastric-cavernosal system. Its success is dependent upon appropriate candidate selection and meticulous surgical technique. This type of surgery is the only treatment modality capable of restoring erectile function without the placement of internal or external penile prosthetics, external mechanical devices, or the use of chronic vasoactive medications. Although success rates have varied in the literature, in optimally selected patients with pure arterial insufficiency without veno-occlusive dysfunction, microvascular penile revascularization provides significant improvement in erectile function and sexual satisfaction with low complication rates. Future prospective studies are needed to further validate these parameters and to assess postoperative penile shortening and hypoesthesia and their prevention.

Microvascular Penile Replantation

Microvascular surgical techniques represent a mainstay in penile replantation. Historically, penile amputation has occurred as a result of self-emasculation, violent assault, and industrial or war injuries [37]. Rarely, improperly performed circumcision has resulted in penile amputation secondary to direct laceration or from excessive use of cautery [38]. Data relating to penile replantation have been accumulated from small series and case reports because of the rarity of this injury. Self-amputation is largely seen in patients who are psychotic or those with severe personality disorders [4, 61, 62]. The former group includes schizophrenic patients in an actively psychotic state. These patients experience hallucinations commanding them to amputate their penis. Continued psychiatric rehabilitative therapy is helpful in preventing them from repeating their actions. Psychiatric treatment is less effective in nonpsychotic patients with severe personality disorders.

Penile replantation should be performed expeditiously to achieve the greatest success rate with regard to viability, erectile function, and voiding parameters [37, 61]. The amputated penis can tolerate prolonged periods of ischemia, so replantation should take place independent of any set time period [37, 39, 61]. Successful penile replantation has occurred after more than 24 h of hypothermic ischemia [42]. At times, a court order may be necessary to proceed with penile replantation in cases of psychotic or noncompetent patients [4].

Initial experience with penile replantation involved a macroscopic approach with corporal and urethral reapproximation without microscopic repair of the dorsal neurovascular structures [64]. Despite this, successful salvage was achieved in the majority of cases. Apparently, proximal corporal cavernosal sinusoid blood supplies the anastomosed distal penile structures prior to collateral vessel neogenesis [37]. Complications have included penile skin and glans slough, necrosis, impotence, and urethral stricture [37–40, 42, 43, 61–63].

In 1976, successful penile replantation was achieved in the United States and Japan by two separate institutions using microsurgical techniques [40, 42]. Microsurgical repair of the dorsal neurovascular structures including both dorsal arteries, the deep dorsal vein, and the dorsal nerve bundle is now the standard of care. It has provided superior results with postoperative erectile function, genital sensation, and penile viability [41, 43].

Technique

First and foremost, the penis must be recovered and the patient stabilized. The amputated penis is cleaned and then preserved using the "bag-within-a-bag" technique [37–38, 41,61]. A saline-soaked gauze is wrapped around the amputated penis and it is placed in a sterile plastic bag if possible. This bag is then placed into a container of ice slush. This hypothermia increases the ischemic tolerance of the severed organ. The amputated penis is not placed directly on the ice slush to avoid skin damage from direct contact [41]. In the operating room, the amputated penis is washed with antibiotic solution [38] (Fig. 13.15).

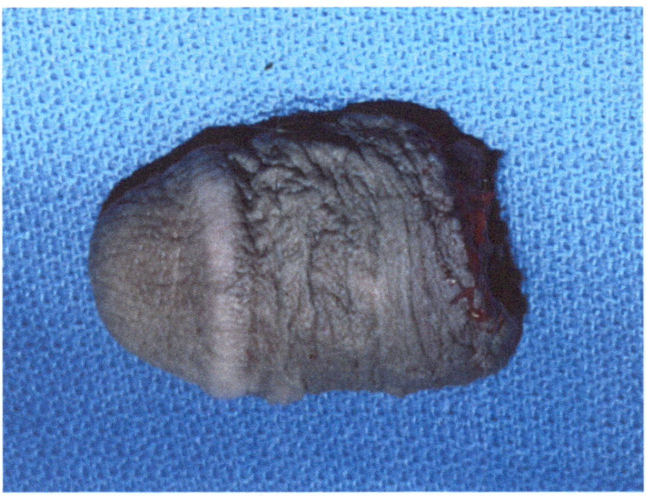

Fig. 13.15 The amputated penis of a 31-year-old male who self-amputated his penis with a kitchen knife. Replantation was started 3 h after injury (photo courtesy of Jack W. McAninch, M.D., F.A.C.S., F.R.C.S. (Hon.), Professor and Vice-Chair Urology, University of California, San Francisco; Chief of Urology, San Francisco General Hospital)

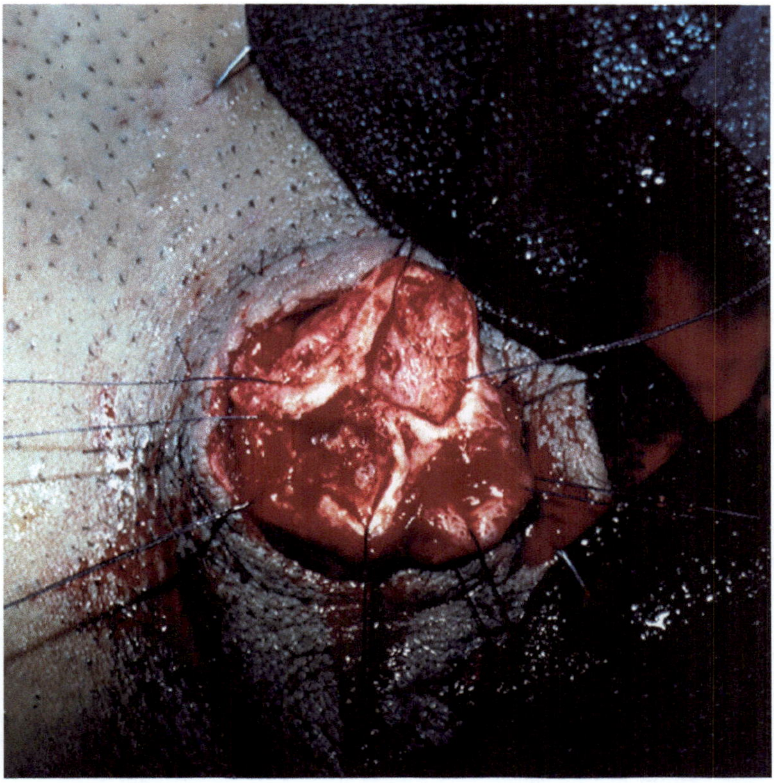

Fig. 13.16 The proximal penile stump of the patient in Fig. 13.15. The corpora cavernosa (whitish tunica albuginea) and the corpora spongiosum are identified. Stay sutures are placed in these structures (photo courtesy of Jack W. McAninch, M.D., F.A.C.S., F.R.C.S. (Hon.), Professor and Vice-Chair Urology, University of California, San Francisco; Chief of Urology, San Francisco General Hospital)

Microsurgical replantation is performed with optical enhanced microscopy. The three corporal bodies and the dorsal neurovascular structures are evaluated and debrided as necessary (Fig. 13.16). The first structure to be reanastomosed is the urethra which provides some stability to the remaining repair [37]. It is spatulated and approximated in two layers. The urethral mucosa is reanastomosed with interrupted 6–0 polydioxanone suture or 6–0 Vicryl. The corpora spongiosum is then reapproximated with 5–0 polydioxanone interrupted sutures. The tunica albuginea of the corpora cavernosa is closed with interrupted 4–0 or 5–0 polydioxanone sutures (Fig. 13.17). The corporal arteries and the autonomic cavernosal nerve branches are not reattached as this has not shown to offer any advantage to the above.

The dorsal neurovascular structures are subsequently reanastomosed [37, 41, 61]. First, both dorsal penile arteries are anastomosed using 11–0 nylon or Prolene interrupted sutures. Then, the deep dorsal vein is approximated using 10–0 nylon or Prolene. Completing the dorsal neurovascular repair, the dorsal nerve bundles

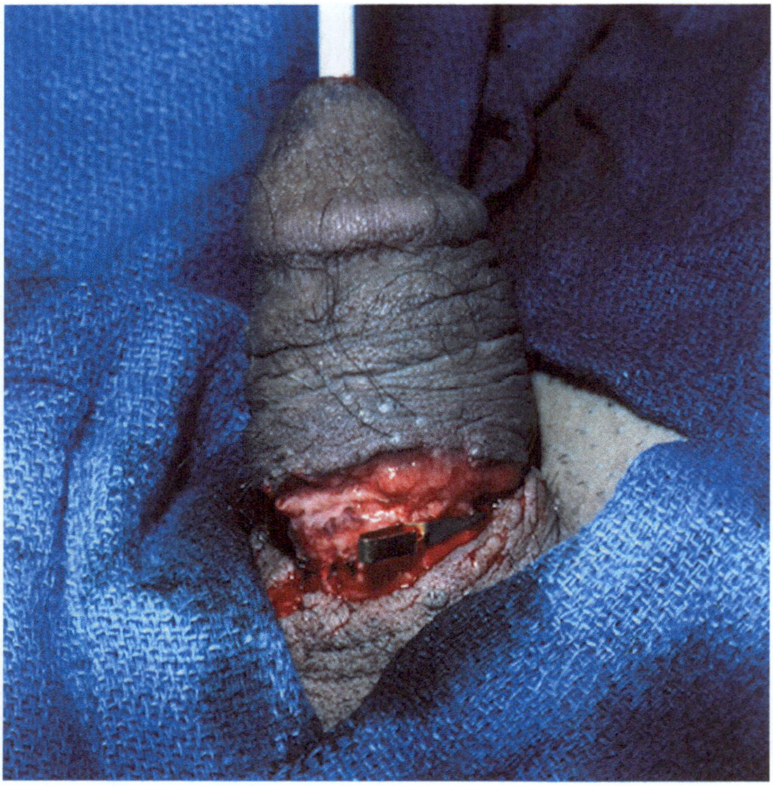

Fig. 13.17 The urethral anastomosis and the anastomosis of the tunica albuginea of the corporal bodies have been performed in the above patient. Two microsurgical clamps are placed on the vessels in preparation of the microanastomosis of the dorsal arteries, vein, and nerves (photo courtesy of Jack W. McAninch, M.D., F.A.C.S., F.R.C.S. (Hon.), Professor and Vice-Chair Urology, University of California, San Francisco; Chief of Urology, San Francisco General Hospital)

are approximated with 10–0 nylon sutures, apposing the epineurium of each side to facilitate fascicular regrowth. The dorsal nerve of the penis is the first branch of the pudendal nerve in Alcock's canal [4, 7]. It supplies sensation to the glans and penile skin.

The dartos fascia is reapproximated using 5–0 Vicryl interrupted sutures. The skin is loosely closed in an interrupted fashion with 6–0 Vicryl sutures (Fig. 13.18). A suprapubic tube is placed for urinary diversion. A small soft silicone catheter is used to stent the urethra. The penis is elevated on the abdomen and immobilized to promote healing and facilitate lymphatic drainage. Doppler ultrasonography can be used intermittently for monitoring. Signs of skin slough and tenuous viability are meticulously documented (Fig. 13.19). A voiding cystogram may be performed by filling through the suprapubic tube and removing the urethral catheter at 3 weeks postoperatively [37, 41, 61]. If no extravasation is seen at the repair site, the suprapubic tube can be plugged and the patient allowed to void spontaneously (Fig. 13.20).

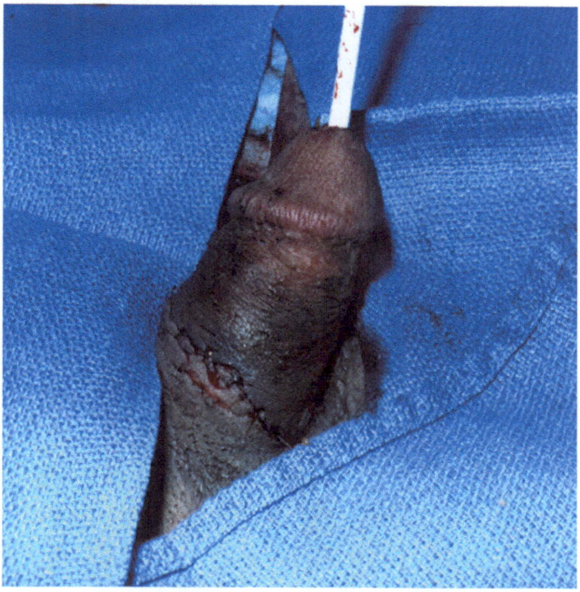

Fig. 13.18 The microneurovascular anastomosis has been completed in the same patient above. The dartos fascia and skin have been closed (photo courtesy of Jack W. McAninch, M.D., F.A.C.S., F.R.C.S. (Hon.), Professor and Vice-Chair Urology, University of California, San Francisco; Chief of Urology, San Francisco General Hospital)

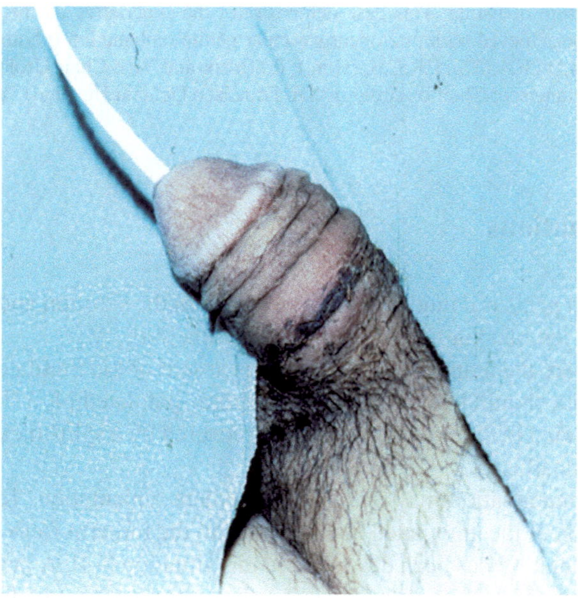

Fig. 13.19 The patient above 1 week postoperatively with the urethral catheter in place. No signs of skin slough (photo courtesy of Jack W. McAninch, M.D., F.A.C.S., F.R.C.S. (Hon.), Professor and Vice-Chair Urology, University of California, San Francisco; Chief of Urology, San Francisco General Hospital)

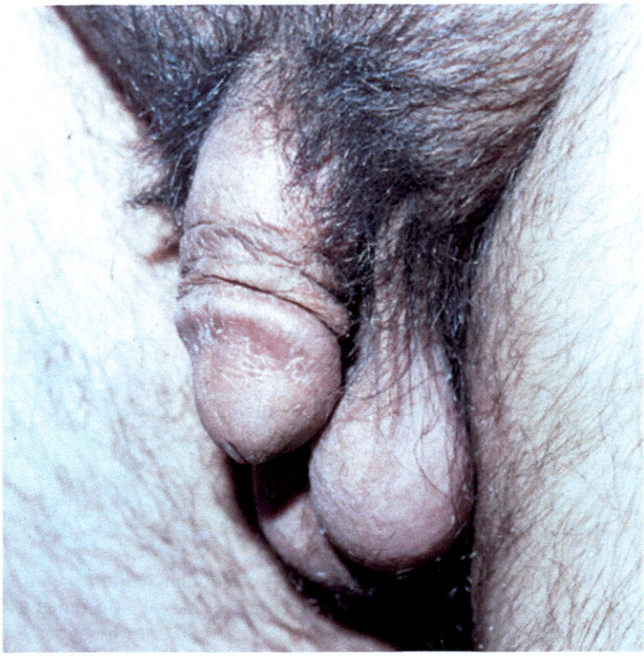

Fig. 13.20 Same patient above 6 months after replantation. The urethral catheter was left in place for 3 weeks postoperatively. The patient was having partial erections and voiding normally without evidence of stricture or fistula. This case demonstrates the superlative cosmetic and functional results that can be achieved with microneurovascular penile replantation (photo courtesy of Jack W. McAninch, M.D., F.A.C.S., F.R.C.S. (Hon.), Professor and Vice-Chair Urology, University of California, San Francisco; Chief of Urology, San Francisco General Hospital)

Special Situations

If the replanted penis is denuded, it may be buried in the scrotum and later liberated by mobilizing scrotal skin flaps or using skin grafts [64].

In cases where the amputated distal penis is absent or too mutilated for replantation, the corpora should be closed and the urethra spatulated [4, 37]. The proximal shaft is then buried in the surrounding skin or covered by a split-thickness skin graft creating a neophallus.

Perineal contamination may preclude immediate replantation. Temporary ectopic implantation of the amputated distal penis into the forearm followed by delayed anatomic replantation has been described in this situation [44]. A perineal urethrostomy may be required when an adequate urethral stump cannot be fashioned.

Complications

The incidence of skin necrosis, glans slough, urethral stricture, penile hypoesthesia, and erectile dysfunction has been reduced with the microvascular approach to replantation [37–40, 42, 43, 61–63].

Several reports document partial or complete erectile function within months after replantation [37, 41]. Those patients with impaired erectile function may respond to erectile dysfunction treatment modalities such as pharmacological agents.

Conclusions

A microsurgical approach to penile replantation offers the best chance to optimize cosmetic and functional results. If microsurgery capabilities are not available, the patient should be transferred to an institution where they are present. If microsurgical repair is not feasible, then the penis should be replanted macroscopically using corporal and urethral approximation.

Although excellent results have been achieved with microsurgical penile replantation, at times nonviability may occur; or the amputated penis may have been discarded, mutilated, or unsuitable for replantation. In these cases, phallic reconstruction represents an efficacious treatment modality in the microsurgical armamentarium (see "Penile Reconstruction" section).

Penile Reconstruction

Novel procedures for phallic creation have ushered in a new era of genitourinary reconstruction. Microvascular techniques play a paramount role in these endeavors.

Neophallus creation may be undertaken for traumatic loss of the penis or female-to-male transsexual surgery.

Autologous tissues for these reconstructive procedures can be transferred as a *graft* or a *flap* [4, 45–49]. A graft is tissue that has been excised from a donor site and transferred to a graft host bed. The transferred graft tissue survives as a result of a new blood supply developing by neovascularization.

A flap is tissue that has been removed and transferred to the recipient area with its blood supply preserved or re-established at the recipient site. As will be discussed below, flaps are the mainstay of penile reconstruction.

Flaps are classified based on *vascularity* or by *elevation technique* [4, 45–49]. With regard to vascularity, flaps can be *random* or *axial*. A random flap lacks a defined cuticular vascular territory. It is based on its dermal or laminar plexus. An axial flap has a defined vessel in its base.

Axial flap types are (1) direct cuticular, (2) musculocutaneous, and (3) fasciocutaneous.

Direct cuticular axial flaps are based on vasculature superficial to the superficial layer of the deep body wall fascia. Musculocutaneous flaps are based on a vessel to the muscle with the overlying skin paddle carried on perforators. Fasciocutaneous flaps have their blood supply carried on the deep and superficial fascia. Similar to the musculocutaneous flap, the overlying skin paddle of the fasciocutaneous flap is based on perforators. If the latter two flaps are transferred without the overlying skin, the skin survives as a random unit.

With regard to elevation technique, flaps can be classified as (1) peninsula, (2) island, and (3) microvascular free flap. Peninsula flaps have the vascular and cutaneous continuity of their base left attached. An island flap has its vascular continuity left intact but its cutaneous attachment is divided elevating it on dangling vessels. A microvascular free flap has both its vascular and cutaneous continuity divided. Its vascular continuity is re-established at the recipient site. A free flap's sensory nerve can be anastomosed via microsurgical techniques to the receptor site to provide sensibility to the flap, resulting in a *sensate free flap* [47]. Erogenous sensibility can be achieved. These flaps form the basis for phallic reconstruction.

The goals of a penile reconstruction procedure should include the following [50] (1) it should be accomplished in a one-stage procedure that can be predictably reproduced, (2) the neophallus should have both tactile and erogenous sensibility, (3) the neophallus should be bulky enough to accommodate and tolerate an external or internal prosthetic stiffener, (4) a neourethra should be fashioned that allows voiding while standing, and (5) an aesthetically acceptable penis.

The main techniques for penile reconstruction were originally pioneered for treating war-injured victims who sustained traumatic penile amputations [4]. Initially, led by [4] the procedures involved delayed formation and transfer of tubed abdominal flaps. Random flaps of skin were utilized to create the tubes in stages. The delay in stages permitted new vascular growth to occur. A "tube-within-a-tube" was formed. The inner tube accommodated a baculum or prosthetic stiffener for intercourse. The outer tube provided skin coverage. The patients voided via a proximal urethrostomy. Modifications of technique occurred over the ensuing decades. These modifications were performed with the eventual creation of sensate phalluses that could be used as urinary conduits and for sexual intercourse. Subsequently, various flaps were utilized culminating in free microneurovascular flaps. Free microneurovascular transfer flaps have included the saphenous flap, tensor fascia lata flap, deltoid flap, and upper medial arm flap [49]. However, many of these flaps have an unpredictable vascular and neural supply. A *dorsalis pedis flap* requires complete dissection of the three major branches of the dorsalis pedis artery and proper elevation of the dorsalis pedis artery off of the tarsal bones, which are extremely tedious [49]. A *lateral upper arm flap* has predictable neurovascular anatomy [49]. Unfortunately, it is often only drained by a single vena comitans which can result in venous insufficiency and congestion with subsequent flap failure.

Presently, the *forearm free flap* is the most pervasive modality for phallic reconstruction [4, 49–51]. It is an axial fasciocutaneous flap based on the radial or ulnar artery, multiple forearm veins, and the antebrachial cutaneous nerves. The radial artery version of the forearm flap was popularized by Chang and Hwang in 1984 [4, 53] and then modified by Biemer in 1988 [4]. A "cricket bat" modification of the radial forearm flap was described by Farrow and Boyd in 1990 [4, 54].

Forearm Flap Technique for Penile Reconstruction [4, 49–51]

The nondominant forearm is usually chosen as the harvest site of the forearm flap. The Allen test is utilized preoperatively to rule out arterial insufficiency. Here, the radial and ulnar arteries are palpated and compressed while the patient makes a tight closed fist. He then opens his hand and the fingers appear pale. When one of the arteries is released by the examiner, the fingers should resume a pink coloration, suggesting that palmar circulation is normal and both arteries are patent. If the fingers remain blanched, compromised circulation may be present. Upper extremity angiography is performed if the Allen test is abnormal or based on patient history to assess the integrity of the radial and ulnar arteries and the palmar arch.

The forearm flap is a fasciocutaneous flap vascularized by the radial and ulnar arteries. Both arteries arise from the brachial artery and vascularize the forearm fascia, skin, and underlying adipose tissue by way of the superficial (antebrachial) forearm fascia (Fig. 13.21). The forearm flap is elevated and transferred on this superficial fascia. The cephalic, basilic, and medial antebrachial veins are included. The venous comitans are evaluated at flap transfer as well to determine which is the dominant drainage system. The lateral and medial antebrachial cutaneous nerves are situated beneath the fascia.

Forearm Flap Modifications

The forearm flap modifications vary in the configuration of the skin island and the position of the urethral paddle relative to the flap skin that will become the shaft.

The *Chang and Hwang Forearm Flap* [4, 53] is composed of a skin island that has two separate paddles. The skin island on the ulnar aspect of the skin paddle is tubed to form the urethra. The radial aspect of the skin paddle forms the shaft coverage. A deepithelialized strip is created between the two skin paddles. The urethral tube is then rolled within the radial tube of skin, creating a tube-within-a-tube. Ischemic stenosis of the reconstructed urethra has been seen with this variant.

In the *Cricket Bat Modification of Forearm Flap* [4,54], the urethral skin island is centered over either the radial or ulnar artery and extends distally. Proximally, a broader portion of the skin paddle forms the shaft coverage. The urethral portion is tubed and rolled into the shaft portion of the skin paddle. Deepithelialized areas lateral to the urethral paddle add bulk to the glans. Placing the urethral portion directly over either the radial or ulnar artery improves vascularity and limits the potential for ischemic stenosis or necrosis of that area.

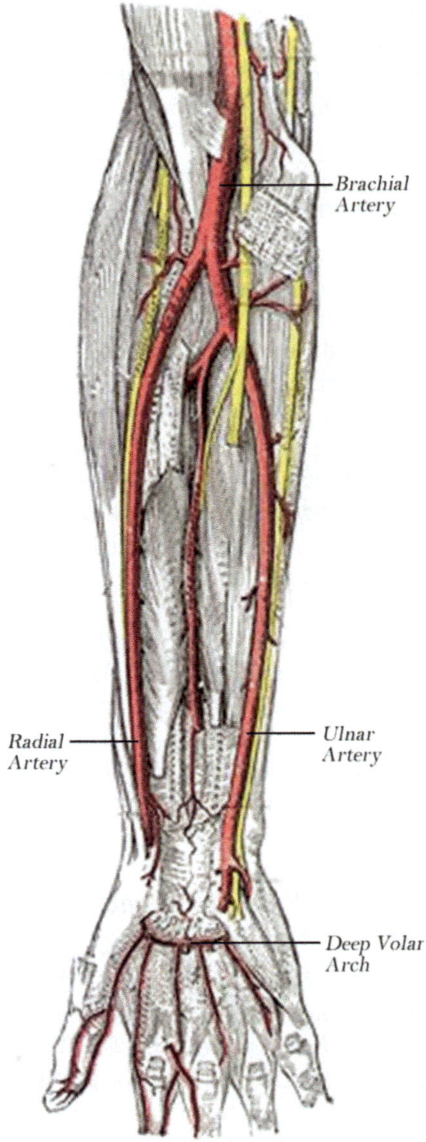

Fig. 13.21 The brachial artery gives rise to the radial and ulnar arteries which anastomose at the volar palmar arch (Gray's Anatomy, 1918). The Allen test is utilized to assess the patency of the radial and ulnar arteries as well as the palmar arch

The *Biemer Modified Forearm Flap* centers the urethral portion of the flap over the radial artery. A vascularized portion of radial bone is included to add rigidity to the neophallus. The incorporation of cartilage and bone has not been predictably successful and rigidity can be achieved by using external or internal prosthetics [4]. The urethral paddle is a midline strip separated from two lateral skin paddles by two deepithelialized strips. The lateral paddles are tubularized to form the shaft while the urethral paddle is tubularized centrally. Glanular reconstruction is achieved using the Puckett and Montie technique where a large distal island is flared back over the tips of the tubed flaps. Jordan et al. [4] perform a modification of the Biemer technique by not including the radial bone, allowing them to elevate the flap on the ulnar artery. They feel it offers the best functional and cosmetic results [56] (Fig. 13.22a–c).

Neural Anastomosis

Microsurgical coaptation of the flap cutaneous nerve(s) to recipient nerve(s) is performed. The flap cutaneous nerves are attached to the dorsal nerves of the penile stump or to the dorsal nerves of the clitoris female-to-male transsexuals. If the dorsal nerves are absent, the flap cutaneous nerves are anastomosed to the pudendal nerve via an interposition nerve graft. Erogenous cutaneous sensibility is achieved. Jordan et al. [4] have coapted the flap's cutaneous nerves to the recipient ilioinguinal nerves, resulting in reasonable erogenous sensibility.

Vascular Anastomosis

Usually, the deep inferior epigastric vessels are anastomosed to the flap's vasculature. As discussed in "Surgical Technique of Microvascular Penile Revascularization" section, the inferior epigastric vessels run on the dorsal aspect of the rectus abdominis muscle and are branches of the iliac system. Two or more venae comitantes accompany the artery. The arteries and veins are directly anastomosed to their respective vessels in an end-to-end fashion. A saphenous vein anastomosis is also used in addition to the above for further venous runoff. When these recipient vessels are unavailable, other modifications have been utilized. However, long-term consequences are unknown [4].

Urethral Anastomosis

Standard techniques apply with regard to creating a tension-free, water-tight anastomosis with absorbable interrupted sutures as discussed in "Microvascular Penile Replantation" section. Various flaps such as gracilis muscle, a bipedicled flap from the penile shaft base, and a tunica dartos flap with tunica vaginalis pedicle have been used to cover the area of the urethral anastomosis [4, 51]. The extra tissue coverage imparts additional vascularity, reducing the incidence of anastomotic strictures and fistulas. A Martius flap can also be used in female-to-male transsexuals. A suprapubic cystotomy tube is placed to divert the urine. The neourethra is stented with a 14 French soft silicone catheter.

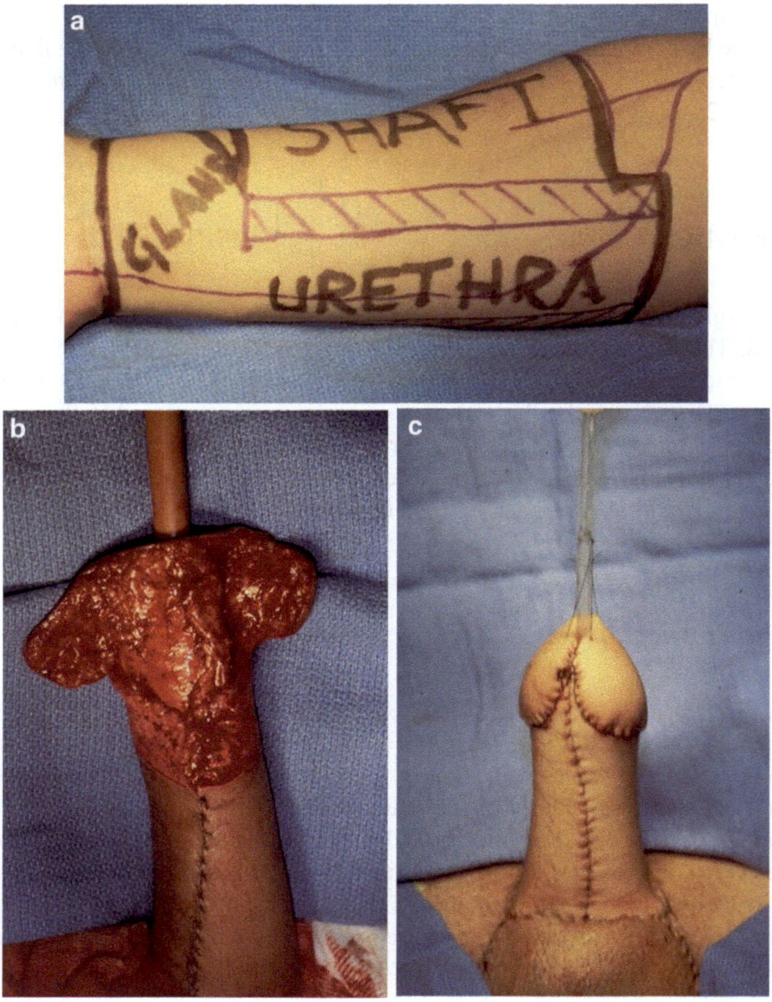

Fig. 13.22 (**a**) The Jordan modification of the Biemer flap elevates the flap on the ulnar artery excluding the radial bone. Placing the urethral portion over the artery improves vascularity and limits the potential for ischemic stenosis and necrosis. The glanular component is a large distal island that will be flared back over the tubed flaps (photo courtesy of Gerald H. Jordan, M.D., F.A.C.S., F.A.A.P. (Hon.), Professor and Fellowship Director, Adult and Pediatric Genitourinary Reconstructive Surgery Program, Eastern Virginia Medical School, Norfolk, VA; Director of the Devine Center for Genitourinary Reconstructive Surgery at Sentara Norfolk General Hospital). (**b**) The flap skin paddles are tabularized. The distal skin island will be flared back over the tubed flaps to accomplish the glanular reconstruction (photo courtesy of Gerald H. Jordan, M.D., F.A.C.S., F.A.A.P. (Hon.), Professor and Fellowship Director, Adult and Pediatric Genitourinary Reconstructive Surgery Program, Eastern Virginia Medical School, Norfolk, VA; Director of the Devine Center for Genitourinary Reconstructive Surgery at Sentara Norfolk General Hospital). (**c**) The constructed neophallus with urethral catheter in place (photo courtesy of Gerald H. Jordan, M.D., F.A.C.S., F.A.A.P. (Hon.), Professor and Fellowship Director, Adult and Pediatric Genitourinary Reconstructive Surgery Program, Eastern Virginia Medical School, Norfolk, VA; Director of the Devine Center for Genitourinary Reconstructive Surgery at Sentara Norfolk General Hospital)

Post-forearm Flap

A voiding cystogram is usually performed after 3 weeks postoperatively. The patient is monitored and seen in follow-up to assess voiding, genital sensation, flap viability, and donor site healing. As nerve regeneration occurs, the neophallus becomes sensate.

This becomes apparent at about 3–4 months postoperatively. Neophallus rigidity for intercourse is accomplished by external or internal prosthetics [4, 50–52]. Implantation of a penile prosthesis is not performed until 1 year postoperatively as sensation must be present. Hydraulic and articulated penile prostheses have been implanted by encasing them in a Gore-Tex® neocorpora [4, 50–52]. The neocorpora is then anchored to the ischial tuberosity and the pubis.

Forearm Flap Penile Reconstruction Complications

Elevating the forearm flap results in a donor site scar and deformity that is highly visible [4, 49]. The donor site can be covered with a full-thickness skin graft from the inguinal crease.

Another disadvantage that can occur is cold intolerance in the hand of the donor side [4, 49]. Jordan et al. [4, 49] previously reconstructed the radial artery with an interposition vein graft. However, they have abandoned this practice in the majority of their cases and have not seen cold intolerance.

Forearm skin can be hirsute [4]. If hair is included in the urethral tube, portion of the flap complications such as stones, strictures, and abnormal voiding can result. This potential problem should be identified preoperatively and the patient referred for epilation.

Neophallus complications can include anastomotic urethral strictures, fistulae, and ischemic necrosis as discussed earlier [4, 50, 51]. Meticulous attention to microneurovascular technique is imperative to limit these sequelae.

Future of Penile Reconstruction

Minimally invasive techniques in urology are growing exponentially. The possibility of laparoscopic- or robotic-assisted harvesting of the deep inferior epigastric vessels for anastomosis has already been realized with regards to penile revascularization [32–34]. This hopefully will limit morbidity and facilitate convalescence with regard to penile reconstruction.

Penile transplantation has been hypothesized and was performed in China in 2006 [55]. The patient was a 44-year-old male who sustained a penile amputation in an accident. The donor was a 22-year-old brain dead male. Reportedly, successful voiding was achieved at 10 days postoperatively. No signs of rejection were apparent. Unfortunately, the transplanted penis was surgically removed because of psychological issues that manifested in the patient and his wife. This case signifies the importance of an interdisciplinary team approach including skilled urologic microsurgeons, transplant immunologists, and psychological professionals.

Recently, tissue engineering in rabbits has been used to create penile erectile tissue as the first functional solid organ produced in this manner [57]. Smooth muscle and endothelial cells were harvested from rabbits' erectile tissue and cultured in the laboratory. The cells were injected into a three-dimensional scaffold of decellularized donor corpora cavernosa that provided support while the cells developed. After implantation into the rabbits, the bioengineered corpora demonstrated structural and functional parameters similar to native tissue. Nitric oxide-induced relaxation was normal as early as 1 month after implantation. The rabbits exhibited normal sexual function and produced offspring. This technology may be useful in the future for patients requiring penile reconstruction.

Conclusion

Microneurovascular techniques are entrenched in the novel reconstructive procedures available for neophallus creation. Creativity fosters successful results and limits morbidity. New technology and minimally invasive techniques continue to optimize the care of these patients. Immunology and regenerative medicine will exponentially facilitate the treatment of even the most complex penile reconstructive cases.

Summary of Microsurgical Penile Revascularization, Replantation, and Reconstruction

This chapter illustrates the pervasiveness of microsurgical techniques within the domains of penile revascularization, replantation, and reconstruction. This array of genital pathology represents a continuum of disorders whose treatments are greatly facilitated by expertise in microsurgery. Microsurgical skills, minimally invasive techniques, and new developments in regenerative medicine will continue to expand the urologist's armamentarium in treating this spectrum of genital disorders.

Acknowledgments The authors would like to acknowledge the scholarly works of Irwin Goldstein, M.D., Ricardo Munarriz, M.D., Gerald Jordan, M.D., and Jack McAninch, M.D. These surgeon scientists represent key thought leaders in their respective subspecialties without whose skills and feedback this chapter would not be possible.

References

1. Devine CJ, Angermeier KW. Anatomy of the penis and male perineum. Part I. AUA Update Series. 1994;13:10–23. Lesson 2.
2. Goldstein AM, Padma-Nathan H. The microarchitecture of the intracavernosal smooth muscle and the cavernosal fibrous skeleton. J Urol. 1990;244:1144–6.
3. Jordan GH. General concepts concerning the use of genital skin islands for anterior urethral stricture. AUA Update Series. 2000;19:66–71. Lesson 9.
4. Jordan GH, Schlossberg SM. Surgery of the penis and urethra. In: Wein AJ, editor. Campbell-Walsh urology. 9th ed. Philadelphia, PA: Saunders Elsevier; 2007. p. 1023–97.
5. Jordan GH. Lower genitourinary tract trauma and male external genital trauma (anatomy, non-penetrating injuries). Part I. AUA Update Series. 2000;19:74–9. Lesson 10.
6. Angermeier KW, Devine CJ. Anatomy of the penis and male perineum. Part II. AUA Update Series. 1994;13. Lesson 3.
7. Brooks JD. Anatomy of the lower urinary tract and male genitalia. In: Wein AJ, editor. Campbell-Walsh urology. 9th ed. Philadelphia, PA: Saunders Elsevier; 2007. p. 38–77.
8. Landwehr P. Penile vessels—erectile dysfunction. In: Wolf K, Fobbe F, editors. Color duplex sonography: principles and clinical applications. New York, NY: Thieme Medical Publishers; 1995. p. 204–16.
9. Goldstein I, Krane RJ, Greenfield AJ, Padma-Nathan H. Vascular diseases of the penis: impotence and priapism. In: Pollack HM, editor. Clinical urography. Philadelphia, PA: WB Saunders; 1990. p. 2231–52.
10. Feldman AS, McDougal WS. Inguinal node dissection for penile carcinoma. AUA Update Series. 2008;27:58–63. Lesson 7.
11. Strasser H, Stenzl A, Hobisch A, Bartsch G, Poisel S. Anatomy and innervation of the male urethra, the rhabdosphincter, and the corpora cavernosa. Part II. AUA Update Series. 2001;20:122–7. Lesson 16.
12. Myers RP. Radical prostatectomy: pertinent surgical anatomy. Atlas Urol Clin North Am. 1994;2:1–18.
13. Goldstein I, Bastuba M, Lurie A, Lubisich J. Penile revascularization. J Sex Med. 2008;5:2018–21.
14. Munarriz R. Microvascular arterial bypass surgery: indications, outcomes, and complications. ScientificWorldJournal. 2010;10:1–9.
15. Munarriz R, Uberoi J, Fantini G, Martinez D, Lee C. Microvascular arterial bypass surgery: long-term outcomes using validated instruments. J Urol. 2009;182:643–8.
16. Montague DK, Jarow JP, Broderick GA, et al. The management of erectile dysfunction: an update. Baltimore, MD: American Urological Association Education and Research; 2005. http://www.auanet.org/content/guidelines-and-quality-care/clinical-guidelines/main-reports/edmgmt/content.pdf. Accessed 23 June 2011.
17. Munarriz R, Mulhall J, Goldstein I. Penile arterial reconstruction. In: Graham Jr SD, Glenn JF, Keane TE, editors. Glenn's urologic surgery. 6th ed. Philadelphia, PA: Lippincott Williams & Wilkins; 2004. p. 573–81.
18. Lewis RW, Munarriz R. Vascular surgery for erectile dysfunction. In: Wein AJ, editor. Campbell-Walsh urology. 9th ed. Philadelphia, PA: Saunders Elsevier; 2007. p. 802–17.
19. Sharaby JS, Benet AE, Melman A. Penile revascularization. Urol Clin North Am. 1995;22(4):821–32.
20. Michal V, Kramar R, Hejhal L. Revascularization procedures of the cavernous bodies. In: Zorgniotti AW, Rossi G, editors. Vasculogenic Impotence: Proceedings of the First International Conference on Corpus Cavernosum Revascularization. Springfield, Illinois: Charles C. Thomas; 1980. pp. 239–55.
21. Virag R, Zwang G, Dermange H, Legman M. Vasculogenic impotence: a review of 92 cases with 54 surgical operations. Vasc Surg. 1981;15:9–16.

22. Furlow WL, Fisher J. Deep dorsal vein arterialization: clinical experience with a new technique for penile revascularization. J Urol. 1988;139:298A. Abstract 543.
23. Licht MR, Lewis RW. Penile venous surgery. In: Graham Jr SD, Glenn JF, Keane TE, editors. Glenn's urologic surgery. 6th ed. Philadelphia, PA: Lippincott Williams & Wilkins; 2004. p. 566–72.
24. Wespes E, Moreira de Goes P, Sattar AA, Schulman C. Objective criteria in the long-term evaluation of penile venous surgery. J Urol. 1994;152:888–90.
25. Ricardo M. Munarriz, MD. Director, Center for Sexual Medicine, Associate Professor of Urology, Boston University School of Medicine. Personal Communication, 7 June 2011.
26. Donatucci LF, Lue TF. Venous surgery: are we kidding ourselves? In: Lue TF, editor. World book of impotence. London: Smith-Gerthdon; 1992. p. 221–7.
27. Lue TF, Broderick GA. Evaluation and nonsurgical management of erectile dysfunction and premature ejaculation. In: Wein AJ, editor. Campbell-Walsh urology. 9th ed. Philadelphia, PA: Saunders Elsevier; 2007. p. 750–87.
28. Goldstein I, Lurie AL, Lubisich JP. Bicycle riding, perineal trauma, and erectile dysfunction: data and solutions. Curr Urol Rep. 2007;8:491–7.
29. Huang V, Munarriz R, Goldstein I. Bicycle riding and erectile dysfunction: an increase in interest (and concern). J Sex Med. 2005;2:596–604.
30. Munarriz R, Huang V, Uberoi J, et al. Only the nose knows: penile hemodynamic study of the perineum–saddle interface in men with erectile dysfunction utilizing bicycle saddles and seats with and without nose extensions. J Sex Med. 2005;2:612–9.
31. Wilkins CJ, Sidhu PS. Diseases of the penis with functional evaluation. In: Baxter GM, Sidhu PS, editors. Ultrasound of the urogenital system. New York, NY: Georg Thieme Verlag; 2006. p. 181–92.
32. Raynor MC, Davis R, Hellstrom WJ. Robotic-assisted vessel harvesting for penile revascularization. J Sex Med. 2010;7:293–7.
33. Lund GO, Winfield HN, Donovan JF. Laparoscopically assisted penile revascularization for vasculogenic impotence. J Urol. 1995;153:1923–6.
34. Trombetta C, Liguori G, Siracusano S, Savoca G, Belgrano E. Laparoscopically assisted penile revascularization for vasculogenic impotence: 2 additional cases. J Urol. 1997;158:1783–6.
35. Hatzichristou D, Goldstein I. Penile microvascular arterial bypass surgery. Urol Clin North Am. 1993;1:39–60.
36. Hatzichristou D, Goldstein I. Arterial bypass surgery for impotence. Curr Opin Urol. 1992;1:114–7.
37. Rosenstein DI, Jordan GH. Penile replantation. In: Graham Jr SD, Glenn JF, Keane TE, editors. Glenn's urologic surgery. 6th ed. Philadelphia, PA: Lippincott Williams & Wilkins; 2004. p. 588–91.
38. Kirkemo A. Complications of penile surgery. In: Smith RB, Ehrlich RM, editors. Complications of urologic surgery: prevention and management. 2nd ed. Philadelphia, PA: WB Saunders; 1990. p. 534–48.
39. Chou EK, Tai YT, Wu CI, Lin MS, Chen HH, Chang SC. Penile replantation, complication management, and technique refinement. Microsurgery. 2008;28:153–6.
40. Cohen BE, May Jr JW, Daly JF, Young HH. Successful clinical replantation of an amputated penis by microneurovascular repair. Plast Reconstr Surg. 1977;59:276–80.
41. Jack W. McAninch, MD. Professor and Vice-Chair Urology, University of California, San Francisco. Chief of Urology, San Francisco General Hospital. Personal Communication, 10 June 2011.
42. Tamai S, Nakamura Y, Motomiya Y. Microsurgical replantation of a completely amputated penis and scrotum. Plast Reconstr Surg. 1977;60:287–91.
43. Carroll PR, Lue TF, Schmidt RA, Trentgrove-Jones G, McAninch JW. Penile replantation: current concepts. J Urol. 1985;133:281–5.
44. Matloub HS, Yousif NJ, Sanger JR. Temporary ectopic implantation of an amputated penis. Plast Reconstr Surg. 1994;93:408–12.

45. Jordan GH. Principles of tissue transfer techniques in urethral reconstruction. Urol Clin North Am. 2002;29:267–75.
46. Jordan GH, Schlossberg SM, McCraw JB. Tissue transfer techniques for genitourinary reconstructive surgery. Part I—principles, definitions, basic techniques and graft techniques. AUA Update Series. 1988;7:65–72.
47. Jordan GH, McCraw JB. Tissue transfer techniques for genitourinary reconstructive surgery. Part II—basic flap definitions and techniques/graft techniques. AUA Update Series. 1988;7:73–80.
48. Jordan GH, McCraw JB. Tissue transfer techniques for genitourinary reconstructive surgery. Part III—local and genital skin flap techniques. AUA Update Series. 1988;7:81–88.
49. Jordan GH, McCraw JB. Tissue transfer techniques for genitourinary reconstructive surgery. Part IV—local myocutaneous flaps and free microvascular transfer flaps. AUA Update Series. 1988;7:89–96.
50. Spindel MR, Gilbert DA, Gilbert D, Winslow BH. Transsexualism. AUA Update Series. 1988;7:1–8.
51. Jordan GH, McCammon KA, Gilbert DA, Schlossberg SM. Transsexualism for the general urologist. AUA Update Series. 1988;7:49–56.
52. Jordan GH, Alter GJ, Gilbert DA, Horton CE, Devine Jr CJ. Penile prosthesis implantation in total phalloplasty. J Urol. 1994;152:410–4.
53. Chang TS, Hwang WY. Forearm flap in one-stage reconstruction of the penis. Plast Reconstr Surg. 1984;74:251–8.
54. Semple JL, Boyd JB, Farrow GA, Robinette MA. The "cricket bat" flap: a one-stage free forearm flap phalloplasty. Plast Reconstr Surg. 1991;88:514–9.
55. Hu W, Lu J, Zhang L, et al. A preliminary report of penile transplantation. Eur Urol. 2006;50:851–3.
56. Gerald H. Jordan, MD, FACS, FAAP (Hon.). Professor and Fellowship Director, Adult and Pediatric Genitourinary Reconstructive Surgery Program, Eastern Virginia Medical School, Norfolk, Virginia; Director of the Devine Center for Genitourinary Reconstructive Surgery at Sentara Norfolk General Hospital. Personal Communication, 14 July 2011.
57. Chen KL, Eberli D, Yoo JJ, Atala A. Bioengineered corporal tissue for structural and functional restoration of the penis. Proc Natl Acad Sci U S A. 2010;107:3346–50.
58. Silber SJ. Microsurgery in clinical urology. Urology. 1975;6:150–3.
59. Crespo E, Soltanik E, Bove D, Farrell E. Treatment of vasculogenic impotence by revascularizing cavernous and/or dorsal arteries using microvascular techniques. Urology. 1982;20:271–5.
60. Goldlust RW, Daniel RK, Trachtenberg J. Microsurgical treatment of vascular impotence. J Urol. 1982;128:821–2.
61. Jordan GH, Gilbert DA. Management of amputation injuries of the male genitalia. Urol Clin North Am. 1989;16:359–67.
62. Greilsheimer H, Groves JE. Male genital self-mutilation. Arch Gen Psychiatry. 1979;36:441–6.
63. Mosahebi A, Butterworth M, Knight R, Berger L, Kaisary A, Butler P. Delayed penile replantation after prolonged warm ischemia. Microsurgery. 2001;21:52–4.
64. McRoberts JW, Chapman WH, Ansell JS. Primary anastomosis of the traumatically amputated penis: case report and summary of the literature. J Urol. 1968;100:751–4.

Index

J.I. Sandlow (ed.), *Microsurgery for Fertility Specialists: A Practical Text*,
DOI 10.1007/978-1-4614-4196-0, © Springer Science+Business Media New York 2013

R

MIX
Papier aus verantwortungsvollen Quellen
Paper from responsible sources
FSC® C105338

If you have any concerns about our products,
you can contact us on
ProductSafety@springernature.com

In case Publisher is established outside the EU,
the EU authorized representative is:
Springer Nature Customer Service Center GmbH
Europaplatz 3, 69115 Heidelberg, Germany

Printed by Libri Plureos GmbH
in Hamburg, Germany